Facial Reconstruction Post-Mohs Surgery

Editor

JAMES B. LUCAS

FACIAL PLASTIC SURGERY CLINICS OF NORTH AMERICA

www.facialplastic.theclinics.com

Consulting Editor
J. REGAN THOMAS

August 2017 • Volume 25 • Number 3

ELSEVIER

1600 John F. Kennedy Boulevard • Suite 1800 • Philadelphia, Pennsylvania, 19103-2899

http://www.theclinics.com

FACIAL PLASTIC SURGERY CLINICS OF NORTH AMERICA Volume 25, Number 3
August 2017 ISSN 1064-7406, ISBN-13: 978-0-323-53229-7

Editor: Jessica McCool
Developmental Editor: Alison Swety

Facial Plastic Surgery Clinics of North America (ISSN 1064-7406) is published quarterly by Elsevier Inc., 360 Park Avenue South, New York, NY 10010-1710. Months of issue are February, May, August, and November. Business and Editorial Offices: 1600 John F. Kennedy Blvd., Suite 1800, Philadelphia, PA 19103-2899. Periodicals postage paid at New York, NY, and additional mailing offices. Subscription prices are $390.00 per year (US individuals), $592.00 per year (US institutions), $445.00 per year (Canadian individuals), $737.00 per year (Canadian institutions), $535.00 per year (foreign individuals), $737.00 per year (foreign institutions), $100.00 per year (US students), and $255.00 per year (foreign students). Foreign air speed delivery is included in all *Clinics* subscription prices. All prices are subject to change without notice. POSTMASTER: Send address changes to *Facial Plastic Surgery Clinics*, Elsevier Health Sciences Division, Subscription Customer Service, 3251 Riverport Lane, Maryland Heights, MO 63043. **Customer service: 1-800-654-2452 (US and Canada); 1-314-447-8871 (outside US and Canada); Fax: 314-447-8029; E-mail: journalscustomerservice-usa@elsevier.com (for print support); journalsonline support-usa@elsevier.com (for online support).**

Reprints. For copies of 100 or more of articles in this publication, please contact the Commercial Reprints Department, Elsevier Inc., 360 Park Avenue South, New York, NY 10010-1710. Tel.: 212-633-3874; Fax: 212-633-3820; E-mail: reprints@elsevier.com.

Facial Plastic Surgery Clinics of North America is covered in *MEDLINE/PubMed* (*Index Medicus*).

Printed in the United States of America.

Contributors

CONSULTING EDITOR

J. REGAN THOMAS, MD, FACS
Mansueto Professor and Chairman,
Department of Otolaryngology–Head and Neck
Surgery, University of Illinois at Chicago,
Chicago, Illinois

EDITOR

JAMES B. LUCAS, MD, FACS
Deputy Commander for Surgical Services,
Director of Facial Plastic and Reconstructive
Surgery, Carl R. Darnall Army Medical Center,
Fort Hood, Texas; Assistant Professor of
Surgery, Uniformed Services University of
Health Sciences, F. Edward Hebert School of
Medicine, Bethesda, Maryland; Fort Hood
Campus Dean, Texas A&M Health Science
Center College of Medicine, Bryan, Texas

AUTHORS

LINDSAY M. BICKNELL, MD
Resident Physician, Department of
Dermatology, Texas A&M Health Science
Center, Baylor Scott & White Health, Temple,
Texas

MICHAEL J. BRENNER, MD, FACS
Associate Professor, Division of Facial Plastic
and Reconstructive Surgery, Department of
Otolaryngology–Head and Neck Surgery,
University of Michigan, Ann Arbor, Michigan

ERIC W. CERRATI, MD
Fellow, Division of Facial Plastic and
Reconstructive Surgery, Department of
Otolaryngology–Head and Neck Surgery,
University of Illinois at Chicago, Chicago, Illinois

GREGORY S. DIBELIUS, MD
Fellow, Division of Facial Plastic and
Reconstructive Surgery, Department of
Otolaryngology–Head and Neck Surgery,
University of Illinois at Chicago, Chicago, Illinois

KATHERINE FIALA, MD
Assistant Professor, Department of
Dermatology, Texas A&M Health Science
Center, Baylor Scott & White Health, Temple,
Texas

GRANT S. HAMILTON III, MD, FACS
Assistant Professor, Department of
Otolaryngology, Mayo Clinic, Rochester,
Minnesota

JOHN E. HANKS, MD
Resident, Department of Otolaryngology–Head
and Neck Surgery, University of Michigan
Health System, Ann Arbor, Michigan

AVRAM HECHT, MD, MPH
Resident, Division of Otolaryngology–Head
and Neck Surgery, Department of Surgery,
University of California, San Diego, San Diego,
California

DANE HILL, MD
Resident Physician, Department of
Dermatology, Texas A&M Health Science
Center, Baylor Scott & White Health, Temple,
Texas

CHAD HOUSEWRIGHT, MD
Assistant Professor, Department of
Dermatology, Texas A&M Health Science
Center, Baylor Scott & White Health, Temple,
Texas

CLINTON D. HUMPHREY, MD
Associate Professor, Division of Facial Plastic
and Reconstructive Surgery, Department of
Otolaryngology–Head and Neck Surgery, The
University of Kansas Medical Center, Kansas
City, Kansas

JOHN DAVID KRIET, MD
Professor, Division of Facial Plastic and
Reconstructive Surgery, Department of
Otolaryngology–Head and Neck Surgery, The
University of Kansas Medical Center, Kansas
City, Kansas

YUNA C. LARRABEE, MD
Fellow, Facial Plastic and Reconstructive
Surgery, Department of Otolaryngology–Head
and Neck Surgery, University of Michigan, Ann
Arbor, Michigan

WILLIAM D. LOSQUADRO, MD
Director of Facial Plastic Surgery, The Mount
Sinai Health System at CareMount Medical,
Katonah, New York

GUANNING NINA LU, MD
Resident, Otolaryngology–Head and Neck
Surgery, The University of Kansas Medical
Center, Kansas City, Kansas

JAMES B. LUCAS, MD, FACS
Deputy Commander for Surgical Services,
Director of Facial Plastic and Reconstructive
Surgery, Carl R. Darnall Army Medical Center,
Fort Hood, Texas; Assistant Professor of
Surgery, Uniformed Services University of
Health Sciences, F. Edward Hebert School of
Medicine, Bethesda, Maryland; Fort Hood
Campus Dean, Texas A&M Health Science
Center College of Medicine, Bryan, Texas

BOBBAK MANSOURI, MD
Resident Physician, Department of
Dermatology, Texas A&M Health Science
Center, Baylor Scott & White Health, Temple,
Texas

JEFFREY S. MOYER, MD, FACS
Associate Professor, Chief, Division of
Facial Plastic and Reconstructive Surgery,
Department of Otolaryngology–Head and Neck
Surgery, University of Michigan, Ann Arbor,
Michigan

MICHAEL D. OLSON, MD
Instructor, Department of Otolaryngology,
Mayo Clinic, Rochester, Minnesota

JESSICA J. PECK, MD
Facial Plastic and Microvascular
Reconstructive Surgery, Otolaryngology–Head
and Neck Surgery, Dwight Eisenhower Army
Medical Center, Fort Gordon, Georgia

RON W. PELTON, MD, PhD
Oculofacial Cosmetic and Reconstructive
Surgery, Colorado Springs, Colorado

LAUREN K. RECKLEY, MD
Division of Otolaryngology–Head and Neck
Surgery, Tripler Army Medical Center,
Honolulu, Hawaii

SCOTTIE B. ROOFE, MD
Associate Professor of Surgery,
Uniformed Services University of the
Health Sciences, Bethesda, Maryland;
Chief, Division of Otolaryngology–Head and
Neck Surgery, Department of Surgery,
Womack Army Medical Center, Fort Bragg,
Georgia

DAVID A. SHERRIS, MD
Chairman, Department of Otolaryngology,
University at Buffalo, Buffalo, New York

MATTHEW SHEW, MD
Department of Otolaryngology–Head and Neck
Surgery, The University of Kansas Medical
Center, Kansas City, Kansas

SIDNEY J. STARKMAN, MD
Otolaryngology Resident, Department of
Otolaryngology, University at Buffalo, Buffalo,
New York

J. REGAN THOMAS, MD, FACS
Mansueto Professor and Chairman,
Department of Otolaryngology–Head
and Neck Surgery, University of Illinois at
Chicago, Chicago, Illinois

DEAN M. TORIUMI, MD
Professor, Division of Facial Plastic and
Reconstructive Surgery, Department of
Otolaryngology–Head and Neck Surgery,
University of Illinois at Chicago, Chicago, Illinois

GREGORY D. WALKER, MD, MBA
Resident Physician, Department of
Dermatology, Texas A&M Health Science
Center, Baylor Scott & White Health, Temple,
Texas

DEBORAH WATSON, MD
Professor of Surgery, Division of
Otolaryngology–Head and Neck Surgery,
Department of Surgery, University of California,
San Diego, San Diego, California

CARSON T. WILLIAMS, MD
Otolaryngology Resident, Department of
Otolaryngology, University at Buffalo,
Buffalo, New York

Contents

Skin is composed of the epidermis, dermis, and adnexal structures. The epidermis is composed of 4 layers—the stratums basale, spinosum, granulosum, and corneum. The dermis is divided into a superficial papillary dermis and deeper reticular dermis. Collagen and elastin within the reticular dermis are responsible for skin tensile strength and elasticity, respectively. The 2 most common kinds of nonmelanoma skin cancers are basal cell and squamous cell carcinoma. Both are caused by a host of environmental and genetic factors, although UV light exposure is the single greatest predisposing factor.

Mohs micrographic surgery is a specialized form of skin cancer surgery in which the Mohs surgeon acts as both surgeon and pathologist. The procedure is characterized by its histopathologic margin control and ability to spare tissue, particularly in cosmetically sensitive locations. Mohs surgery is known for both limiting the size of the final defect and its high cure rate. In this review, the authors highlight indications for the procedure, detail the technique itself, discuss cutaneous tumors for which Mohs micrographic surgery is indicated, and present the economic benefit of Mohs surgery.

Facial skin defects created by Mohs micrographic surgery are commonly reconstructed using local cutaneous flaps from surrounding skin. To provide optimal survival and aesthetic outcomes, the cutaneous surgeon must command a thorough understanding of the complex vascular anatomy and physiology of the skin as well as the imperative physiologic and biomechanical considerations when elevating and transferring tissue via local skin flaps.

In many cases of complex facial defects, because of advanced cutaneous malignancies, primary wound closure is impossible. In these instances, ideal results can be obtained through recruitment of adjacent tissue with the use of local flaps. Advances in local flap techniques have raised the bar in facial reconstruction; however, acceptable results to the surgeon and patient require high levels of planning and surgical technique. Defects resulting from Mohs surgery and other traumatic injuries can typically be repaired with local flaps. A well-planned and executed local flap can lead to excellent cosmetic results with minimal distortion of the surrounding facial landmarks.

A mastery of advancement flap design, selection, and execution greatly aids the surgeon in solving reconstructive dilemmas. Advancement flaps involve carefully planned incisions to most efficiently close a primary defect in a linear vector. Advancement flaps are subcategorized as unipedicle, bipedicle, V-to-Y, and Y-to-V flaps, each with their own advantages and disadvantages. When selecting and designing an advancement flap, the surgeon must account for primary and secondary movement to prevent distortion of important facial structural units and boundaries.

Paramedian forehead and melolabial flaps are the most common examples of interpolated flaps used by facial plastic surgeons and are excellent options for reconstruction of the midface after Mohs surgery. They provide superior tissue match in terms of thickness, texture, and color, while leaving minimal defects at the tissue donor sites. The main advantage of interpolated flaps is the robust blood supply, which can be either axial of randomly based, and the maintenance of the integrity of facial landmarks. The main disadvantage is the frequent need for a multistage procedure, which eliminates some patients from consideration.

Skin and composite grafting provide effective resurfacing and reconstruction for cutaneous defects after excision of the malignancy. The goal is to restore a natural appearance and function while preventing distortion of the eyelid, nose, or lips. With careful planning and attention to aesthetic subunits, the surgeon can camouflage incisions and avoid blunting aesthetically sensitive sulci. The surgical plan is also informed by the pathology, as basal or squamous cell carcinomas removed by Mohs micrographic excision have different prognostic and logistical considerations from melanoma. Skin and composite grafting are useful as stand-alone procedures or may complement local flaps and other soft tissue reconstructions.

Scalp and forehead reconstruction after Mohs micrographic surgery can encompass subcentimeter defects to entire scalp reconstruction. Knowledge of anatomy, flap design, and execution will prepare surgeons who operate in the head and neck area to confidently approach a variety of reconstructive challenges in this area.

Eyelid defects disrupt the complex natural form and function of the eyelids and present a surgical challenge. Detailed knowledge of eyelid anatomy is essential in evaluating a defect and composing a reconstructive plan. Numerous reconstructive techniques have been described, including primary closure, grafting, and a variety of local flaps. This article describes an updated reconstructive ladder for eyelid defects that can be used in various permutations to solve most eyelid defects.

Repairing defects of the auricle requires an appreciation of the underlying 3-dimensional framework, the flexible properties of the cartilages, and the healing contractile tendencies of the surrounding soft tissue. In the analysis of auricular defects and planning of their reconstruction, it is helpful to divide the auricle into subunits for which different techniques may offer better functional and aesthetic outcomes. This article reviews many of the reconstructive options for defects of the various auricular subunits.

Mohs micrographic surgery has become the standard of care for the treatment of cutaneous malignancies. Reconstructing cutaneous defects of the nose can be challenging, as form and function must be respected to the greatest extent possible. A wide range of reconstructive techniques are used. Secondary intent, primary closure, skin grafts, local flaps, and the interpolated workhorse flaps represent the spectrum of options, each with specific advantages and disadvantages. Vigilant postoperative care, including judicious use of adjunctive procedures, can improve outcomes. A subunit approach to reconstruction aids with surgical planning in order to achieve the best possible results.

Reconstruction of defects of the lips after Mohs micrographic surgery should encompass functional and aesthetic concerns. The lower lip and chin compose two-thirds of the lower portion of the face. The focus of this article is local tissue transfer for primarily cutaneous defects after Mohs surgery. Various flaps exist for repair. For small defects, elliptical excision with primary closure is a viable option. During reconstruction of the lip, all of the involved layers need to be addressed, including mucosa, muscle, and the vermillion or cutaneous lip. It is especially important to realign the vermillion border precisely for optimal results.

Successful reconstruction of the cheek following excision for cutaneous malignancy requires careful consideration of defect location, size, and depth in relation to the anatomic properties of the affected cheek unit. Various reconstructive options are available to the surgeon, ranging from simple excisions to complex cervicofacial advancements to meet the needs for functional and aesthetically pleasing reconstructive outcomes. The surgeon must prevent distortion of mobile structures, such as the eyelid, nose, and lips; respect aesthetic subunits; and avoid blunting natural creases. This discussion covers choice of flap, techniques, and technical

FACIAL PLASTIC SURGERY CLINICS OF NORTH AMERICA

RELATED INTEREST

Oral and Maxillofacial Surgery Clinics, February 2017 (Vol. 29, No. 1)
Emerging Biomaterials and Techniques in Tissue Regeneration
Alan S. Herford, *Editor*
Available at: http://www.oralmaxsurgery.theclinics.com/

THE CLINICS ARE AVAILABLE ONLINE!
Access your subscription at:
www.theclinics.com

Preface
In Pursuit of Perfection: The Art of Facial Restoration

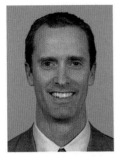

James B. Lucas, MD, FACS
Editor

One of the common traits that inspire young surgeons to pursue a calling in the reconstructive arts is a passion for restoration. The ability to restore balance and harmony to the human form, to re-create function and beauty in an area where it has been lost or compromised, is one of the requisite fundamental skills that all plastic surgeons seek to acquire and perfect throughout their career. It is the sine qua non in the art of aesthetic and reconstructive surgery.

Facial defects created by Mohs micrographic surgery provide reconstructive surgeons with outstanding opportunities to enhance the lives of their patients by returning what has been taken from them…a sense of normalcy. While providing the most conservative yet definitive form of surgical extirpation for most types of skin cancer, Mohs surgery can nonetheless create tremendously disfiguring cutaneous defects. These wounds often result in significant emotional distress for patients who wonder if they will ever look like themselves again. The ability to restore form and function during this vulnerable time in their lives, even if only approximate, is one of the great rewards of the profession. Their expressions of gratitude provide ample professional satisfaction and motivation to further refine one's surgical skills in the pursuit of excellence.

Of course, to achieve the type of outcomes that will result in a happy patient and a happy surgeon, a thorough mastery of the essentials is an imperative, allowing the surgeon to apply a knowledgeable analysis of the "reconstructive ladder" to their surgical decision-making process. This issue of *Facial Plastic Surgery Clinics* was designed with the intent of providing a thorough review of the science and art of facial reconstruction post-Mohs surgery, a review that it is hoped will be a valuable resource not only to a budding facial plastic surgeon but also to the most seasoned of reconstructive surgeons.

Our contributing authors were each chosen for their distinguished knowledge and expertise in the fields of facial reconstructive surgery and dermatology. I am deeply grateful for their insightful contributions to this project and am honored to have been able to work with each of them. It is our collective hope that you, the reader, will find this tome to be a useful tool in your armamentarium of surgical resources. If we have, in any way, contributed to better surgical outcomes for our patients, then we count this endeavor a resounding success.

James B. Lucas, MD, FACS
Carl R. Darnall Army Medical Center
36065 Santa Fo Avenue
Fort Hood, TX 76544, USA

Uniformed Services University of Health Sciences
F. Edward Hebert School of Medicine
Bethesda, MD 20814, USA

E-mail address:
jlucasfprs@gmail.com

Facial Plast Surg Clin N Am 25 (2017) xiii
http://dx.doi.org/10.1016/j.fsc.2017.06.001
1064-7406/17/© 2017 Published by Elsevier Inc.

Anatomy of the Skin and the Pathogenesis of Nonmelanoma Skin Cancer

William D. Losquadro, MD

KEYWORDS

• Skin • Epidermis • Dermis • Basal cell carcinoma • Squamous cell carcinoma

KEY POINTS

- Skin is composed of 2 layers: the epidermis and dermis. Beneath it lays the hypodermis or subcutaneous tissue.
- The epidermis is composed of 4 layers: the stratum basale, spinosum, granulosum, and corneum.
- The dermis is composed of a thin, looser papillary dermis and a thicker, denser reticular dermis.
- The most commonly diagnosed nonmelanoma skin cancers are basal cell carcinoma and squamous cell carcinoma.
- Basal cell and squamous cell carcinomas are caused by a host of environmental and genetic factors.

Skin consists of 2 basic layers, the epidermis and dermis. The epidermis is primarily composed of keratinocytes but also contains melanocytes, Langerhans cells, and Merkel cells. It is divided into 4 layers or strata that are traversed by skin appendages such as pilosebaceous units and sweat glands. The dermis is divided into a papillary and reticular layer. Within the dermis resides the skin's neurovascular supply. The subcutaneous tissue beneath the skin contains the superficial fascia and subcutaneous fat.

EPIDERMIS

The epidermis is the outermost layer of skin (**Fig. 1**). It is responsible for skin color, texture, and moisture. Epidermal thickness is relatively constant throughout the head and neck region. The primary cell type within the epidermis is the keratinocyte, and the 4 epidermal layers represent the maturation of keratinocytes from the deep to superficial layer. This process of keratinization allows for the development of keratin, a protein filament.

The deepest layer of the epidermis is the stratum basale, or basal layer. It is composed of stem cells called basal cells. The basal layer is often 1 cell thick, but can be 2 or 3 cells thick. Basal cells divide to form keratinocytes, which then begin migrating superficially.

The next layer is the spinous layer or stratum spinosum. Keratinocytes in this layer form intercellular attachments via protein channels called desmosomes. The attachments are responsible for this layer's spiny appearance beneath the microscope. Lipid-containing lamellar granules first become visible here within the keratinocytes.[1]

Keratinocytes then migrate to the granular layer or stratum granulosum, so named for the visible keratohyalin granules. Fillagrin forms within these granules from its precursor protein, profillagrin. Keratin filaments then begin to aggregate into complex structures via fillagrin.

Cells within the granular layer gradually lose their organelles and become more compact. They form the outermost epidermal layer, the stratum corneum. Here, keratinization is completed. The keratinocytes attach to one another via desmosomes in

The Mount Sinai Health System at CareMount Medical, 111 Bedford Road, Katonah, NY 12533, USA
E-mail address: wlosquad@cmmedical.com

Facial Plast Surg Clin N Am 25 (2017) 283–289
http://dx.doi.org/10.1016/j.fsc.2017.03.001

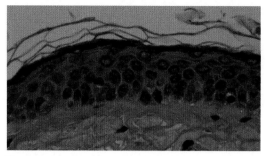

Fig. 1. Epidermis. (*Courtesy of* Kim Ruska, MD, Mount Kisco, New York.)

a bricklike pattern and are surrounded by lipids secreted from the lamellar granules. This construct is responsible for the skin's function as a both a protective and a moisture-control barrier.

Cells

The keratinocyte is the primary cell type within the epidermis, but other cell types reside there as well. Melanocytes are confined to the basal layer. Their primary function is to produce melanin, a pigment that protects cellular nuclei from UV radiation-induced injury. Melanin-containing vesicles called melanosomes are secreted from the melanocyte dendritic processes and taken up by adjacent keratinocytes. The melanin pigment is then distributed over the nuclei to maximize the protection of DNA. Variations in skin color are not due to the number of melanocytes but rather to their activity level and volume of melanin production.

Langerhans cells are antigen processing and presenting cells found in the stratum spinosum, stratum granularum, and the dermis. Electron microscopy reveals racket-shaped granules called Birbeck granules. Langerhans cells have dendritic processes similar to melanocytes. Langerhans cell numbers decrease with UV radiation exposure, and the consequent decrease in skin immunologic activity may create a more permissive environment for carcinoma development.[2]

Another epidermal cell type is the Merkel cell. Merkel cells reside in the basal layer and contain secretory granules whose contents are similar to those in other neuroendocrine cells. Groups of Merkel cells associated with peripheral nerve endings form specialized structures called tactile discs, which most likely facilitate fine sensation. They are predictably dense within and around highly sensitive locations and structures such as the lips, oral cavity, and hair follicles.

Dermal-Epidermal Junction

The basal layer of the epidermis is connected to the dermis below by a basement membrane called the dermal-epidermal junction. Two distinct layers of this junction are visible on electron microscopy. The more superficial layer, the lamina lucida, is composed of anchor filaments connecting hemidesmosomes within the basal cell plasma membrane to the deeper, more compact layer known as the lamina densa. The lamina densa is connected to the underlying dermis via collagen-anchoring fibrils.

DERMIS

The dermis lies between the epidermis and subcutaneous tissue and is responsible for the regional variation in skin thickness (**Fig. 2**). It is composed primarily of collagen, but also contains elastin, blood vessels, nerves, and sweat glands. The primary dermal cell type is the fibroblast, and it produces collagen, elastin, and other proteins. The dermis is further divided into the papillary and reticular dermis. The papillary dermis is located beneath the dermal-epidermal junction and contains a loose mixture of fibrocytes, collagen, and blood vessels. Below it lays the much thicker reticular dermis. It contains fewer fibrocytes but a denser collection of collagen. Dermal thickness within the head and neck ranges from less than 1 mm on the eyelids to 2.5 mm on the scalp.[3]

Collagen

Collagen is a family of proteins found throughout the skin and connective tissue of the human body. There are 18 different subtypes, 11 of which are present in the skin.[4] Type I collagen comprises approximately 80% of the dermis and endows skin with tensile strength. Type III collagen makes up approximately 15% of the dermis and is responsible for the skin's pliability. It is the predominate form of collagen in the developing fetus and is

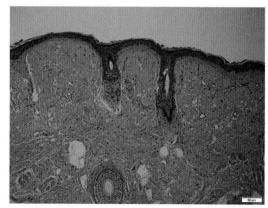

Fig. 2. Epidermis and dermis. (*Courtesy of* Kim Ruska, MD, Mount Kisco, New York.)

often referred to as fetal collagen. Type V collagen comprises approximately 4% to 5% of dermal collagen, and its function is unknown. Types IV and VII form a structural lattice and anchoring fibrils, respectively, within the dermal-epidermal junction.

Collagen is synthesized within fibroblasts from its precursor procollagen. Each type of collagen is composed of 3 chains twisted to form a triple helix. The procollagen triple helix is secreted from the fibroblasts and then modified by collagen peptidases into tropocollagen. Tropocollagen polymerizes to form collagen fibrils. Fibrils may further aggregate to form collagen fibers.

Elastin

Elastin fibers confer elasticity to the skin. Elastin is formed from the precursor protein tropoelastin in the fibroblasts. Thinner elastin fibers termed oxytalan are found primarily in the papillary dermis perpendicular to the dermal-epidermal junction. Thicker fibers called elaunin are more horizontally oriented within the reticular dermis, and still larger elastin fibers are found deeper within the reticular dermis.

Neurovascular Anatomy

The skin vasculature consists of a deep dermal/subcutaneous plexus and a superficial plexus (**Fig. 3**). The deep plexus supplies vessels to the pilosebaceous units and the superficial plexus; the superficial plexus originates vascular loops within the papillary dermis. Nutrients diffuse into the epidermis because no vessels cross the dermal-epidermal junction. Venous and lymphatic systems exist in a similar arrangement.

Both afferent and efferent nerve endings are present in the skin, and both myelinated and unmyelinated afferent nerve endings are found in the dermis (**Fig. 4**). Unencapsulated or "free" nerve endings within the papillary dermis sense pain; free nerve endings interacting with Merkel cells sense light touch. Encapsulated Meissner corpuscles in the papillary dermis also mediate light touch. Pacinian corpuscles in the deeper dermis sense vibration and pressure. Efferent nerves connect to the arrector pili muscles, apocrine glands, and eccrine glands.

Subcutaneous Tissue

The subcutaneous tissue, or hypodermis, is the tissue bridging the skin with deeper tissues such as muscle and bone. It contains the subcutaneous fat, superficial fascia, perforating blood vessels, and nerves. The relative contribution of the subcutaneous fat and superficial fascia to the overall soft tissue coverage of the facial skeleton varies within each regional unit.

SKIN APPENDAGES

Multiple appendages traverse both the dermis and the epidermis throughout the head and neck. Each hair follicle and its associated sebaceous gland, arrector pili muscle, and nerve endings form a pilosebaceous unit (**Fig. 5**). This unit is involved in skin maintenance, temperature regulation, and sensation. Sebaceous glands secrete a complex lipid onto follicles called sebum. Sebum protects the surrounding skin from desiccation and is a barrier against harmful bacteria. The small arrector pili muscle attaches obliquely from the hair follicle to the papillary dermis. Sympathetic input causes muscle contraction and the hairs to rise vertically; this in turn creates a thicker thermal air barrier. Nerve endings around the hair follicle enhance overall skin sensation.

Eccrine and apocrine sweat glands reside with the deep dermis and subcutaneous tissue while their ducts traverse the epidermis. Ecrrine glands are most abundant in the forehead, whereas apocrine glands are found in the eyelids (Moll glands) and external auditory canals. Eccrine glands produce cholinergically mediated sweat essential to temperature regulation; they empty directly onto the skin surface. Apocrine glands secrete onto the hair shaft. Their secretions release an odor when acted upon by bacteria; the secretion's function is unknown.

NONMELANOMA SKIN CANCER

Nonmelanoma skin cancer primarily refers to basal cell and squamous cell carcinoma. There are other, much less common forms of nonmelanoma skin cancer including Merkel cell carcinoma, primary cutaneous B-cell lymphoma, Kaposi sarcoma, and dermatofibrosarcoma protuberans. Basal cell carcinoma is the most common form of skin cancer and is 3 to 5 times more common than squamous cell carcinoma in many populations.[5] It is almost twice as common in men and found most commonly in the head and neck region. Squamous cell carcinoma is also more common in elderly men. A majority occur in the head and neck region, with the ear being the most common site in men.

Basal Cell Carcinoma

Basal cell carcinoma is the most commonly diagnosed skin cancer in the United States each

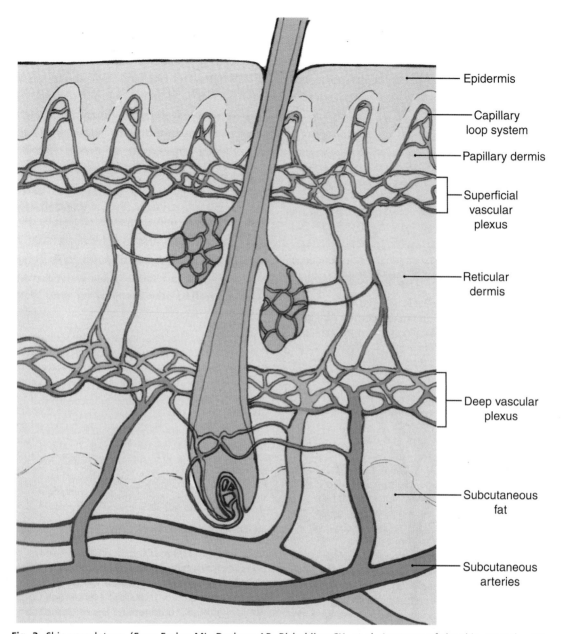

Epidermis

Capillary loop system

Papillary dermis

Superficial vascular plexus

Reticular dermis

Deep vascular plexus

Subcutaneous fat

Subcutaneous arteries

Fig. 3. Skin vasculature. (*From* Frohm ML, Durham AB, Bichakjian CK, et al. Anatomy of the skin. In: Baker SR, editor. Local flaps in facial reconstruction, 3rd edition. Philadelphia: Elsevier; 2014; p. 3–13; with permission.)

year, with 70% arising on the head. It arises from the basal cell layer of the epidermis. Basal cell carcinomas rarely metastasize but are locally destructive. Timely treatment minimizes their morbidity.

The most common cause of basal cell carcinoma is exposure to UV light, particularly UVB light.[6] Short durations of intense exposure during youth may be more important than cumulative lifetime doses. UV light may cause mutations in the *p53* tumor suppressor gene, which then disables programmed cell death and permits damaged cells to replicate. UV light from other sources such as tanning beds and photochemotherapy (with psoralens and UVA, or PUVA) also damages cells.

Heritable genetic mutations also cause basal cell carcinoma. Autosomal dominant causes include nevoid basal cell carcinoma syndrome (or Gorlin syndrome) and Rombo syndrome. Bazek syndrome is an X-linked dominant condition that causes multiple basal cell carcinomas. Xeroderma

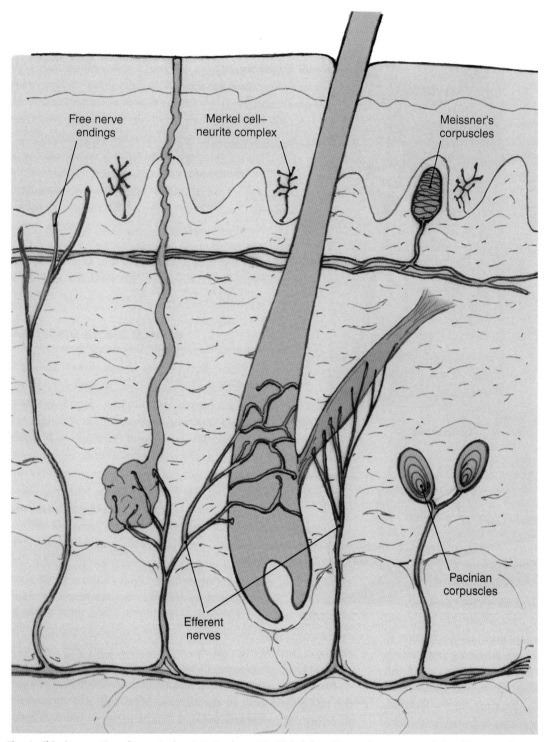

Free nerve
endings

Merkel cell–
neurite complex

Meissner's
corpuscles

Pacinian
corpuscles

Efferent
nerves

Fig. 4. Skin innervation. (*From* Frohm ML, Durham AB, Bichakjian CK, et al. Anatomy of the skin. In: Baker SR, editor. Local flaps in facial reconstruction, 3rd edition. Philadelphia: Elsevier; 2014; p. 3–13; with permission.)

pigmentosa is an autosomal recessive condition characterized by an inability to repair UV damaged DNA and the subsequent development of multiple skin cancers.

Other causes of basal cell carcinoma include ionizing radiation, immunosuppression, and toxin exposures. Radiation was an early therapy for benign skin conditions such as acne and hirsutism.

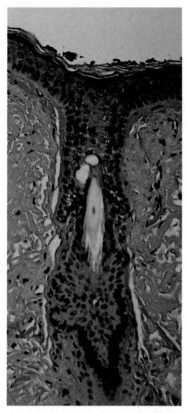

Fig. 5. Pilosebaceous unit. (*Courtesy of* Kim Ruska, MD, Mount Kisco, New York.)

Basal cell carcinoma often develops many years later in these seemingly undamaged tissue beds. Immunosuppression plays an unclear role in basal cell carcinoma development, although transplant recipients and patients with leukemia have a slight increase in the amount of basal cell carcinomas. Arsenic exposure from contaminated well water, medications, or heavy industry can also cause basal cell carcinomas.

Squamous Cell Carcinoma

Squamous cell carcinoma is the most common skin cancer after basal cell carcinoma. It develops from epidermal keratinocytes, and it is much more common in men than women.[7] As with basal cell carcinomas, prompt treatment minimizes local destruction. Delayed treatment is more dangerous because squamous cell carcinoma is more likely to recur or metastasize.

Environmental and genetic factors contribute to the development of squamous cell carcinoma. Higher cumulative lifetime doses of both UVB light and, to a lesser degree, UVA light are the primary risk factors for developing squamous cell carcinoma. UVB causes DNA damage that is generally repaired, but some escapes detection and produces mutations. P53 tumor suppressor gene mutations then allow mutated cells to escape apoptosis and propagate. UVA from sunlight or PUVA therapy impairs the ability of suppressor T cells to attack mutated cells, thus allowing them to propagate.

The most common precursor lesion to squamous cell carcinoma is the actinic keratosis. Actinic keratoses are rough, scaly lesions with ill-defined borders that develop from UV light exposure. The risk of an individual lesion developing into squamous cell carcinoma is low, although the risk that an individual patient develops squamous cell carcinoma over time is greater than 10% because multiple lesions are often present.

Sites of chronic scarring and inflammation may also predispose to squamous cell carcinoma. Marjolin ulcers are squamous cell carcinomas that develop in settings of chronic scarring or ulceration, including osteomyelitis sinuses, burn scars, and radiation dermatitis. Chronic inflammatory conditions such as lichen planus and lupus erythematosus also predispose to squamous cell carcinoma many years later, although the exact mechanism is unclear.

Finally, human papillomavirus (HPV) leads to squamous cell carcinoma. Proteins produced by high-risk HPV strains inhibit *p53* and other apoptotic pathways independent of *p53*. Immunocompromised patients are especially susceptible to HPV-induced squamous cell carcinoma.

SUMMARY

Skin is composed of the epidermis, dermis, and adnexal structures. The epidermis is composed of 4 layers: the strata basale, spinosum, granulosum, and corneum. The dermis is divided into a superficial papillary dermis and deeper reticular dermis. Collagen and elastin within the reticular dermis are responsible for skin tensile strength and elasticity, respectively. The 2 most common kind of nonmelanoma skin cancers are basal cell and squamous cell carcinoma. Both are caused by a host of environmental and genetic factors, although UV light exposure is the single greatest predisposing factor.

REFERENCES

1. Baumann L, Saghari S. Basic science of the epidermis. In: Baumann L, editor. Cosmetic dermatology. 2nd edition. New York: McGraw-Hill; 2009. p. 3–7.
2. Leithauser LA, Collar RM, Ingraffea A. Structure and function of the skin. In: Papel ID, Frodel JL, Holt GR, et al, editors. Facial plastic and reconstructive surgery. 4th edition. New York: Thieme; 2016. p. 1–5.

3. Frohm ML, Durham AB, Bichakjian CK, et al. Anatomy of the skin. In: Baker SR, editor. Local flaps in facial reconstruction. 3rd edition. Elsevier; 2014. p. 3–13.

4. Baumann L, Saghari S. Basic science of the dermis. In: Baumann L, editor. Cosmetic dermatology. 2nd edition. New York: McGraw-Hill; 2009. p. 8–13.

5. Eide MJ, Weinstock MA. Epidemiology of skin cancer. In: Rigel DS, Robinson JK, Ross M, et al, editors. Cancer of the skin. 2nd edition. Elsevier; 2011. p. 44–55.

6. Cockerell CJ, Tran KT, Carucci J, et al. Basal cell carcinoma. In: Rigel DS, Robinson JK, Ross M, et al, editors. Cancer of the skin. 2nd edition. Elsevier; 2011. p. 99–123.

7. Bhambri S, Dinehart S, Bhambri A. Squamous cell carcinoma. In: Rigel DS, Robinson JK, Ross M, et al, editors. Cancer of the skin. 2nd edition. Elsevier; 2011. p. 124–39.

Mohs Micrographic Surgery for the Management of Cutaneous Malignancies

Bobbak Mansouri, MD, Lindsay M. Bicknell, MD,
Dane Hill, MD, Gregory D. Walker, MD, MBA,
Katherine Fiala, MD*, Chad Housewright, MD

KEYWORDS

- Mohs • Mohs micrographic surgery • Skin cancer • Appropriate use criteria

KEY POINTS

- The practice of Mohs surgery has become increasingly widespread among the dermatologic surgery community and is now considered the treatment of choice for many common and uncommon cutaneous neoplasms.
- In Mohs surgery, the blade is oriented at a 45° angle to the skin, which is referred to as beveling. Beveling of the scalpel blade allows for proper alignment of the peripheral edges and examination of nearly 100% of the specimen margins.
- National guidelines, or "appropriate use criteria (AUC)," were created for Mohs surgery in 2012 based on the characteristics of an individual tumor, anatomic location, and unique patient characteristics.
- In general, locally aggressive tumors, tumors arising in locations that necessitate tissue sparing, and patients at highest risk of aggressive tumor abnormality or recurrence are ideal candidates for Mohs surgery.
- Mohs surgery is highly effective for most nonmelanoma skin cancers, is cost-effective, and has become the standard of care for many cutaneous tumors.

INTRODUCTION

Mohs micrographic surgery (MMS) is a specialized form of skin cancer surgery in which cure rates close to 100% are achieved with minimal tissue removal. The procedure was pioneered by Dr Frederic E. Mohs in the 1930s. In the late 1960s, Dr Mohs, along with Dr Theodore Tromovitch, introduced the fresh-frozen tissue technique used today.[1–3]

The method of MMS is unique in that the Mohs surgeon acts as both surgeon and pathologist.[1] In most cases, the tumor is removed, histopathology is interpreted, and the defect is repaired, all in the same day. Since Dr Mohs' initial work in the 1930s, the practice of Mohs surgery has become increasingly widespread among the dermatologic surgery community and is now considered the treatment of choice for many common and uncommon cutaneous neoplasms.[1,2,4]

HISTORY

Dr Frederic E. Mohs devised the technique of Mohs surgery during his time as a medical student.[4,5] Although working as a cancer research

Disclosure Statement: The authors have nothing to disclose.
Department of Dermatology, Baylor Scott and White Health and Texas A&M Health Science Center, 409 West Adams Avenue, Temple, TX 76501, USA
* Corresponding author.
E-mail address: Katherine.fiala@bswhealth.org

Facial Plast Surg Clin N Am 25 (2017) 291–301
http://dx.doi.org/10.1016/j.fsc.2017.03.002
1064-7406/17/Published by Elsevier Inc.

assistant, he found that application of a zinc chloride solution to cancer tissue in vitro led to tumor necrosis with maintenance of tumor histopathology, as if the tissue had been preserved in formalin. He extrapolated this finding to in vivo skin cancers. In his initial experiments, a 20% zinc chloride solution was applied to a skin cancer, allowed to fix overnight, and then the lesion was excised with narrow margins the next day. The specimen was prepared in slides via paraffin embedding and evaluated with light microscopy. If tumor cells were noted at the margin of the specimen, this process was repeated until margins were clear.[1,2] Because of extensive wound bed damage caused by the zinc chloride solution, the only option for repair after tumor extirpation was healing by secondary intention. Although this led to surprisingly pleasing cosmetic results, the healing process was lengthy, and the procedure itself quite painful for patients.[1] Although Dr Mohs started his work in what he coined "chemosurgery" in the 1930s, his findings were not published until 1941.[5] He continued to modify his method, and in 1953, he performed the first "fresh frozen section," which is the technique used today.[2]

Dr Mohs discovered the benefits of fresh-frozen sectioning quite by mistake. While filming an educational video about chemosurgery in the 1960s, he was forced to complete the procedure in 1 day.[1,2,4] Unable to allow his fixative to sit overnight, he removed an eyelid tumor using local anesthesia and prepared his slides using fresh-frozen sectioning. He found this technique caused less destruction to surrounding normal tissue, and he maintained his impressive 100% 5-year cure rate. Mohs presented his data, a cohort of 70 basal cell carcinomas (BCCs) on the eyelid removed with the fresh-frozen technique, in 1969.[3] The following year, Dr Theodore Tromovitch published a series of an additional 75 cases successfully treated with the fresh-frozen technique.[6] These findings further validated the efficacy of this method.

The fresh-frozen tissue technique quickly became the standard of care, and in 1987, the American College of Chemosurgery was renamed the American College of Mohs Surgery and Cutaneous Oncology to reflect this practice.[2] Despite numerous changes to the original method, MMS remains one of the few methods of treating cutaneous malignancies with a cure rate nearing 100%.

MOHS MICROGRAPHIC SURGERY: PREOPERATIVE CONSIDERATIONS

MMS is typically performed as an outpatient procedure under local anesthesia in a dermatology office. As with any surgical procedure, a careful review of the medical record is performed. Specific considerations include antibiotic prophylaxis in compliance with the American Heart Association (AHA),[7] American Academy of Orthopedics, and American Dental Association guidelines,[8] careful review of implantable devices (as electrodessication devices may cause interference),[9] verification of prescription or nonprescription anticoagulants, HIV and hepatitis C status, allergies, and oxygen requirements.

Antibiotic Prophylaxis

In 2007, the AHA published revised guidelines on the use of antibiotics for endocarditis prophylaxis before minor procedures.[7] Their current recommendations indicate that endocarditis prophylaxis is only necessary in cases involving infected skin or in patients with prosthetic implants, a history of endocarditis, cardiac valve disease after cardiac transplant, or history of cyanotic congenital heart disease. In addition, prophylaxis may be given to patients who have received an orthopedic implant in the 2 years before their procedure or any patient with a history of a previously infected joint.[8]

For patients requiring antibiotic prophylaxis, the AHA recommends 2 g amoxicillin administered by mouth 30 to 60 minutes before their procedure, because it allows antibiotics to be in the bloodstream at the time of incision and in the wound coagulum at the time of procedure completion.[7,10] Alternative antibiotic choices include cephalexin 2 g by mouth or, for penicillin-allergic patients, clindamycin 600 mg by mouth.[8] If the preprocedure antibiotic dose was missed inadvertently, the medication may be given up to 2 hours after the procedure.

Anticoagulants

In the authors' practice, they recommend patients continue their anticoagulant medications during MMS because most cutaneous and subcutaneous bleeding is easily managed with electrodessication. For patients receiving warfarin, a prothrombin time and international normalized ratio are obtained 1 week preoperatively. Surgery should be avoided in patients with supratherapeutic anticoagulation.

Implantable Devices

The use of electrodessication to achieve hemostasis is of particular concern in patients with a pacemaker and/or defibrillator as well as other implanted electrical devices, including deep brain stimulators and pain pumps. Traditionally, the use of electric current is contraindicated in these patients because of risk of device malfunction from electromagnetic interference.[9] Device destruction, reprogramming, or battery depletion may also occur.[11] More recent in vitro studies indicate that electrodessication with a hyfrecator on maximal settings may be used safely beyond a 3-cm radius around the implanted device or beyond a 1-cm radius with standard settings.[9] Use of short, 1-second bursts of electricity, as opposed to longer bursts, further improves the safety of hyfrecator use in the setting of implanted devices.[11] In oxygen-dependent patients, oxygen flow is temporarily discontinued while using electrical means of hemostasis because the spark could ignite a fire.

MOHS MICROGRAPHIC SURGERY: SURGICAL TECHNIQUE

MMS is customarily performed in a nonsterile, minor procedure room. Studies have shown that clean, nonsterile gloves are safe and effective for this procedure without altering infection rates during tumor extirpation.[12] In fact, a recent systematic review and large meta-analysis showed that no difference was found in the rate of postoperative surgical site infections between outpatient surgical procedures performed with sterile versus nonsterile gloves.[13]

Obtaining informed consent before MMS is unique and nuanced in comparison to other dermatologic procedures. The final defect size and subsequent repair are estimated before the procedure. There exists a high likelihood that the tumor may extend beyond what is evident to the naked eye, referred to as subclinical extension. Factors associated with subclinical extension include tumors greater than 1 cm in diameter, recurrent tumors, and tumors with fibrosis noted on initial biopsy.[14] It is essential to discuss expectations of final defect sizes and potential repair options with the patient.

Once informed consent is obtained, the biopsy site is identified. In an effort to avoid wrong site surgery, biopsy site confirmation is of the utmost importance. This identification, however, can present a challenge. Small biopsy specimens are frequently sampled, resulting in a small wound or scar. Lag time between the biopsy and surgery in addition to background actinic damage compounds the issue. Furthermore, patient confusion can play a role as they may have had multiple procedures (on separate tumors) scheduled on the same day. Since the exact site is not always readily visible, patients can point to the precise biopsy site with a cotton tip applicator while holding a hand-held mirror. Multiple studies have shown, though, that the patient may identify the incorrect site of the biopsy.[15–17] One such study revealed that 16.6% of patients and 5.9% of physicians incorrectly identify biopsy sites.[15] When preoperative photographs were available in this study, the correct site was always identified. As such, photography at the time of biopsy is perhaps the best way to ensure that the biopsy site is evident at the time of surgery.

Several additional strategies may be used to aid in the identification of the correct site. Rubbing the site with cotton gauze produces hyperemia and/or superficial abrasions in the biopsy site. In addition, visualization of the area with a dermatoscope can assist in revealing residual tumor or scar tissue. A patient may argue that if the tumor is not clinically visible, there is no need to proceed with surgery. However, although residual tumor was clinically observed in only 12% of patients, histologically apparent tumor was present in 69% of cases.[18]

Procedure Preparation

Once the site is confirmed, the patient is placed in a recumbent position, and the area is cleansed with an antiseptic, such as chlorhexidine. Before injecting local anesthesia, a surgical ink pen is used to delineate clinically evident tumor or boundaries of the biopsy scar. Marking the site before injection of local anesthesia is preferred because the fluid's tumescence distorts the site and obscures clear delineation of the scar/tumor margins.

Once anesthetized, a reusable curette is used to gently scrape the tumor. Curettage debulks the tumor to allow for proper fixation of the peripheral edges of the specimen by the histotechnicians. Bulky, thick specimens are more technically challenging to process. In addition, data have shown that the use of curettage reduces the number of stages needed to clear the tumor, because it helps to delineate the margins of the tumor.[19]

Following curettage, a 1-mm (mm) peripheral margin is marked with the surgical ink pen. Reference marks are placed at the 12, 3, 6, and 9 o'clock positions to ensure precise orientation (Fig. 1). Some surgeons choose to create superficial nicks or reference marks with the blade versus the surgical ink pen. All methodologies for specimen marking are to properly orient the specimen and allow anatomic triangulation of any residual tumor based on histopathologic interpretation.

Excision of the First Layer

In most cutaneous excisions, the blade is oriented at a 90° angle to the skin in order to more closely approximate the skin during repair. In MMS, the

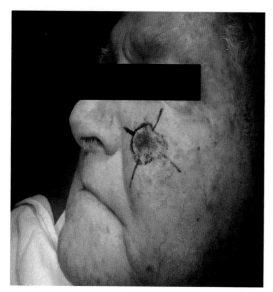

Fig. 1. Reference marks at the 12, 3, 6, and 9 o'clock positions to assist with orientation.

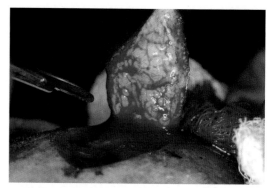

Fig. 3. Removal of a Mohs stage in a flat horizontal plane.

blade is oriented at a 45° angle to the skin, which is referred to as beveling (**Fig. 2**). Beveling of the scalpel blade allows for proper alignment of the peripheral edges of the tissue specimen during preparation of the histologic specimen.

Once the Mohs surgeon scores the skin in a beveled fashion, the tumor is excised with careful attention to remove a thin specimen in a flat, horizontal plane immediately below the depth of previous curettage (**Fig. 3**). Obtaining a flat, disc-shaped specimen is imperative, because it helps ensure proper processing of the specimen onto slides in a horizontal plane. Hemostasis is obtained with electrodessication, and the patient is temporarily bandaged. During slide preparation and evaluation, the patient is free to wait in a comfortable waiting area.

The tissue is placed on surgical gauze with careful attention to maintain the anatomic orientation of the specimen. The tissue is transported to the histology laboratory, where the MMS map is produced (**Fig. 4**). The map is an essential tool that correlates the surgical site, tissue specimen, and histologic slides produced. Extreme care is taken to maintain precise orientation of the specimen and map, because the map serves to guide future stages of tumor removal should the margins be involved in the first or subsequent stages.

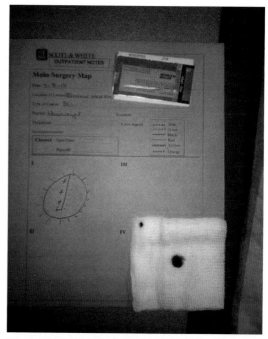

Fig. 4. The first Mohs stage is oriented on the gauze to match the Mohs map. The map indicates date, tumor location, tumor type, name of the Mohs surgeon, and the plan for inking the first stage.

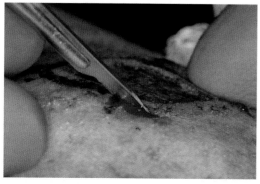

Fig. 2. The number 15 blade beveled at a 45° angle to the underlying skin during the first Mohs stage.

Processing of the Surgical Specimen

The first stage is inked and mapped with a drawn representation on the Mohs map (**Fig. 5**). The inked tissue is cut into appropriately sized blocks to fit onto a glass slide. The specimen is flattened, often by using relaxing shallow cuts parallel to the epidermal edge, in order for the epidermis to lie evenly in the same plane as the deep margin. This step is crucial and allows the epidermis and the subcutaneous fat to both be visualized by the Mohs surgeon on the glass slide with the goal of examining 100% of the specimen's margin.

The practice of examining the entire margin is one of the key advantages of MMS and differs from the traditional "bread-loafing" technique used by pathologists on excisional specimens, which slices tissue specimens vertically at 2- to 4-mm intervals to check for tumor at the margins.[2] Thus, in excisional specimens, less than 1% of the surgical margin is examined with standard vertical sectioning techniques.[20] Once the tissue is frozen in the cryostat and fixed with optimal cooling temperature embedding medium, approximately 6 to 9 wafers of tissue initially coming from the deepest margin are placed onto the glass slide. The slides are stained, most commonly with hematoxylin and eosin, which takes 10 minutes on average using an automated stainer (**Fig. 6**). Complete sections of tissue containing 100% or a 360° representation of the peripheral and deep margins are examined by the Mohs surgeon who serves as the pathologist and determines residual skin cancer or clearance. Each wafer of tissue should contain complete areas of epidermis, dermis, and subcutis.

There is considerable variability in the practice of Mohs surgeons and their definitions of a tumor-free margin.[21] Based on the practices of the average Mohs surgeon, if 4 or more wafers of

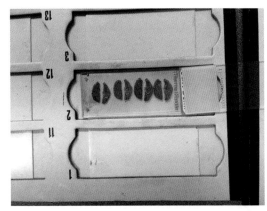

Fig. 6. Glass slide (micrograph) of Mohs specimen showing tissue mounted with deep and peripheral margins within the same plane. Four wafers of the first stage are placed on the first slide in this example.

tissue are tumor free, then the tumor excision is complete, and the margins are considered clear. If the epidermal edge contains tumor within the first 4 wafers, then a second layer is taken, which widens the defect. If the deep dermis or subcutis contains tumor, then the second layer deepens the defect in the corresponding anatomic location. Each subsequent layer taken with small (1–2 mm) margins is marked on the Mohs map, and the processing is repeated (**Fig. 7**). Once clear margins are confirmed, the Mohs surgeon prepares for reconstruction.

INDICATIONS FOR MOHS MICROGRAPHIC SURGERY

In 2012, the American Academy of Dermatology (AAD), American College of Mohs Surgery, American Society for Dermatologic Surgery Association, and American Society for Mohs Surgery

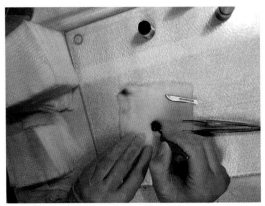

Fig. 5. The Mohs surgeon inks the first stage in the laboratory.

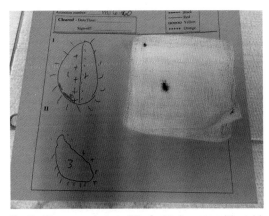

Fig. 7. The second stage (II) of a Mohs map with residual tumor removed from the area of prior tumor positivity and mapped as stage II.

devised a set of guidelines to help clinicians select the most appropriate neoplasms for treatment with MMS.[22] These guidelines, or "appropriate use criteria (AUC)," were based on the characteristics of an individual tumor, anatomic location, and unique patient characteristics (**Table 1**). In general, locally aggressive tumors, tumors arising in locations that necessitate tissue sparing, and patients at highest risk of aggressive tumor abnormality or recurrence are ideal candidates for MMS.

The AAD generated a Smartphone application that aids in the determination of an individual lesion's appropriateness for MMS according to these AUC guidelines. Although this tool is not intended to replace the physician's clinical judgment, it may aid in clinical decision making.

Tumor Characteristics

Important factors in determining the appropriateness of MMS for certain cutaneous tumors include tumor type, histologically aggressive growth patterns, tumor size, and a positive margin on a prior curative excision (see **Table 1**).

The most common nonmelanoma skin cancers treated with MMS are basal cell and squamous cell carcinomas (SCCs). In addition, due to its unique histologic margin control and subsequent limitation of final defect size, MMS is considered appropriate for the extirpation of a variety of less common cutaneous neoplasms, including adenocystic carcinoma, adnexal carcinoma, apocrine/eccrine carcinoma, atypical fibroxanthoma, dermatofibrosarcoma protuberans, extramammary Paget disease, leiomyosarcoma, malignant fibrous histiocytoma, Merkel cell carcinoma, microcystic adnexal carcinoma, mucinous carcinoma, and sebaceous carcinoma,[22] and may be appropriate for porocarcinoma.[23] MMS is also considered appropriate for the surgical removal of primary or recurrent lentigo maligna and melanoma in situ (MIS) in certain anatomic locations. Furthermore, MMS has been shown to be an effective treatment of invasive melanoma with a 0.72% recurrence rate for primary invasive melanomas and a 5.1% recurrence rate for recurrent invasive melanomas with a mean follow-up time of 3.73 years,[24] although many Mohs surgeons do not regularly treat melanocytic lesions.

Aggressive histologic growth patterns indicate that a lesion may have a higher risk of recurrence, and MMS is appropriate.[22] For BCCs, these growth patterns include morpheaform, fibrosing, sclerosing, infiltrating, perineural, keratotic, and micronodular. For SCCs, histologically aggressive growth patterns include sclerosing, basosquamous, small cell, poorly or undifferentiated, perineural,

perivascular, spindle cell, pagetoid, infiltrating, keratoacanthoma type (central facial), single cell, clear cell, lymphoepithelial, and sarcomatoid.

Breslow depth 2 mm or greater and Clark level IV or greater are also indications of aggressive SCCs.[22] In general, as cutaneous tumors become larger, they become more appropriate for MMS. In fact, tumors larger than 2 cm are generally considered appropriate for MMS, regardless of tumor type or anatomic location.[1,22]

Patient Characteristics

Patients who are immunocompromised, diagnosed with a genetic syndrome that increases risk of skin cancer (eg, basal cell nevus syndrome or xeroderma pigmentosum), have been previously treated for an aggressive skin cancer, or have received adjuvant radiation for a skin cancer are typically considered good candidates for MMS.[22]

Areas of the Body

MMS has been shown to reduce the size of final surgical defects[25] and, as such, is most appropriate for functionally and cosmetically sensitive anatomic locations.[1] The AUC divides the body into 3 areas: H, M, and L. Area H includes the central portion of the face (eyelids, nose, lips, and chin), ears, genitalia, hands, feet, nails, ankles, and nipples (see **Table 1**). Neoplasms in these anatomic locations are considered highly appropriate candidates for Mohs surgery because of the need for tissue preservation.

Area M includes the cheeks, forehead, scalp, neck, jawline, and pretibial surface. Area L includes the trunk and extremities, but excludes the pretibial surface, hands, feet, nail units, and ankles. For neoplasms in areas M and L, other characteristics, including the aforementioned tumor and patient characteristics, must be taken into consideration to determine a patient's candidacy for treatment with MMS.

EFFECTIVENESS OF MOHS MICROGRAPHIC SURGERY FOR CUTANEOUS TUMORS
Basal Cell Carcinoma

BCC is the most common cutaneous malignancy.[26] BCCs are typically slow-growing and only locally destructive, and metastases and mortality associated with these tumors are extremely rare.[27–29]

Recurrence rates for primary BCCs treated with standard excision versus MMS are 10% and 1%, respectively.[30–32] Five-year recurrence rates for recurrent BCCs with standard excision are 5% to 40% compared with those treated with MMS, which are 3% to 8%.[30,31,33,34] In a randomized

Table 1		
Mohs appropriate use criteria		
Areas of the body		
H	Central face (eyelids, nose, lips, chin) Ears Genitalia Hands Feet Nails Ankles Nipples	
M	Cheeks Forehead Scalp Neck Jawline Pretibial surface	
L	Trunk Extremities, excluding sites listed above	
Patient characteristics		
Immunocompromised		
Genetic predisposition to skin cancer development		
History of aggressive cutaneous neoplasm		
History of adjuvant radiation for cutaneous neoplasm		
Tumor characteristics		
Positive margins on prior excision		
Aggressive histopathology		
BCC	Morpheaform, fibrosing, or sclerosing Infiltrative growth pattern Perineural invasion Metatypical or keratotic growth pattern Micronodular Recurrent	
SCC	Sclerosing Basosquamous Small cell Poorly differentiated or undifferentiated Perineural or perivascular invasion Spindle cell morphology Pagetoid spread Infiltrative growth pattern Keratoacanthoma type Single cell Clear cell Lymphoepithelial Sarcomatoid Recurrent	
Size		
Less than or equal to 0.5 cm	Highly appropriate for Mohs surgery in areas H and M, or if aggressive tumor features are noted. Exception is superficial BCC In areas L, appropriateness determined by presence of aggressive tumor features	

(continued on next page)

Table 1 (continued)	
0.6 to 2 cm	Highly appropriate for Mohs surgery in areas H and M, or if aggressive tumor features are noted In areas L, appropriateness determined by presence of aggressive tumor features
Greater than 2 cm	Highly appropriate for Mohs surgery in areas H, M, or L, particularly if aggressive features are noted. Exception is superficial BCC

Adapted from Ad Hoc Task F, Connolly SM, Baker DR, et al. AAD/ACMS/ASDSA/ASMS 2012 appropriate use criteria for Mohs micrographic surgery: a report of the American Academy of Dermatology, American College of Mohs Surgery, American Society for Dermatologic Surgery Association, and the American Society for Mohs Surgery. J Am Acad Dermatol 2012;67(4):531–50; with permission.

clinical trial of patients with BCC on the face, 10-year cumulative probabilities for recurrence in primary BCCs were 12.2% versus 4.4% with standard excision and MMS, respectively, and 13.5% and 3.9% for recurrent BCCs treated with standard excision versus MMS, respectively.[35] Furthermore, larger tumors and tumors in anatomically challenging locations can have lower cure rates. For example, BCCs larger than 3 cm in diameter have a 93% cure rate as opposed to the 99% cure rate for lesions smaller than 3 cm,[1] whereas periocular and perioral BCCs have a cure rate of 98%.[36]

Squamous Cell Carcinoma

SCC is the second most common skin malignancy. They are typically graded as well-, moderately-, or poorly differentiated neoplasms. Unlike BCCs, SCCs have significant metastatic potential.[37] SCCs are considered to be more aggressive in the presence of perineural or perivascular involvement, high mitotic rate, sclerotic stroma, pagetoid spread of cells into the epidermis, and spindle cell morphology, among other factors. High-risk SCCs are characterized by moderate to poor cellular differentiation, larger size (greater than 2 cm in diameter or 2 mm in thickness), anatomic location on the face, ear, periauricular, genitalia, hands, or feet, perineural invasion, immunosuppression, and local recurrence.[38,39] As such, they are more likely to be locally aggressive or metastasize.

For SCCs smaller than 2 cm in diameter, there is a 5-year cure rate of 99% with MMS.[2] Tumors between 2 and 3 cm in diameter have an 82% 5-year cure rate, whereas tumors larger than 3 cm have a 59% cure rate. Of important note, 95% of SCCs that recur locally or metastasize do so in the first 5 years after surgery.[40]

Melanoma in Situ and Malignant Melanoma

MIS and malignant melanoma may exhibit significant subclinical spread as well as local and distant metastases. MIS is confined to the epidermis and does not invade past the basement membrane into the dermis, whereas malignant (or invasive) melanomas invade into the dermis and have a higher malignant potential. Because of the locally extensive nature of melanoma, some debate exists regarding appropriate margins of excision, and many melanocytic neoplasms require wider than recommended margins to clear.[41,42]

MMS is ideal for such tumors and provides evidence for appropriate excision margins. A recent study by Stigall and colleagues[43] showed that only 83% of MIS of the trunk and proximal extremities were cleared with 6-mm margins. In order to achieve a 97% clearance rate, 9-mm margins were needed. In their retrospective review of 882 patients who had MIS treated with MMS, only one patient had local recurrence and only one patient had distant metastases. For MIS of the head and neck, 65% of lesions required margins greater than 5 mm.[44]

RECONSTRUCTION

Following complete clearance of the tumor, the Mohs surgeon prepares for reconstruction of the surgical defect. Mohs surgeons use a variety of techniques when closing both simple and more complex skin defects, including complex linear closures, skin flaps, and skin grafts. Anatomic location of the defect, depth of the wound, reservoir of nearby skin, and adjacent anatomic structures are all taken into consideration while planning defect repair, as they all affect function and aesthetics.[45]

Mohs surgeons use local anesthesia for the closure of most defects. However, in the case of larger head or neck defects, the use of tumescent anesthesia may reduce the risk of lidocaine toxicity.[46] Delaying repair is an additional consideration for larger defects but can present complications with wound care as well as deformity of nearby structures.[45] For patients with larger defects, general anesthesia may be necessary given the limits of local anesthesia and the risk of discomfort and toxicity to the patient.[1]

Although dermatologic surgeons are trained to perform complex closures involving the nose, eyelid, and ears, larger and more complicated defects involving these areas may be better served by collaboration with otolaryngology, ophthalmology, or plastic surgery. For example, periocular defects involving greater than 50% of the cosmetic subunit and nasal lesions that involve the nasal sinuses may be better served by referral to an appropriate specialist.[45] Surgeons should certainly consider patient preference and comorbidities with regards to referral.[1]

COST OF MOHS MICROGRAPHIC SURGERY

The cost of MMS was previously thought to be comparable to standard surgical excision.[47] More recently, Ravitskiy and colleagues[48] examined more than 400 tumors treated in the United States. There was a decreased cost using MMS for skin cancer removal versus standard excision at an average cost of $805 per tumor treated. Standard surgical excision in the office setting with permanent margins ($1026) was more expensive than MMS but less expensive than standard surgical excision with frozen margins ($1200). Standard surgical excision with frozen margins in an ambulatory surgical center was the most expensive ($2507) type of skin cancer treatment. The cost savings of treating skin cancers with MMS is a result of bundling payments, because the Mohs surgeon acts as both the surgeon and the pathologist on the case.

European studies have demonstrated to a lesser degree the cost-effectiveness of MMS when compared with standard surgical excision.[49,50] In these studies, however, separate pathology-trained physicians interpret the histopathology, and their billing is not included in the Mohs surgical calculation. Adjusting for this variable would likely yield results similar to those seen in the United States.

SUMMARY

MMS is a form of skin cancer surgery in which the Mohs surgeon acts as both surgeon and pathologist. The procedure is characterized by its histopathologic margin control and ability to spare tissue, particularly in cosmetically sensitive locations. MMS is highly effective for most nonmelanoma skin cancers, is cost-effective, and has become the standard of care for many cutaneous tumors.

REFERENCES

1. Dim-Jamora KC, Perone JB. Management of cutaneous tumors with Mohs micrographic surgery. Semin Plast Surg 2008;22(4):247–56.
2. Shriner DL, McCoy DK, Goldberg DJ, et al. Mohs micrographic surgery. J Am Acad Dermatol 1998; 39(1):79–97.
3. Mohs FE. Cancer of eyelids. Bull Am Coll Chemosurgery 1970;3:10–1.
4. Mohs FE. Mohs micrographic surgery. A historical perspective. Dermatol Clin 1989;7(4):609–11.
5. Mohs FE. Chemosurgery: a microscopically controlled method of cancer excision. Arch Surg 1941;42(2): 279–95.
6. Tromovitch TA, Stegeman SJ. Microscopically controlled excision of skin tumors. Arch Dermatol 1974;110(2):231–2.
7. Wilson W, Taubert KA, Gewitz M, et al. Prevention of infective endocarditis: guidelines from the American Heart Association: a guideline from the American Heart Association Rheumatic Fever, Endocarditis, and Kawasaki Disease Committee, Council on Cardiovascular Disease in the Young, and the Council on Clinical Cardiology, Council on Cardiovascular Surgery and Anesthesia, and the Quality of Care and Outcomes Research Interdisciplinary Working Group. Circulation 2007; 116(15):1736–54.
8. American Dental Association, American Academy of Orthopedic Surgeons. Antibiotic prophylaxis for dental patients with total joint replacements. J Am Dent Assoc 2003;134(7):895–9.
9. Weyer C, Siegle RJ, Eng GG. Investigation of hyfrecators and their in vitro interference with implantable cardiac devices. Dermatol Surg 2012;38(11): 1843–8.
10. Classen DC, Evans RS, Pestotnik SL, et al. The timing of prophylactic administration of antibiotics and the risk of surgical-wound infection. N Engl J Med 1992;326(5):281–6.
11. Taheri A, Mansoori P, Sandoval LF, et al. Electrosurgery: part II. Technology, applications, and safety of electrosurgical devices. J Am Acad Dermatol 2014; 70(4):607.e1–2 [quiz: 619–20].
12. Rhinehart MB, Murphy MM, Farley MF, et al. Sterile versus nonsterile gloves during Mohs micrographic surgery: infection rate is not affected. Dermatol Surg 2006;32(2):170–6.
13. Brewer JD, Gonzalez AB, Baum CL, et al. Comparison of sterile vs nonsterile gloves in cutaneous surgery and common outpatient dental procedures: a systematic review and meta-analysis. JAMA Dermatol 2016;152(9):1008–14.
14. Breuninger H, Dietz K. Prediction of subclinical tumor infiltration in basal cell carcinoma. J Dermatol Surg Oncol 1991;17(7):574–8.

15. McGinness JL, Goldstein G. The value of preoperative biopsy-site photography for identifying cutaneous lesions. Dermatol Surg 2010;36(2):194–7.

16. Ke M, Moul D, Camouse M, et al. Where is it? The utility of biopsy-site photography. Dermatol Surg 2010;36(2):198–202.

17. Nijhawan RI, Lee EH, Nehal KS. Biopsy site selfies–a quality improvement pilot study to assist with correct surgical site identification. Dermatol Surg 2015; 41(4):499–504.

18. Palmer VM, Wilson PR. Incompletely excised basal cell carcinoma: residual tumor rates at Mohs re-excision. Dermatol Surg 2013;39(5):706–18.

19. Ratner D, Bagiella E. The efficacy of curettage in delineating margins of basal cell carcinoma before Mohs micrographic surgery. Dermatol Surg 2003; 29(9):899–903.

20. Davidson TM, Nahum AM, Haghighi P, et al. The biology of head and neck cancer. Detection and control by parallel histologic sections. Arch Otolaryngol 1984;110(3):193–6.

21. Cartee TV, Monheit GD. How many sections are required to clear a tumor? Results from a web-based survey of margin thresholds in Mohs micrographic surgery. Dermatol Surg 2013;39(2):179–86.

22. Ad Hoc Task F, Connolly SM, Baker DR, et al. AAD/ACMS/ASDSA/ASMS 2012 appropriate use criteria for Mohs micrographic surgery: a report of the American Academy of Dermatology, American College of Mohs Surgery, American Society for Dermatologic Surgery Association, and the American Society for Mohs Surgery. J Am Acad Dermatol 2012;67(4): 531–50.

23. Tolkachjov SN, Hocker TL, Camilleri MJ, et al. Treatment of porocarcinoma with Mohs micrographic surgery: the Mayo Clinic experience. Dermatol Surg 2016;42(6):745–50.

24. Valentin-Nogueras SM, Brodland DG, Zitelli JA, et al. Mohs micrographic surgery using MART-1 immunostain in the treatment of invasive melanoma and melanoma in situ. Dermatol Surg 2016;42(6): 733–44.

25. Muller FM, Dawe RS, Moseley H, et al. Randomized comparison of Mohs micrographic surgery and surgical excision for small nodular basal cell carcinoma: tissue-sparing outcome. Dermatol Surg 2009;35(9):1349–54.

26. Robinson JK. Mohs micrographic surgery. Clin Plast Surg 1993;20(1):149–56.

27. Raszewski RL, Guyuron B. Long-term survival following nodal metastases from basal cell carcinoma. Ann Plast Surg 1990;24(2):170–5.

28. Christian MM, Murphy CM, Wagner RF Jr. Metastatic basal cell carcinoma presenting as unilateral lymphedema. Dermatol Surg 1998;24(10):1151–3.

29. Berti JJ, Sharata HH. Metastatic basal cell carcinoma to the lung. Cutis 1999;63(3):165–6.

30. Swanson NA. Mohs surgery. Technique, indications, applications, and the future. Arch Dermatol 1983; 119(9):761–73.

31. Robins P. Chemosurgery: my 15 years of experience. J Dermatol Surg Oncol 1981;7(10):779–89.

32. Rowe DE, Carroll RJ, Day CL Jr. Long-term recurrence rates in previously untreated (primary) basal cell carcinoma: implications for patient follow-up. J Dermatol Surg Oncol 1989;15(3):315–28.

33. Menn H, Robins P, Kopf AW, et al. The recurrent basal cell epithelioma. A study of 100 cases of recurrent, re-treated basal cell epitheliomas. Arch Dermatol 1971;103(6):628–31.

34. Rowe DE, Carroll RJ, Day CL Jr. Mohs surgery is the treatment of choice for recurrent (previously treated) basal cell carcinoma. J Dermatol Surg Oncol 1989; 15(4):424–31.

35. van Loo E, Mosterd K, Krekels GA, et al. Surgical excision versus Mohs' micrographic surgery for basal cell carcinoma of the face: a randomised clinical trial with 10 year follow-up. Eur J Cancer 2014; 50(17):3011–20.

36. Downes RN, Walker NP, Collin JR. Micrographic (MOHS') surgery in the management of periocular basal cell epitheliomas. Eye (Lond) 1990;4(Pt 1):160–8.

37. Goldman GD. Squamous cell cancer: a practical approach. Semin Cutan Med Surg 1998;17(2):80–95.

38. Haisma MS, Plaat BE, Bijl HP, et al. Multivariate analysis of potential risk factors for lymph node metastasis in patients with cutaneous squamous cell carcinoma of the head and neck. J Am Acad Dermatol 2016;75(4):722–30.

39. Burton KA, Ashack KA, Khachemoune A. Cutaneous squamous cell carcinoma: a review of high-risk and metastatic disease. Am J Clin Dermatol 2016;17: 491–508.

40. Marks R. Squamous cell carcinoma. Lancet 1996; 347(9003):735–8.

41. Nagi C, O'Grady TC, Izadpanah A. Mohs micrographically controlled surgery and the treatment of malignant melanoma. Semin Oncol 2002;29(4): 336–40.

42. Harris TJ, Hinckley DM. Melanoma of the head and neck in Queensland. Head Neck Surg 1983;5(3): 197–203.

43. Stigall LE, Brodland DG, Zitelli JA. The use of Mohs micrographic surgery (MMS) for melanoma in situ (MIS) of the trunk and proximal extremities. J Am Acad Dermatol 2016;75:1015–21.

44. Felton S, Taylor RS, Srivastava D. Excision margins for melanoma in situ on the head and neck. Dermatol Surg 2016;42(3):327–34.

45. Gladstone HB, Stewart D. An algorithm for the reconstruction of complex facial defects. Skin Therapy Lett 2007;12(2):6–9.

46. Acosta AE. Clinical parameters of tumescent anesthesia in skin cancer reconstructive surgery. A

review of 86 patients. Arch Dermatol 1997;133(4):
451–4.

47. Cook J, Zitelli JA. Mohs micrographic surgery: a
cost analysis. J Am Acad Dermatol 1998;39(5 Pt
1):698–703.

48. Ravitskiy L, Brodland DG, Zitelli JA. Cost analysis:
Mohs micrographic surgery. Dermatol Surg 2012;
38(4):585–94.

49. Smeets NW, Krekels GA, Ostertag JU, et al. Surgical
excision vs Mohs' micrographic surgery for basal-
cell carcinoma of the face: randomised controlled
trial. Lancet 2004;364(9447):1766–72.

50. Essers BA, Dirksen CD, Nieman FH, et al. Cost-
effectiveness of Mohs micrographic surgery vs surgical excision for basal cell carcinoma of the face.
Arch Dermatol 2006;142(2):187–94.

The Physiology and Biomechanics of Skin Flaps

James B. Lucas, MD[a,b,*]

KEYWORDS

- Cutaneous vascular anatomy • Skin physiology • Local skin flaps • Cutaneous flap physiology
- Vascular delay • Skin flap biomechanics • Mohs reconstruction

KEY POINTS

- The skin is an incredibly complex organ system responsible for the 3 main functions of protection, thermoregulation, and sensation.
- The vascular anatomy of the skin comprises an intricate network of vascular plexuses that are responsible for maintaining the vitality of the cutaneous structures and facilitating the use of local skin flaps in Mohs reconstruction.
- Local skin flaps are categorized based on their vascular supply and include random cutaneous flaps, axial or direct cutaneous flaps, and fasciocutaneous flaps.
- Significant physiologic changes occur within the skin during flap elevation and transfer, enhancing and promoting flap survival. These changes can be further leveraged using the concepts of vascular delay.
- An understanding of the biomechanical properties of nonlinearity, anisotropy, and viscoelasticity is critical in the design and execution of local skin flap reconstruction.

INTRODUCTION

The closure of skin defects created by Mohs micrographic surgery routinely requires the use of cutaneous flaps borrowed from the surrounding skin to produce an aesthetically pleasing result. Flap creation results in tissue stresses that can have a significant impact on survival of the flap by potentially compromising the neurovascular supply to the cutaneous structures. With these stresses in mind, cutaneous surgeons must command a full knowledge and understanding of the vascular patterns, physiology, and biomechanics of skin flaps. That a skin flap is able to survive such insults is a direct result of these redundant and complex systems providing vitality and survivability to the flap when correctly designed. A full understanding of the physiology of integumentary structures and the biomechanics involved in tissue transfer results in improved flap survival and outcomes.

VASCULAR ANATOMY AND PHYSIOLOGY OF THE SKIN

The skin is a complex organ system comprising the epidermis, the dermis, and the subcutaneous tissues. It is the body's largest organ system, responsible for 3 main functions: sensation, protection, and thermoregulation. The thermoregulatory function and nutritional support of the integument result from the unique configuration

Disclosure Statement: The author has nothing to disclose.
[a] Facial Plastic and Reconstructive Surgery, Carl R. Darnall Army Medical Center, 36065 Santa Fe Avenue, Fort Hood, TX 76544, USA; [b] Department of Surgery, Uniformed Services University of Health Sciences, 4301 Jones Bridge Road #A3007, Bethesda, MD 20814, USA
* 36065 Santa Fe Avenue, Fort Hood, TX 76544.
E-mail address: james.b.lucas12.mil@mail.mil

and rheology of the blood supply to the skin. Although the sensory and barrier functions of the skin are of obvious and of vital importance, the main focus of this discussion is on the blood supply and thermoregulatory function of the skin.

Vascular Anatomy

The vascular supply to the skin is extraordinarily complex. It receives contributions from a variety of sources, coupled with a dizzying network of anastomosing vessels that forms several extensive and highly interconnected vascular plexuses at differing levels within the architecture of the skin. A fair degree of variance exists in the literature when describing the vascular anatomy, with certain terms used interchangeably by different investigators. To help alleviate any confusion, an attempt is made to simplify the anatomic descriptions and maintain consistency in the application of this terminology.

There are 3 main locoregional conduits of blood flow to the skin: musculocutaneous arteries, direct cutaneous arteries, and septocutaneous arteries. Musculocutaneous arteries are perforators from deeper muscular arteries that pass through their corresponding muscle tissue and enter the subcutaneous fat to ultimately drain into the subdermal and dermal plexuses. Less common than their musculocutaneous counterparts, direct cutaneous arteries are generally specific, named arteries or branches of named arteries that run through the subcutaneous tissues in a plane parallel to the skin. They have been described as confined to specific areas of the body[1] and are generally accompanied by veins known as venae comitantes. Although they may branch off septocutaneous arteries, they are generally named branches of larger arteries. Examples include the parietal and frontal branches of the superficial temporal artery, the posterior auricular artery, the occipital artery, the supratrochlear artery, and the supraorbital artery.[1] Septocutaneous arteries course through the fascial septa dividing the individual muscle segments to provide blood flow to the skin. The fasciocutaneous component of these arteries runs parallel to the skin surface atop and/or deep to the superficial muscular fascia, and they are also generally accompanied by a pair of veins.[2] The direct cutaneous and septocutaneous arteries are responsible for supplying larger, more diffuse regions of skin, whereas the areas supplied by musculocutaneous arteries are generally smaller and more discrete in distribution. All 3 arterial sources drain into components of the rich network of plexuses that exist within the superficial soft tissues. It is particularly relevant that there is often more than one source of blood supply to a particular area of the skin,[3] which contributes significantly to the hardiness of the cutaneous flaps commonly used in facial reconstruction.

As many as 5 different vascular plexuses within the skin and superficial soft tissues have been described in the literature, including the dermal, subdermal, subcutaneous, prefascial, and subfascial networks.[3] The dermal and subdermal networks are sometimes considered a single unit, referred to as the dermal-subdermal plexus. The prefascial and subfascial networks are formed from the fasciocutaneous system off the septocutaneous arteries. The subcutaneous plexus is probably the least consistent and least described of the skin plexuses. **Fig. 1** represents the manner in which all these vascular webs are extensively interconnected, creating a vast and elaborate system of collateral blood flow. This rich collateral blood flow, facilitated by the various plexuses, provides an impressive breadth of vascular redundancy to the cutaneous structures. It is this redundancy of flow that provides not only the mechanism for the thermoregulatory function of the skin but also the critical nutrient flow, allowing for cutaneous flap survival and optimal healing. These robust vascular networks form the foundation for the complex circulatory physiology of the skin.

Physiology of the Skin

Due to the important role of the integument in corporeal thermoregulation and homeostasis, the skin has a remarkable hemodynamic ability to vary the rate and quantity of flow through its vascular plexuses. Even under normal circumstances, the

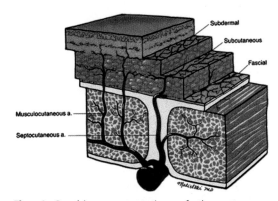

Fig. 1. Graphic representation of the cutaneous vascular plexuses as an extension of the musculocutaneous and septocutaneous perforating arteries. (*From* Larrabee WF, Makielski KH, Henderson JL. Surgical anatomy of the face. Second edition. Philadelphia: Lippincott Williams & Wilkins; 2004; p. 97; with permission.)

blood supply provided to the skin is far greater than that needed for its nutrient support. It has been estimated that the rate of flow through the skin at normal temperatures is approximately 10 times greater than the minimal requirement for adequate tissue nutrition.[4] As the body is heated, cutaneous vasodilatation increases to such an extent that the flow through the cutaneous plexuses can elevate as high as 6 L/min to 8 L/min during periods of hyperthermia.[5] Likewise, hypothermia or extreme local skin cooling can induce a thermoregulatory vasoconstriction in skin that can reduce blood flow rates to levels that are barely adequate to completely inadequate for cutaneous cellular nutrition. These autonomic vasoconstrictive and vasodilatory mechanisms also significantly contribute to reflex control of systemic blood pressure.[5]

The variability of blood flow to and through the skin is the result of arterioles that serve as regulatory sphincters under conditions of adequate systemic pressure, controlling flow through the cutaneous subdermal and dermal networks. The dermal networks are divided into 2 main segments that are responsible for the primary functions of the integumentary circulation. The reticular dermis contains a capillary network that is responsible for nutrient flow to the skin. The arterioles serving as precapillary sphincters control flow through this intricate endothelial web and are chiefly responsive to conditions of hypoxemia and increased metabolic demand, resulting in sphincter dilation to increase local blood flow.[2] Conversely, the papillary dermis contains a network of looping arteriovenous shunts (**Fig. 2**) that allow for the thermoregulatory and hemodynamic functions of the skin. The arterioles serving as preshunt sphincters respond primarily to local autonomic release of norepinephrine or acetylcholine to either decrease or increase flow through the papillary network in response to the thermal or systemic pressure changes affecting the skin locally or the body globally. Other factors, such as inflammation, cytokines, nitric oxide, free radicals, tissue edema, and toxins, such as tobacco smoke, can also have a profound impact on cutaneous blood flow. Several of these factors are discussed in more detail, as the discussion broadens to include cutaneous flap physiology.

LOCAL CUTANEOUS FLAPS

Cutaneous flaps of the head and neck region are generally broken down into 2 categories: random pattern flaps and axial pattern flaps. A third category considered is the fasciocutaneous flap, which also has relevant applications in facial reconstruction. **Fig. 3** illustrates the anatomic differences between the differing flaps.

Random Flaps

Random pattern flaps, also known as local cutaneous or random cutaneous flaps, are frequently

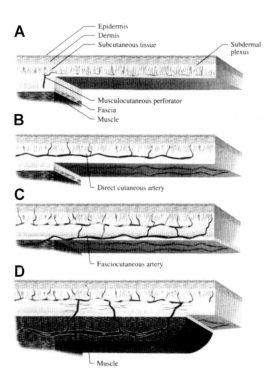

Fig. 3. Illustration of the various types of flaps. (*A*) Local cutaneous (random) flap. (*B*) Direct cutaneous (axial) flap. (*C*) Fasciocutaneous flap. (*D*) Musculocutaneous flap. (*From* Honrado CP, Murakami CS. Wound healing and physiology of skin flaps. Facial Plast Surg Clin North Am 2005;13(2):212; Figure 10; with permission.)

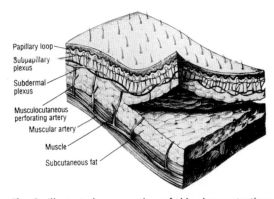

Fig. 2. Illustrated cross-section of skin demonstrating the papillary loops of the dermal plexus. (*From* Honrado CP, Murakami CS. Wound healing and physiology of skin flaps. Facial Plast Surg Clin North Am 2005;13(2):211; Figure 9; with permission.)

used in reconstruction of facial skin defects. Dissection of these flaps occurs in the subcutaneous tissue plane, and they can be classified into advancement, transposition, and rotation flaps based on their geometric design. The vascular supply to random cutaneous flaps is through musculocutaneous perforators located near the base of the flap. Blood flow to the body, margins, and tip of the flap are supplied via the dermal-subdermal plexus. The maximal survival length of these flaps is reliant on the vascular perfusion pressure. In the past, a length-to-width ratio no greater than 3:1 had been advocated for random cutaneous flaps. This rule of thumb is now generally regarded as inaccurate. The vascular perfusion pressure of a random flap can be unpredictable based on several variables. Ultimately, if the perfusion pressure at any portion of the flap falls below the arteriole closing pressure, the distal soft tissues becomes ischemic and ultimately results in necrosis of that portion of the flap. Recruiting more vessels into the base of the flap does not change the perfusion pressure of those vessels, thus providing no change in the maximal survival length of the flap[2] (**Fig. 4**).

Axial Flaps

Axial pattern flaps (also known as direct cutaneous or arterial cutaneous flaps) in the head and neck differ from random flaps in that their arterial supply is based off a direct cutaneous artery that is located beneath the long axis of the flap, thus providing a more definitive and easily described blood supply. Survival lengths of the flap are directly related to the length of the cutaneous artery supplying the flap. Skin extending beyond the arterial component of these flaps is the essential equivalent of a random pattern flap, with perfusion of the distal soft tissues provided solely via the dermal-subdermal plexus.[2] Although these flaps are not as common as random pattern flaps in facial reconstruction, they are advantageous because of the longer flap lengths that can be achieved without compromising survival. The paramedian forehead flap is an axial pattern flap that is frequently used in nasal reconstruction. Based off the supratrochlear artery and vein(s), the axial arterial supply of this flap allows for flap lengths that can be rotated from the upper limits of the forehead down to the nasal tip and columella. The axial configuration also facilitates rotation of the paramedian flap by minimizing pedicle width while maintaining adequate perfusion to the distal tip of the flap.

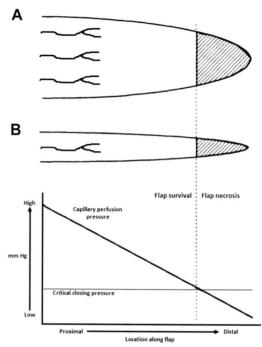

Fig. 4. Distal flap perfusion depends on capillary perfusion pressure as opposed to flap width. Flaps *A* and *B* represent flaps of equal length but differing base width. (*From* Gaboriau HP, Murakami CS. Skin anatomy and flap physiology. In: Baker SR, editor. Local flaps in facial reconstruction. Philadelphia: Mosby; 1995. p. 19; with permission.)

Fasciocutaneous Flaps

The third type of flap is the fasciocutaneous flap. These flaps are based on the fasciocutaneous system of vessels branching off the septocutaneous arteries running in the fascia between muscle bellies. This system forms the subfascial and prefascial plexuses (discussed previously). Branches and perforators off of these networks connect with the dermal-subdermal plexus to supply the skin and subcutaneous tissues. These fascial plexuses typically have an element of directionality,[3] so flap orientation is important and is generally axial in nature. There seems some debate within the literature[1,2,6] over whether the paramedian forehead flap is best categorized as a direct cutaneous flap or a fasciocutaneous flap, owing to the supratrochlear artery described as both a direct cutaneous artery and a fasciocutaneous artery. A dilemma in flap nomenclature occurs when a flap is based on a vessel that feeds a fascial plexus with a predominant directionality, such as the supratrochlear artery and its accompanying fascial plexus.[1] Although the paramedian flap might be more aptly considered an axial fasciocutaneous flap, the confusion seems mostly a matter of semantics with little to no practical impact. When designed with a skin component, the temporoparietal flap is also properly classified as a fasciocutaneous flap. A versatile flap, it can be used for coverage of auricular, orbital, and other defects of the upper two-thirds of the face.

BASIC CUTANEOUS FLAP PHYSIOLOGY

What are the physiologic changes that occur within the skin and surrounding soft tissue when flap elevation occurs? What effect do these physiologic changes have on the potential for flap survival or demise? Without question, the most obvious and profound physiologic insult to occur with elevation of a cutaneous flap is the significant reduction in blood flow to the involved skin due to the partial transection of the vascular supply. The ability of a properly designed flap to survive in light of the resulting ischemia serves as a testament not only to the low nutrient requirements of the skin but also to the importance of collateral flow provided by the intricate vascular networks within the skin. This collateral flow can be further augmented by applying the concepts of vascular delay when appropriate. Additional factors to consider in blood flow alterations to the skin flap include the effects of sympathetic denervation, local inflammatory changes, and the neovascularization of the flap within its recipient bed.

Vascular Compromise

When a cutaneous flap is elevated, the most direct blood flow to that segment of skin is interrupted. The disruption of flow results in a drop in the perfusion pressure to the involved skin. In random pattern flaps, the elevated skin is reliant on the vascular supply from the base of the flap. Perfusion pressures are further diminished as the distance from the base of the flap increases.[2] Widening the base may recruit more feeding arteries into a random flap; however, the perfusion pressures at the base of the flap remain unchanged.[7,8] As discussed previously, once the perfusion pressure falls below critical closing pressures of the arterioles within the dermal-subdermal plexus, nutrient flow to the distal tissues ceases. This ultimately results in necrosis to the distal portion of the flap unless flow can be re-established to the critically ischemic areas. Kerrigan and Daniel[9] used a porcine model to demonstrate that arterial (axial) and random flaps tolerate an average of 13 hours of complete avascularity before tissue viability is irreversibly compromised. It can be logically extrapolated that this viability would be significantly lengthened if perfusion was reduced rather than eliminated. Fortunately, extensive collateral flow through the interconnected vascular networks within the cutaneous structures provides adequate support from adjacent tissues to the more poorly perfused areas. This allows the majority of flaps the ability to survive until more complete vascular flow can be re-established to the transposed tissues. An additional factor to consider as it pertains to vascular compromise is the interruption of venous outflow. Although complete venous occlusion of a flap has the potential to be more damaging than inadequate arterial perfusion, the subdermal plexus alone is usually adequate for venous outflow.[2]

Vascular Delay

When discussing the subject of vascular compromise, it is also important to address the topic of vascular delay, also known as the delay phenomenon. Briefly, vascular delay occurs when a portion of the vascular supply to a flap is divided before it is definitively elevated and transferred. Surgical delay can be accomplished in several ways, including

- Making only the incisions needed to create the flap without elevating any tissues
- Initially elevating a bipedicled flap
- Elevating only a portion of a planned single pedicle flap

After the delay procedure, the flap is then fully elevated and transferred at a later time, typically within 5 days to 14 days. Holzbach and colleagues[10] demonstrated an ideal delay time of 5 days in an exquisitely designed rat model; conversely, numerous investigators[11–15] have advocated for a delay of 2 weeks, allowing for full development of neovascular channels within the flap. Although it is difficult to draw definitive conclusions based on the disparate nature of these findings, it indicates that there is likely a fairly broad sweet spot as it applies to the timing of flap elevation and transfer after a delay procedure.

It is well known that delay results in improved viability and survival of skin flaps. What is less well known are the exact mechanisms responsible for the beneficial effect on flap viability. Several mechanisms that are generally agreed on include the loss of sympathetic tone (with the ultimate depletion of vasoconstrictive substances) and the axial reorientation and dilation of vascular channels and choke vessels within the flap.[16] The existence of choke vessels arose from the concept of angiosomes first described by Taylor and Palmer[17] and further refined by Taylor and others in later research.[18–21] In short, choke vessels ordinarily regulate collateral blood flow between neighboring vascular territories (angiosomes). Vascular delay causes choke vessels along the longitudinal axis of the flap to irreversibly dilate through a process of hypertrophy and hyperplasia of the cells within the walls of the choke artery.[18,21] This process seems maximal at 7 days. A delay of 14 days allows for neovascularization to occur. Additionally, metabolic factors that have yet to be well described are also likely factors in the enhanced viability of delayed flaps.

Sympathetic Denervation

As discussed previously, flap creation results not only in disruption of the cutaneous sensory innervation but also in the sympathetic innervation of the involved tissues. Sympathetic nerve division results in the release of catecholamines from the nerve terminal and impairs neurotransmitter reuptake, resulting in a relative hyperadrenergic state and local vasoconstriction.[22] This vasoconstriction is clearly a part of the elaborate homeostatic mechanisms within the body, minimizing blood loss after a penetrating injury. Unfortunately, it also contributes to diminished nutritive blood flow within the already flow-compromised skin flap.[23] Once the adrenergic neurotransmitter levels have diminished after 24 hours to 48 hours,[24] the loss of sympathetic tone results in vasodilation of the vascular networks supplying the flap. As discussed previously, this rebound vasodilation after sympathectomy is one of the mechanisms leveraged to enhance flap viability via the delay phenomenon.

Inflammatory Changes

When soft tissue is injured, as in skin flap elevation, an inflammatory response reliably ensues. This response is acutely mediated by the extracellular release of inflammatory mediators, such as histamine, serotonin, and kinins. These substances cause an increase in microvascular permeability, with a subsequent elevation in the concentration of inflammatory cells and proteins within the extracellular milieu.[2] The resulting tissue edema can further reduce perfusion of the compromised flap in the acute phase. The inflammatory response, however, ultimately leads to the initiation of prostaglandin synthesis which, among other functions, results in local vasodilation. Thus, the effects of inflammation can have both positive and negative effects on the overall viability of cutaneous flaps.

Neovascularization

After a flap is transposed to its recipient bed, blood flow reliably and gradually improves after the first few days as a result of neovascularization of the flap. This process begins at approximately days 3 to 4 and is generally robust enough after day 7 that the flap pedicle can be transected if appropriate.[2,25] The exact mechanisms through which neovascularization occur are complex but likely involve both angiogenic (new microvessels sprouting from a preexisting capillary network) and vasculogenic (new vessel formation from marrow-derived endothelial progenitor cells) processes.[15] In the presence of tissue ischemia, release of growth factors, such as basic fibroblast growth factor and vascular endothelial growth factor, stimulate endothelial cells and endothelial progenitor cells to proliferate and form new capillary channels.[15] This capillary neovascularization is characterized by vessel ingrowth of the flap from the surrounding tissues, down the ischemic gradient, and toward the angiogenic source. New capillary growth toward an angiogenic stimulus occurs at rate of approximately 0.2 mm per day, ultimately spanning distances of 2 mm to 5 mm.[2]

There are a significant number of additional factors that can impede or enhance flap viability. Some of the most commonly discussed and studied include reperfusion/free radical injury, alterations of rheology, increased nitric oxide production, hyperbaric oxygen use, tissue irradiation, and tobacco use. Although these factors are all notable for their potential effects on flap survival, further elaboration on these subjects is beyond the scope of this discussion.

SKIN FLAP BIOMECHANICS

Valued as a close companion to an understanding of the vascular supply and physiology of the skin, a thorough mastery of the biomechanics of soft tissue is a critical element in the proper design of robust, viable skin flaps to repair facial defects. A reconstructive surgeon must fully comprehend the importance of the 3 main mechanical properties of the skin: nonlinearity, anisotropy, and viscoelasticity. Consideration of these properties is imperative when designing a skin flap, because they have a profound impact on flap blood flow, viability, and aesthetic healing.

Nonlinearity

To adequately explain the concept of nonlinearity, a brief discussion of the mechanical quantities of stress, strain, and the stress/strain ratio must be undertaken. Stress is a measure of the force applied to a material per unit of its cross-sectional area; strain is a measure of the change in length of a material placed under stress, divided by its original length. Accordingly, the stress/strain ratio is a measurement of the dynamic relationship of an applied force and the resulting change in material length caused by that force for a given cross-sectional area.[26] Many of the common, more homogeneous materials used in engineering applications have a linear stress/strain ratio. Simply put, this means that the greater the force applied to the material, the greater the change in its length.

Skin, on the other hand, behaves differently from these uniform, linear materials. The construct of the integument is heterogeneous; its composition includes collagen and elastic fibers, blood vessels, lymphatics, nerve fibers, and ground substance, all within the dermis. The collagen fibers are arranged throughout the dermis in thick and thin bundles that extend in multiple directions with numerous interconnections. This complex mesh of collagen also has elastin fibers integrated throughout. These elastin fibers provide memory to the bundles, allowing collagen that is stretched to return to its original, relaxed state.[26] Because of the heterogeneous construct of the skin, it behaves in a distinctly nonlinear manner when placed under stress.

Fig. 5 demonstrates the nonlinear stress/strain relationship of the skin.[27] The graph demonstrates that the mechanical response of skin to an applied force can be broken down into 3 stages:

1. An initial flat stage showing a significant degree of strain (lengthening) in response to a minimal amount of stress (force)
2. An intermediate or transition stage, where a rapidly increasing amount of force is required to achieve a smaller degree of lengthening

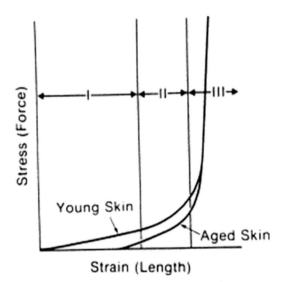

Fig. 5. The stress/strain curve. (*From* Honrado CP, Murakami CS. Wound healing and physiology of skin flaps. Facial Plast Surg Clin North Am 2005;13(2):213; Figure 12; with permission.)

3. A terminal stage where continuously increasing, maximal force results in little to no additional lengthening of the skin

Histologic evaluation of these stages of stress/strain on the skin renders a clear account of the microanatomic changes that determine this nonlinear response to stress. When an initial stress is applied, the haphazardly arranged collagen and elastin fibers stretch along the vector of the applied force with limited resistance to deformation. This results in a stress/strain ratio (stage 1) that is essentially linear and elastic.[26] As the force and resulting deformation progress (stage 2), additional collagen fibers are recruited into a load-bearing role, causing rapid increases in resistance to further deformation.[1] Stage 2 is the strain at which many of the collagen fibers within the skin transition from a non–load-bearing role to one that is wholly load bearing. Finally, as stress loads rapidly increase to extremes (stage 3), essentially all the dermal collagen fibers are aligned in the direction of the applied force. When collagen is fully oriented in one direction, it becomes inextensible and resists further deformation. This allows for preservation of the structural integrity of skin during unexpected, high-level stresses.[26] Although increasing tension on the skin may not cause further deformation, it can have an extremely deleterious effect on the blood flow to the skin or skin flap. At a certain point, increasing skin tension compromises the vascular supply to a skin flap, ultimately resulting in necrosis of the involved portion of the flap.[28]

Anistropy

An understanding of the variations in extensibility and tension of the skin is vitally important to the concepts of skin biomechanics. Skin tension varies significantly from one location on the body to another. Each of these locations can display significant variance in the directionality of cutaneous movement. The term, anisotropy, refers to the directional qualities of the skin. Tension on the skin exists in every direction in most locations of the body; however, the greatest degree of skin tension runs parallel to lines in the skin known as relaxed skin tension lines (RSTLs).[29,30] An incision placed at a right angle to the RSTL results in a widely gaping defect that commonly results in a widened or hypertrophic scar.[1,26] The lines of maximal extensibility (LMEs) are imaginary lines within the skin that run perpendicular to the RSTLs. Closure of skin defects in parallel with the LMEs produce the least amount of tension on the skin edges.[31] Accordingly, every attempt should be made to place incisions parallel to

RSTLs, whereas local skin flaps should be designed to ensure that donor site closure is parallel to the LMEs.[27]

Viscoelasticity

As discussed previously, skin behaves in an essentially elastic manner in the earliest stage of low-stress deformation. A material is considered elastic when the stress/strain relationship does not vary with time.[26] Thus, at low stress levels, the deformation of the skin is rapidly reversible when the stress is removed. The same low-level stress repeated multiple times continues to result in the same degree of deformation followed by rapid return to the resting state. At higher stress loads, however, skin assumes a more viscoelastic property. Viscoelasticity results when strain (lengthening) is a function of both stress and time. Due to the nonlinear nature of skin, further lengthening at higher stress loads does not occur acutely because of the load-bearing nature of wholly aligned collagen bundles. When skin is held under high stress for a period of time, however, additional lengthening ultimately occurs. This time-dependent viscoelasticity is further defined by the properties of creep and stress relaxation.

The biomechanical property of creep occurs when skin lengthens further than the original length observed when the skin is placed under a constant tension or stress. A small degree of lengthening can be rapidly achieved when the skin is placed under extremely high stress loads for a short period of time. This slight lengthening is a result of the displacement of interstitial fluids that are loosely bound to the extracellular matrix,[26] and it is sometimes referred to as mechanical creep. It is the basis for the practice of rapid, intraoperative tissue expansion. Further lengthening can be achieved in skin placed under constant load for longer periods of time. This lengthening is thought to be due to further histologic changes occurring within the skin and is sometimes referred to as biologic creep. It is the basis for more conventional tissue expansion techniques.

The property of stress relaxation is closely related to creep. It refers to the decline in stress on the skin when it is placed under tension at a constant strain over time. The relationship to creep is due to stress relaxation occurring as a result of creep. The prolonged tension on the skin causes a slow, progressive elongation of the skin (creep), which ultimately leads to a lessening of the stress placed on the skin (relaxation). This viscoelastic characteristic of skin allows surgeons to use serial excisions to remove lesions that are in relatively inelastic locations of the body.[1]

SUMMARY

An intimate knowledge of the vascular anatomy and basic physiology of skin allows the reconstructive surgeon to accurately predict and explain the physiologic changes that can affect the viability of local skin flaps used to repair facial defects created by Mohs surgery or other mechanisms of trauma. The biomechanical properties of skin are also vitally important to consider when designing skin flaps, because these properties also have an impact on the survivability and utility of the flap. Although an attempt is made to be as concise and consistent yet thorough as possible in this brief review of the topic, readers are encouraged to further explore this vast and fascinating subject to broaden and refine their confidence in using many of the modalities of skin repair, as discussed in the following articles of this review on facial reconstruction techniques.

REFERENCES

1. Honrado CP, Murakami CS. Wound healing and the physiology of skin flaps. Facial Plast Surg Clin North Am 2005;13:203–14.
2. Hom DB, Goding GS. Skin flap physiology. In: Baker SR, editor. Local flaps in facial reconstruction. Philadelphia: Mosby Elsevier; 2007. p. 15–30.
3. Robertson K. Fasciocutaneous flaps. Medscape 2015. Available at: http://emedicine.medscape.com/article/1284631-overview. Accessed October 3, 2016.
4. Hauben DJ, Zijlstra FJ. Prostacyclin formation in delayed pig flank flaps. Ann Plast Surg 1984;13:304.
5. Charkoudian N. Skin blood flow in adult human thermoregulation: how it works, when it does not, and why. Mayo Clin Proc 2003;78(5):603–12.
6. Gaboriau HP, Murakami CS. Skin anatomy and flap physiology. Otolaryngol Clin North Am 2001;34(3):555–69.
7. Cutting C. Critical closing and perfusion pressures in flap survival. Ann Plast Surg 1982;9(6):524.
8. Cutting C, Ballantyne D, Shaw W, et al. Critical closing pressure, local perfusion pressure, and the failing skin flap. Ann Plast Surg 1982;8(6):504–9.
9. Kerrigan CL, Daniel RK. Critical ischemia time and the failing skin flap. Plast Reconstr Surg 1982;69(6):986–9.
10. Holzbach T, Neshkova I, Vlaskou D, et al. Searching for the right timing of surgical delay: angiogenesis, vascular endothelial growth factor and perfusion changes in a skin-flap model. J Plast Reconstr Aesthet Surg 2009;62(11):1534–42.
11. Milton SH. The effects of the "delay" on the survival of experimental pedicled skin flaps. Br J Plast Surg 1969;22(3):244–52.

12. Milton SH. Pedicled skin-flaps: the fallacy of the length:width ratio. Br J Surg 1970;57(7):502–8.

13. Pang CY, Forrest CR, Neligan PC, et al. Augmentation of blood flow in delayed random skin flaps in the pig: effect of length of delay period and angiogenesis. Plast Reconstr Surg 1986;78(1):68–74.

14. Boyd JB, Markland B, Dorian D, et al. Surgical augmention of skin blood flow and viability in a pig musculocutaneous flap model. Plast Reconstr Surg 1990;86(4):731–8.

15. Ghali S, Butler PEM, Tepper OM, et al. Vascular delay revisited. Plast Reconstr Surg 2007;119(6): 1735–44.

16. Hamilton K, Wolfswinkel E, Weathers WM, et al. The delay phenomenon: a compilation of knowledge across specialties. Craniomaxillofac Trauma Reconstr 2014;7(2):112–8.

17. Taylor GI, Palmer JH. The vascular territories (angiosomes) of the body: experimental study and clinical applications. Br J Plast Surg 1987;40:113–41.

18. Dhar SC, Taylor GI. The delay phenomenon: the story unfolds. Plast Reconstr Surg 1999;104(7): 2079–91.

19. Taylor GI, Chubb DP, Ashton MW. True and "choke" anastomoses between perforator angiosomes: part I. Anatomical location. Plast Reconstr Surg 2013; 132(6):1447–56.

20. Chubb DP, Taylor GI, Ashton MW. True and "choke" anastomoses between perforator angiosomes: part II. Thermographic identification. Plast Reconstr Surg 2013;132(6):1457–64.

21. Callegari PR, Taylor GI, Caddy CM, et al. An anatomic review of the delay phenomenon: I. Experimental studies. Plast Reconstr Surg 1992;89(3): 397–407.

22. Pearl RM. A unifying theory of the delay phenomenon: recovery from the hyperadrenergic state. Ann Plast Surg 1981;7(2):102–12.

23. Pang CY, Neligan PC, Forrest CR, et al. Hemodynamics and vascular sensitivity to circulating norepinephrine in normal skin and delayed and acute random skin flaps in the pig. Plast Reconstr Surg 1986;78(1):75–84.

24. Jurell G. Adrenergic nerves and the delay phenomenon. Ann Plast Surg 1986;17(6):493–7.

25. Tsur H, Daniller A, Strauch B. Neovascularization of skin flaps: route and timing. Plast Reconstr Surg 1980;66(1):85–93.

26. Larrabee WF, Bloom DC. Biomechanics of skin flaps. In: Baker SR, editor. Local flaps in facial reconstruction. Philadelphia: Mosby Elsevier; 2007. p. 31–40.

27. Larrabee WF Jr. Immediate repair of facial defects. Dermatol Clin 1989;7(4):661–76.

28. Larrabee WF Jr, Holloway GA, Sutton D. Wound tension and blood flow in skin flaps. Ann Otol Rhinol Laryngol 1984;93(2 Pt 1):112–5.

29. Borges AF. Relaxed skin tension lines. Dermatol Clin 1989;7:169–77.

30. Borges AF. Relaxed skin tension lines (RSTL) versus other skin lines. Plast Reconstr Surg 1984;73(1): 144–50.

31. Borges AF. The rhombic flap. Plast Reconstr Surg 1981;67(4):458–66.

Flap Basics I
Rotation and Transposition Flaps

Sidney J. Starkman, MD, Carson T. Williams, MD, David A. Sherris, MD*

KEYWORDS

- Mohs • Reconstruction • Rotation flap • Transposition flap • Bilobe • Rhombic

KEY POINTS

- Local facial flaps offer a good option for repair of Mohs micrographic surgery for cutaneous lesions.
- Rotation flaps are curvilinear in nature and rotate adjacent tissue into a defect.
- Transposition flaps are linear and pivot toward a defect over an incomplete bridge of tissue.
- Rhombic and bilobe flaps incorporate components of transposition and rotation flaps and serve as the workhorse flaps of Mohs reconstruction.
- Local facial flaps are hearty, only suffering rare, mild complications.

BACKGROUND

Modern evolution in techniques of facial reconstruction have dramatically increased the possibilities for repair of facial defects. The need for advanced facial reconstruction has grown significantly since the advances of Mohs micrographic surgery, which represents the gold standard for malignancies of the face and neck.[1] Use of immediate fresh tissue fixation allows for Mohs surgical excisions to be performed quickly, facilitating expedient repair. In many cases of complex facial defects resulting from the extirpation of advanced cutaneous malignancies, primary wound closure is impossible. In these instances, ideal results can be obtained through recruitment of adjacent tissue with the use of local and regional flaps. Advances in local flap techniques have raised the bar in facial reconstruction; however, acceptable results to both the surgeon and the patient require high levels of planning and surgical technique.

Defects resulting from Mohs surgery and other traumatic injuries can typically be repaired with grafts or local flaps. Between these options, local flaps are often preferred because of their superior color match and texture. A well-planned and executed local flap can lead to excellent cosmetic results with minimal distortion of the surrounding facial landmarks. Local flaps used for facial reconstruction are classified by a variety of methods, including blood supply, flap contents, and the method of transfer. Rotation flaps are curvilinear flaps that pivot into the defect. Transposition flaps are linear and pivot toward the defect over an incomplete bridge of skin. This is in contrast to interpolation flaps, which pivot toward defects over intact bridges of skin. The rhombic flap, bilobe flap, O-T/O-Z flap, and note flap are types of transposition flaps, some of which include both transposition and rotation components.

ROTATION FLAPS

Rotation flaps are designed with curvilinear orientation in the direction of the defect that they pivot toward. Although these flaps are rotational in their direction, they also span the defect by stretching the elastic tissues. This leads to the points of greatest wound closure tension occurring along the distal border of the flap rather than along the length of the flap.[2] The secondary defect that occurs following execution of a rotational flap is determined by the size of the flap, with a larger-rotation flap leading to a narrower and longer

Disclosure: The authors have nothing to disclose.
Department of Otolaryngology, University at Buffalo, 1237 Delaware Avenue, Buffalo, NY 14209, USA
* Corresponding author.
E-mail address: dsherris@buffalo.edu

Facial Plast Surg Clin N Am 25 (2017) 313–321
http://dx.doi.org/10.1016/j.fsc.2017.03.004

secondary defect. A narrower secondary defect will lead to less tension on closure of the wound; however, this exists only up to a certain point. Larrabee and Galt[3] demonstrated there is minimal benefit to extending the arc of rotation flaps beyond 90° from the axis of the defect.

The ideal defect for rotation flaps are triangular in shape. The height-width ratio of the triangle ideally should be 2:1. The arc of rotation extending from the base of the triangle should be a symmetric curve, with the radius of the curve being 1 to 2 times the height of the triangle (**Fig. 1**A). For optimal results with rotation flaps, the defects can be modified into triangular shapes via conservative excision of normal tissue.[4] Burow triangles are often used to assist with closing the secondary defect. The length of the flap should be 4 times the width of the base of the triangular defect (see **Fig. 1**B, C). This ratio obviates the need for excision of a Burow triangle to equalize the defects. Enlarging the flaps beyond the 4:1 ratio does not significantly decrease the wound closure tension; however, a longer flap can be useful in areas of limited skin mobility.[5]

Wide undermining is performed to allow for pivoting of the flap toward the defect. Undermining can also reduce the extent of standing cutaneous deformity by shifting the deformity slightly away from the flap's base. When a standing cutaneous deformity persists in spite of these techniques, secondary excision of the deformity is warranted. In most instances, a standing cutaneous deformity will flatten over 6 weeks postoperatively. Additionally, close attention must be paid to the closure of deep layers, ensuring close approximation at the points of maximal tension and meticulous eversion of the skin edges.

Rotation flaps have several significant advantages in the repair of facial defects. There is a great amount of flexibility in the planning and orientation of the arc of the flap.[6] This can allow for orientations that promote lymphatic drainage, and also that minimize vascular and nervous disruption. The flap is very robust with strong vascular flow due to its broad-based design. The surgeon can also often position the single long arc of the flap within a relaxed skin tension line (RSTL) or aesthetic unit for greater scar camouflage.

The rotation flap has utility for many types of facial defects; however, because of the curved incision of the flap, it sometimes does not lie cleanly within an RSTL. In cases in which the incision does not lie within an RSTL, the scar can be less camouflaged and more noticeable than in other methods of repair. Because of the degree of rotation, these flaps often develop standing cutaneous deformities at their base. These deformities cannot be initially excised, as that would compromise the vascular supply to the tissues.

Rotation flaps are not the optimal choice in repair of central cheek defects or most nasal defects. In men, the rotation flap can distort the hair-bearing skin of the sideburn medially toward the malar eminence. The skin of the nasal tip is very inelastic, making recruitment difficult. Additionally, the donor site scars along the nose do not typically fall cleanly between the nasal aesthetic subunits. Most nasal defects are better repaired with other flaps, such as the bilobe or rhombic flap.

BILOBE FLAP

The bilobe flap is generally considered one of the "workhorse" flaps of facial reconstruction. Classified as both rotational and transpositional, the bilobe flap is a transposition flap because it is elevated and mobilized toward an adjacent defect and transposed over an incomplete bridge of skin, and a rotational flap because it pivots around a specific point and maintains its radius.[7] It is

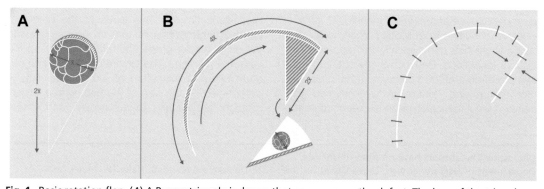

Fig. 1. Basic rotation flap. (*A*) A Burow triangle is drawn that encompasses the defect. The legs of the triangle are approximately twice the diameter of the defect. (*B*) The arc of the rotation flap measures 4 times the defect diameter. (*C*) The final outcome of the basic rotation flap.

particularly useful when a single transposition flap exerts too much tension on the closure. The bilobe flap is able to more effectively transfer tension across a greater angle of rotation and therefore distributes the load both more equally and with a larger component being placed away from the primary defect.

Originally described for nasal tip reconstruction by Esser in 1918, the bilobe flap continues to serve the facial plastic surgeon during post-Mohs micrographic surgery defect repair.[8] Although the use of the bilobe flap can be used in many parts of the body, its utility is greatest in areas that need to minimize tension in the area directly adjacent to the primary defect, like the nasal dorsum, sidewall, and tip subunits (**Fig. 2**).[7,9]

As described previously, this flap is best used for defects of the nasal tip, dorsum, and sidewall equal to or less than 1.5 to 2.0 cm.[10] Extension to the nasal ala reduces this flap's efficacy as the scarring that occurs will many times cause cephalic elevation, retraction, and/or distortion of the alar rim leading to lesser cosmetic outcomes.[11] The Zitelli-modified bilobe flap is designed with a total arc of rotation 100° or less, with each limb of the flap rotating 45 to 50°.[12] The flap is routinely based medially along the nasal dorsum or laterally along the nasofacial groove, with laterally based flaps resulting in better concealed scars. The bilobe flap is most successful when the skin is elevated in the subcutaneous plane and the raised lobes closely match the thickness of the defect area. When there is a considerable mismatch, a delayed closure may be beneficial by allowing a deeper defect time to granulate in its base. This allows for a flap that may not need much alteration and produces a more even level to the healed flap and surrounding skin.

When designing a bilobe flap, first measure the radius of the defect. Once obtained, mark a point to the side of the defect, preferably laterally, equal to the radius of the defect. Next, measure 2 arcs: one equal to 2 times radius and the other 3 times the radius, spanning the entire area of the defect and planned area for flap rotation. Once the 2 arcs are marked, use the diameter distance of the defect to measure the base of the first lobe along the first arc immediately adjacent to the defect, ensuring the middle of the lobe is 45 to 50° from the center of the defect. The height of the first lobe should extend to the line of the second arc, therefore making its height equal to the radius of the defect. Next, again measuring along the first arc line, the second lobe should be a distance slightly smaller than the first lobe, and again 45 to 50° from the middle of the first lobe or 90 to 100° away from the middle of the defect. Its height is a distance twice that of the first lobe, and of a slightly more triangular shape. Finally, mark the standing cutaneous deformity between the edge of the defect and the initial mark placed equal to 1 radius of the defect (**Fig. 3**).[11]

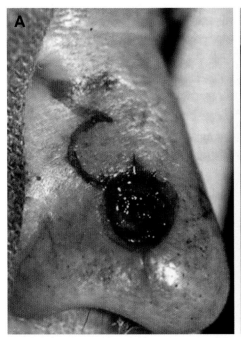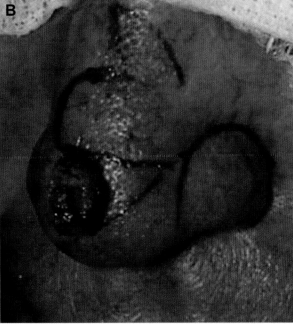

Fig. 2. (*A*) Bilobe flap of the right nasal sidewall. (*B*) Bilobe flap of the left nasal sidewall to reconstruct a nasal tip defect.

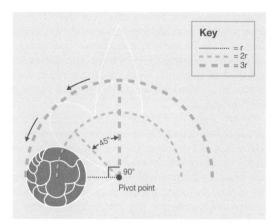

Key
.... = r
– – – – = 2r
▪ ▪ ▪ ▪ = 3r

45°
90°
Pivot point

Fig. 3. Schematic of the ideal bilobe flap. Note the first lobe is approximately the same size as the defect and the center of which is 45° from the center of the defect. The second lobe is approximately half the size of the first lobe, is 90° from the center of the defect, and is more triangular in shape.

It is important to remember, when lesions are excised using the Mohs technique, they have a resulting edge that is beveled inward. To aid in proper inset of the flap with good eversion, it is necessary to first bevel the edges outward before laying the flap into position. Once the flap has been precisely designed, incisions along the lobes are performed. Wide undermining is crucial to ensure adequate mobilization of the 2 lobes and for tension-free closure. The defect created by lifting and mobilizing the second lobe should be fully closed first. Only after it has been closed, the first lobe should then be sutured into place covering the initial defect. At this point, the standing cutaneous deformity is determined and it is resected to relieve tension and provide close skin approximation. Finally, the second lobe is trimmed to size and sutured into position within the defect created by the first lobe (**Fig. 4**).

Suture selection should consist of a permanent monofilament appropriate for the size of the defect, most often 6-0 prolene or nylon. The area should have a light compression dressing placed for 24 to 48 hours following the procedure and sutures removed 5 to 7 days postoperatively.

Although the bilobe flap is extremely versatile in facial reconstruction, it is not without its downsides. Because of its curvilinear incisions not lying parallel to the RSTLs, a potential downside to the use of the bilobe flap is its risk of trapdoor deformity.[12] Careful preoperative planning and design, along with close attention to tension-free closure and good skin eversion are usually successful in preventing this. Nevertheless, dermabrasion of the entire area 6 to 8 weeks following the initial procedure is often advocated to conceal the slight scar when one seeks additional cosmesis.

O-T/O-Z FLAP

Mohs micrographic surgery leaves circular defects, making their closure in certain areas of the face a challenge to the reconstructive surgeon. Rearrangement of tissues to convert the circular defect to one that more closely approximates the natural RSTLs is beneficial for acceptable cosmetic healing.

The O-T flap converts a circular defect to one that is approximately "T" shaped once closure is completed (**Fig. 5**). Incorporating rotation and advancement, it is able to recruit adjacent tissue from a specific area around the defect while leaving one of its borders undisturbed. This is important in facial regions like the forehead, temple, and lips, where distortion created by closure and scar contracture lead to unsatisfactory results.

This flap is commonly used in the temple region abutting the hairline. The undisturbed border, the top of the "T," should be placed along the hairline in a vertical fashion. The circular defect and a standing cutaneous deformity are resected simultaneously in a "V" shape. Next, the area of rotation and advancement is widely undermined in a subcutaneous plane above the facial nerve and the

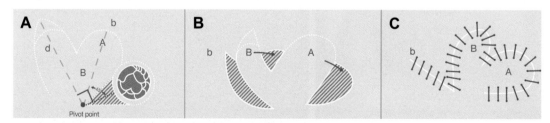

Fig. 4. Bilobe flap elevation, mobilization, and inset. (*A*) Design of a bilobe flap. (*B*) Resection of the defect and standing cutaneous deformity and elevation and mobilization of the 2 lobes toward the defect. (*C*) Closure of a bilobe flap. The second lobe should be trimmed and sutured into the first lobe defect initially, followed by closure of the second lobe defect, and finally the initial defect closed with the first lobe after appropriate trimming.

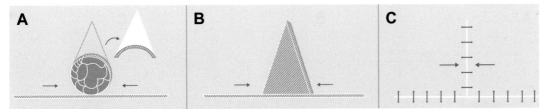

Fig. 5. O-T flap. (*A*) The defect is converted from nearly circular to triangular in shape with the broad base of the triangle lying perpendicular to the straight limb. (*B*) Resultant defect and direction of movement. (*C*) Resultant appearance after closure.

skin edges are prepared for closure. The opposing edges from the resected area are closed, primarily forming the bottom portion of the "T." The top of the "T" runs adjacent to the hairline and all edges are closed using nonabsorbable monofilament sutures, being certain to relieve tension at all points and produce good wound edge eversion.

Because of the formation of the "T" shape, this flap inherently creates a scar perpendicular to the RSTLs of the facial subunits. Knowing this, utilization of the O-Z flap, or double rotation flap, can be beneficial. Like the O-T, this flap also has rotational and advancement components and is usually used in similar areas, like the cheek and temple. The versatility of the O-Z flap comes from its ability to minimize distortion of important structures because the tension vectors are primarily parallel to the limbs of the repair (**Fig. 6**).[13]

Here, adjacent flaps are based on opposing sides, which creates scars that run more obliquely to one another and allows them to more closely approximate the RSTLs. Resection of the lesion leaves a circular defect, and 2 lines from opposite sides of the periphery as mirror arcs of one another are drawn. Incisions along these lines are made down to the subcutaneous plane and wide undermining is performed for increased tissue mobility. Once adequate tissue mobility has been achieved, the skin flaps are advanced and rotated into the defect and the edges of the flaps are sutured to one another creating the middle portion of the "Z." Next, the remaining wound edges are closed in an interrupted manner with nonabsorbable monofilament sutures.

NOTE FLAP

Roughly resembling the musical eighth note, the aptly named note flap is a simple transposition flap (**Fig. 7**). An adjacent "V," or triangular, shaped area of skin is used to cover the defect and the skin edges of the donor site are simply closed primarily. To create this flap, a point approximately equal to radius of the defect is marked away from the defect and 2 lines are marked from opposite sides of the perimeter of the defect coursing back to the marked point. This represents the "V"-shaped area to be excised. Next, a similar-sized V-shaped area is marked next to this with a long limb of each intersecting one another at their ends. Once marked, the defect and standing cutaneous deformity are resected and the entire area is widely undermined in a subcutaneous plane. The second V-shaped area is transposed over the triangular bridge of skin and set into the defect area. The defect created by raising the flap is first closed primarily and then the flap is trimmed and sutured into place. Opposite the standing cutaneous deformity "V" of resected tissue, a small Burow triangle may be necessary to avoid skin excess and to accomplish better wound eversion and closure.

RHOMBIC FLAP

The rhombic flap is another "workhorse" flap for many of the smaller cutaneous defects of the head and neck. It is a transposition flap and pivots over an incomplete bridge of skin (**Fig. 8**). The

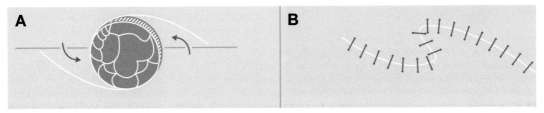

Fig. 6. O-Z flap. (*A*) Double opposing rotation flaps are raised and rotated into the skin defect. (*B*) Resultant appearance after closure.

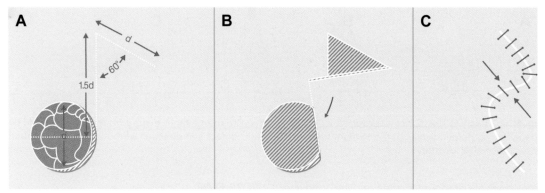

Fig. 7. Note flap. (*A*) Design of an ideal note flap. The vertical tangential limb is approximately 1.5 times the diameter of the defect and the second limb lies at approximately 60° from the first limb and is approximately the length of the defect diameter. (*B*) Note flap elevation and mobilization. (*C*) Closure of the note flap.

rhombic flap uses specifically engineered vectors and results in a predictable scar and point of maximum tension. The traditional rhombic flap used the Limberg design, based around a defect with 60-degree and 120-degree angles and limbs of equal length (**Fig. 9**A).[14] A first limb is then extended outwardly from the short axis of the rhomboid defect, equal in length to one side of the defect. A second limb of equal length is then extended from the end of the first limb, back toward the primary defect at a 60° angle. The point of maximum tension (58%) corresponds to distal end of the closure of the secondary defect (see **Fig. 9**B, C).[15] Because the resultant scars from closure of a rhombic flap run in multiple directions,

it is not possible to orient all of them within RSTLs. Therefore, the flap orientation is dictated by the lines of maximal extensibility. The vectors of maximum tension are designed to lie within these lines of maximal extensibility to minimize wound tension. A disadvantage of the Limberg flap is the amount of discarded normal tissue needed to convert a defect into a geometric rhombus.[16]

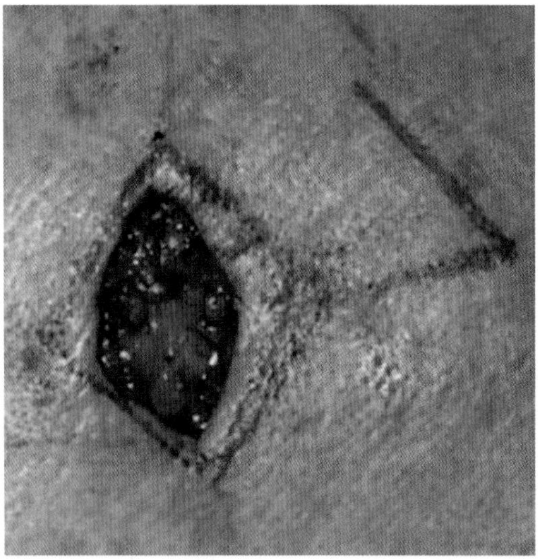

Subsequently, modifications, including the Dufourmentel and Webster designs, were introduced to address the pitfalls of the Limberg design. Dufourmentel adjusted the design to accommodate defects that were squarer, and the Webster modification uses a rhombic flap with 30° edges that transposes a narrower flap into the defect.[17] Theoretically, this minimizes the risk of "dog ear" deformity. The narrower Webster flap distributes the wound tension more evenly around the flap, and decreases the amounts of distortion to the surrounding facial structures. Furthermore, the use of Z-plasties has expanded the potential applications of the rhombic flap for larger effects of the face. The Z-plasty allows for greater mobilization of the flap at the expense of a longer scar.

For closure of larger facial defects, bilateral rhombic flaps can be used. The main utility of these flaps is for large defects of the nasal tip and dorsum, offering acceptable color and texture match. Bilateral rhombic flaps use identical geometry and principles as single rhombic flaps, except 2 locations adjacent to the defect are used for tissue recruitment instead of 1. The use of 2 flaps allows for each individual flap to be smaller, as each must cover only half of the defect. However, this technique does result in additional scar limbs. When designing the flaps symmetrically positioned on either side of the nose, the wound closure tensions are identical. Repair of a defect over the nasal dorsum often slightly elevates the

Fig. 8. Rhombic flap. A nearly circular defect is converted to a rhomboid and planned incisions are marked.

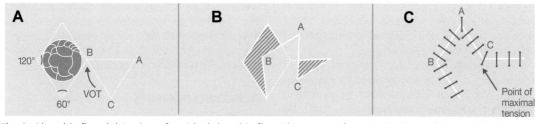

Fig. 9. Rhombic flap. (*A*) Design of an ideal rhombic flap. The vector of tension is the B-C limb in this schematic and not an incision line. (*B*) Elevation and mobilization of rhombic flap into position. (*C*) Closure of the defect with the rhombic flap. The point of maximal tension should be approximated first followed by the remaining flap closure.

nasal tip, which is particularly useful in patients with tip ptosis. The medial corners of the rhombic flaps overlap in the middle of the defect and redundant tissue is carefully excised.

WOUND CARE

Following inset and closure of the local flap, meticulous wound care is critical to optimizing the viability and outcome of the facial reconstruction. Topical antibiotic ointment is applied to the incision lines and a nonadhesive dressing is placed over the surgical site. With a topical adhesive, a compression dressing is placed over the defect for 24 hours following the surgical repair, after which the surgical site is left open to air. All patients are instructed to avoid strenuous exercise, as well as direct exposure to sunlight, for 4 to 6 weeks postoperatively. All undermined skin and incisions are more prone to early tanning and burning. Sutures are removed from the face 5 to 7 days postoperatively.

On an outpatient basis, patients are instructed to clean their incisions twice daily with hydrogen peroxide, followed by a moisturizing ointment. Hydrogen peroxide serves to remove crust from the surgical incisions, and also helps minimize the width of the scarring. Hydrogen peroxide is applied for 3 days postoperatively, after which the incisions can be cleaned with mild soap and water. Continued moist coverage with topical ointment during the duration of wound healing is critical to ideal cosmetic outcomes.

COMPLICATIONS

Like most other areas of surgery and medicine, preventing complications is far superior to managing them postoperatively. Therefore, prevention begins with a detailed patient history focusing on aspects that may predispose to poor wound healing or postoperative wound care adherence. Preoperatively, cigarette smoking is the single greatest risk

factor for microvascular compromise and poor wound healing. Other medical conditions, such as uncontrolled hypertension, collagen disorders, diabetes mellitus, and previous irradiation, should be approached with caution and detailed conversations with the patient should be had to highlight these conditions' ability to compromise wound healing.

Thorough flap design preoperatively cannot be overemphasized. When determining the correct flap for the defect in question, one must consider surrounding immobile structures, adequate areas of tissue recruitment, RSTLs, facial aesthetic subunits, and the resultant scar. Areas such as the nose possess complex topography and are the focal point of facial anatomy requiring attention to small details of defect analysis and flap design.

Overall, complications of local facial flaps are mild.[11] Although the face has an extremely vigorous vascular supply, most complications of facial flaps are secondary to the inflow or outflow of blood to the flap. Venous congestion is most common and can significantly affect flap healing. Usually caused by compression of the veins, signs of this condition reflect trapped venous blood. Warmth, edema, and dark discoloration that blanches with digital pressure, lend evidence the flap is congested. A pinprick should reveal dark, venous blood. Management is aimed at relieving the compression. Simply removing several sutures to allow expansion may be enough to relieve the congestion. Release of any tight dressings or bolsters should occur immediately. If unrelieved by these simple maneuvers, consider the use of transcutaneous leech therapy or hyperbaric oxygen therapy.

Arterial ischemia is a rare, but arguably more serious threat to flap health than venous congestion. Characterized by a pale-colored, cool, flat flap that does not blanch with pressure, ischemic flaps do not bleed with pinprick due to impaired perfusion. Microvascular disease at baseline significantly increases the chance of ischemia, but with a thorough preoperative assessment with careful patient selection and education about smoking cessation, the chances of encountering this complication are lessened.

Acute management of flap ischemia involves pharmacologic agents administered to vasodilate and thin the blood. Subcutaneous heparin, with or without additional dipyridamole, should be given at the first signs of flap ischemia. Hyperbaric oxygen therapy has also shown benefits, however, its utility in the acute setting is less effective.

Other complications like hypertrophic scarring, flap pin-cushioning, and discoloration plague the facial plastic surgeon's attempt at an aesthetically pleasing Mohs reconstruction. Again, good preoperative evaluation of the patient's skin type and history of unsightly scarring may encourage one type of flap over another. Certain factors, like the patient being younger than 60 years, Fitzpatrick skin type 3 or higher, nasal defects, and superiorly based rhombic, glabellar, nasolabial, and bilobe flaps are associated with higher rates of complications.[11] However, if one does develop scarring, postoperative injections of triamcinolone acetate may reduce scar volume. Scar revision with removal and repeat closure, followed by additional injections of triamcinolone acetate may repair the hypertrophic scars. Dermabrasion approximately 6 to 8 weeks later may help even out the skin of the defect and donor areas and further conceal the scar. Hypopigmentation or hyperpigmentation is usually transient in nature if the skin covering the defect is of the same general characteristics. During the acute healing process, incision lines commonly present with darker and deeper red coloration than the surrounding skin. This is more common in the skin of those who tan easily and do not avoid sun exposure during the healing process. Educating the patient about avoiding direct sunlight to these areas with protective clothing and high UVA/UVB protective sunscreens is very important.[18] In patients who have hyperemia of the incision lines and desire intervention before final wound maturity, selective photothermolysis to the area occurring after approximately 12 weeks of wound healing may be performed to lessen the color differences.[11]

SUMMARY

Here, some local flap basics have been introduced to the reader. With advancements made to tissue-sparing excision of lesions, the role of the reconstructive surgeon has evolved. With the myriad of local cutaneous facial flaps, defects of nearly every shape and size can be managed. Thorough understanding of the unique characteristics of each type of flap, along with the specifics of facial subunit reconstruction, will continue to offer patients a safe, functional, and aesthetically pleasing outcome of post-Mohs reconstruction.

ACKNOWLEDGMENTS

The authors gratefully acknowledge the work of Amanda Widzinski for her illustrations of the flaps included in this article.

REFERENCES

1. Mohs FE. Chemosurgery, a microscopically controlled method of cancer excision. Arch Surg 1941;42:279.
2. Larrabee WF Jr. Design of local skin flaps. Otolaryngol Clin North Am 1990;23:899.
3. Larrabee WF Jr, Galt JA. A finite element model of skin deformation. III, The finite element model. Laryngoscope 1986;96:413.
4. Rageer B, Anuja MS. Geometric considerations in the design of rotation flaps in the scalp and forehead region. Plast Reconstr Surg 1988;81:900.
5. Buckingham ED, Quinn FB, Calhoun KH. Optimal design of the O-Z flaps for closure of facial skin defects. Arch Facial Plast Surg 2003;5:92.
6. Golumb FM. Closure of the circular defect with double rotation flaps and Z-plasties. Plast Reconstr Surg 1984;74:813.
7. Sherris DA, Larrabee WF. Nose. Principles of facial reconstruction: a subunit approach to cutaneous repair. New York: Thieme; 2009. p. 102–59.
8. Baker SR. Bilobe flaps. Local flaps in facial reconstruction. 2nd edition. Philadelphia: Mosby; 2007. p. 189–211.
9. Grosfeld EC, Smit JM, Krekels GA, et al. Facial reconstruction following Mohs micrographic surgery: a report of 622 cases. J Cutan Med Surg 2014;18:265–70.
10. Ibrahim AMS, Rabie AN, Borud L, et al. Common patterns of reconstruction for Mohs defects in the head and neck. J Craniofac Surg 2014;25:87–92.
11. Sclafani AP, Sclafani JA, Sclafani AM. Successes, revisions, and postoperative complications in 446 Mohs defect repairs. Facial Plast Surg 2012;28: 358–66.
12. Papel ID, Park SS. Local and regional cutaneous flaps. Facial plastic and reconstructive surgery. 3rd edition. New York: Thieme; 2009. p. 528–48.
13. Jewett BS, Baker SR. Complications of local flaps. Local flaps in facial reconstruction. 2nd edition. Philadelphia: Mosby; 2007. p. 691–722.
14. Limberg AA. The planning of local plastic operations on the body surface: theory and practice. Toronto: Cullamore Press; 1984.

15. Larrabee WF Jr, Trachy R, Sutton D. Rhomboid flap dynamics. Arch Otolaryngol 1981;107:755–7.

16. Lister GD, Gibson T. Closure of the rhomboid skin defects: the flaps of Limberg and Dufourmentel. Br J Plast Surg 1972;25:300.

17. Webster RF, Davidson TM, Smith RC. The thirty-degree transposition flap. Laryngoscope 1978;88:85.

18. Regula CG, Liu A, Lawrence N. Versatility of the O-Z flap in the reconstruction of facial defects. Dermatol Surg 2016;42:109–14.

Flap Basics II
Advancement Flaps

Matthew Shew, MD, John David Kriet, MD, Clinton D. Humphrey, MD*

KEYWORDS

• Advancement flap • Unipedicle • Bipedicle • H-plasty • T-plasty • Cervicofacial advancement flap

KEY POINTS

- A mastery of advancement flap design, selection, and execution greatly aids the surgeon in solving reconstructive dilemmas.
- Advancement flaps involve carefully planned incisions to most efficiently close a primary defect in a linear vector.
- Advancement flaps are subcategorized as unipedicle, bipedicle, V-to-Y, and Y-to-V flaps, each with their own advantages and disadvantages.
- When selecting and designing an advancement flap, the surgeon must account for primary and secondary movement to avoid distortion of important facial structural units and boundaries.

DEFINITIONS AND CORE CONCEPTS

Local flaps, including advancement flaps, are useful for closing a wide range of skin defects in the head and neck. Although most wounds and primary defects in the head and neck region are a result of using micrographic surgical techniques (Mohs), removal of benign lesions and traumatic injuries can also result in defects that are too large to close primarily. The surgeon must consider secondary intention healing, skin grafting, or local flaps, to address the wound in these situations. The advantages of local flaps over secondary intention healing or skin grafting include superior match of skin color and texture along with minimal wound contraction. Many of the local cutaneous flaps in the head and neck include an advancement component. The simplest "advancement flap" is the linear closure of an incisional wound (**Fig. 1**). Adjacent tissue is advanced from both sides to close the defect primarily. A wide range of advancement flaps that are variations on this basic technique are useful for closing defects throughout the head and neck. A mastery of advancement flap design, selection, and execution greatly aids the surgeon in solving reconstructive dilemmas.

Advancement flap design, like all local flaps, involves carefully planned incisions to most efficiently close a primary defect. Advancement flaps are defined as having a linear vector. The flap is incised, undermined, and "slides" forward to cover the primary defect. Because of this design, advancement flaps rely heavily on skin elasticity and its ability to stretch into the defect. By stretching and advancing local tissue in a linear vector into the defect, maximum wound tension exists along that linear vector at the distal border of the flap. The vector of wound tension is taken into account during flap design with attention to surrounding facial structures susceptible to distortion. Facial subunits and relaxed skin tension lines (RSTLs) are additional considerations.

When designing advancement flaps, one must anticipate 2 types of movement to achieve an optimal outcome that minimizes distortion of surrounding facial aesthetic structures. *Primary*

Department of Otolaryngology Head and Neck Surgery, The University of Kansas Medical Center, 3901 Rainbow Boulevard, MS 3010, Kansas City, KS 66160, USA
* Corresponding author.
E-mail address: chumphrey@kumc.edu

Facial Plast Surg Clin N Am 25 (2017) 323–335
http://dx.doi.org/10.1016/j.fsc.2017.03.005
1064-7406/17/© 2017 Elsevier Inc. All rights reserved.

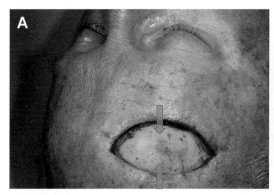
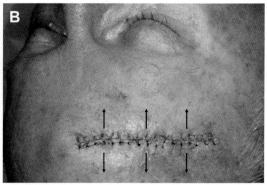

Fig. 1. Cutaneous forehead defect followed by repair. The most basic advancement flap is simple linear closure. (*A*) Large blue arrows demonstrate anticipated primary movement. (*B*) Simple linear closure of defect. The adjacent tissue was undermined and advanced to close the defect primarily. Incision lines were purposefully placed within the natural crease of the forehead. The small black arrows demonstrate the secondary movement from closure.

movement refers to the "sliding" and/or advancement of tissue into the defect (see **Fig. 1**; **Fig. 2**). *Secondary movement* refers to displacement of surrounding skin directed toward the central defect from wound closure tension (see **Figs. 1** and **2**). Secondary movement can result in unfavorable distortion of mobile facial structures, such as the vermillion border, nostril, brow, eyelid, and ear lobule. Conversely, minimal secondary movement is seen along facial boundaries with strong underlying attachments. Undermining and selecting an appropriate site where maximum tension occurs help the surgeon favorably control secondary movement. Broad undermining around both the flap and the defect minimizes and distributes circumferential secondary movement. Locating maximum tension vectors next to tissue with a strong underlying bony attachment or the use of an "anchoring stitch" to secure the flap to

periosteum adjacent to the distal cutaneous defect minimizes secondary movement.

Advancement flaps are subcategorized as unipedicle, bipedicle, V-to-Y, and Y-to-V flaps. Bipedical flaps can be further divided into T-plasty (O-T, A-T plasty) and H-plasty. Common to all these advancement flaps is that the advancing border of the flap represents the margin of the cutaneous defect. When using advancement flaps, surgeons must be conscious of the wound tension vector and place incision lines to lie along RSTLs whenever possible.

ANATOMY AND PHYSIOLOGY: VASCULAR SUPPLY

Understanding both the vascular supply and the process of neovascularization is essential for successful local cutaneous flap design. The vascular

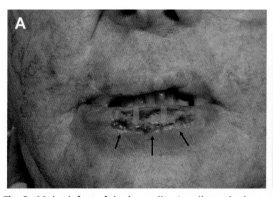
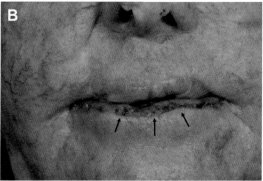

Fig. 2. Mohs defect of the lower lip. A unilateral advancement flap was used to advance the posterior lip mucosa into the distal border of the defect along the vermillion border. (*A*) Large blue arrows demonstrate primary movement, whereas the small black arrows demonstrate anticipated secondary movement. (*B*) Unilateral advancement flap closure of lower lip. The black arrows demonstrate the secondary movement vectors. Differential undermining was used to help minimize secondary movement.

supply to the cutaneous skin serves 2 primary functions, nutrition and thermoregulation. The nutrition role is most pertinent to local flap design and survival. The 2 main sources of cutaneous circulation are the musculocutaneous and septocutaneous arteries. First, the musculocutaneous arteries pass through muscle into the cutaneous dermis to supply smaller skin regions. Second, septocutaneous arteries, also known as direct cutaneous arteries, follow a path through fascial septa that separate and divide muscle segments. These septocutaneous vascular networks typically run parallel to the cutaneous skin within the fascia below the subcutaneous fat and supply most of the nutritional and vascular support to the skin. Once the vascular supply reaches the cutaneous skin, these larger vessels empty into the complex system of interconnected dermal and subdermal plexuses.

Flaps are classified based on their arterial supply as arterial or random cutaneous flaps. Arterial cutaneous flaps incorporate a septocutaneous artery within the flap axis, offering greater survival and length compared with random cutaneous flaps. One example of an arterial cutaneous flap in the head and neck is the paramedian forehead flap. Conversely, advancement flaps are random cutaneous flaps. Random cutaneous flaps derive their vascular supply from the interconnecting dermal and subdermal plexuses originating from the flap base. Other local flaps, including rotation, transposition, and tubed flaps, also rely on this "random" but typically reliable blood supply.

Following local flap transfer, perfusion through the dermal and subdermal plexuses continues until neovascularization provides the blood supply and nourishment. Local flap perfusion from the base of the flap to its most distal tip is determined by the following: the intravascular resistance, or intrinsic properties of the supplying vessels, and the perfusion pressure.[1] Distal perfusion pressure is the most important factor for flap viability on days 0 to 3 following flap transfer. Perfusion pressure decreases with increasing distance from the base of the flap secondary to distance traveled and stretch applied through advancement. Distally, there is ultimately a critical juncture where closing pressure of the arterioles within the subdermal plexus exceeds the perfusion pressure. At this juncture, the arterioles will collapse and perfusion ceases. A flap will be ischemic beyond this juncture. Arterial closing pressure is typically between 5 and 10 mm Hg. Early hypotheses of flap survival mandated that specific length-to-width ratios would ensure flap perfusion and viability. This thinking is flawed. Although wider-based flaps will capture more of the subdermal

plexus that feeds the flap, the wider base will not increase distal perfusion pressure. Therefore, even designing a very widely based flap will not maintain distal perfusion pressure and viability in flaps of excessive length.[2,3]

Although distal perfusion pressure is important at the beginning, neovascularization is essential for continued flap viability and flap integration with the tissue surrounding a defect. A complex interaction between vascular endothelial cells and stimulating angiogenic factors drives neovascularization that is typically complete by day 3 to 7 following flap transfer. During the first 48 hours after flap transfer, a fibrin layer forms between the adjacent tissues to provide a pathway for communication. The interaction of stimulating angiogenesis growth factors and vascular endothelial cells results in vessel dilation, increased permeability of the basement membrane and cell junctions, and finally, endothelial proliferation and sprouting. With continued growth, these capillary outgrowths form capillary loops that undergo rearrangement to form new capillary beds. Neovascularization then occurs through inosculation, the joining of capillaries with preexisting flap vessels, and direct ingrowth into recipient vessels. Both animal and human models have shown that neovascularization is complete by about 7 days and can typically stimulate growth from 2 to 5 mm in length.[4–6]

UNIPEDICLE ADVANCEMENT FLAP

A unipedicle flap is a single cutaneous pedicle flap that is advanced directly into a defect. Unipedicle flaps are created by making 2 parallel incision lines that isolate the flap. The adjacent defect margin forms the flap's distal border (**Fig. 3**). Subcutaneous undermining of the flap and the surrounding skin facilitates flap movement. A typical ratio of defect-to-flap length is 1:3. A unipedicle flap is also known as a U-plasty based on the appearance following closure. Two parallel incisions facilitate sliding movement of the tissue in a single direction toward the defect (see **Fig. 3**).

Unipedicle advancement flaps create redundancy of the adjacent tissue lateral to the borders of the flap along its long axis (see **Fig. 3**). Unequal lengths of the borders of the wound once the flap is advanced and inlayed into the defect result in 2 standing cutaneous deformities or standing cones. The flap incision length plus the cutaneous defect length will always be longer than the length of the flap itself. Incorporating a Burow triangle anywhere along each of the lateral incisions will eliminate the cutaneous redundancy or standing cones (see **Fig. 3**). A Burow triangle is a method of triangular skin excision that allows for

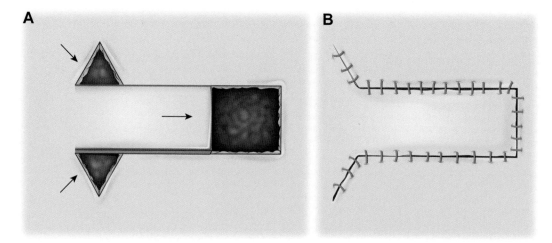

Fig. 3. Unipedicle advancement flap. (*A*) Two incision lines isolate a linear cutaneous flap. The arrows demonstrate the unilateral advancement vector over the cutaneous defect. The triangles demonstrate Burow triangle excision of the standing cutaneous deformities. (*B*) Closure following unipedicle advancement flap.

shortening of the peripheral border to ultimately achieve equal lengths of the peripheral skin and flap edges. The ability to incorporate the Burow triangles anywhere along the length of the flap is an advantage of unipedicle advancement flaps. This flexibility ultimately allows better cosmetic incorporation of skin incisions into RSTLs or along facial subunits. Conversely, standing cutaneous defects for pivotal flaps must be excised at the point of flap rotation, which is not always aesthetically ideal. When cutaneous redundancy lateral to the flap is mild, an alternative to using Burow triangles is the halving suture technique. By halving the length of wound repair in a systematic fashion, surgeons can evenly distribute the redundant tissue throughout the entire length of the flap.

Many cutaneous defects following Mohs excision are round or oval in nature. Advancing a rectangular flap into a round or oval defect results in tissue distortion. It is important when designing unipedicle advancement flaps to match the flap design to the defect by either "squaring off" the defect or "rounding off" the advancement flap. The authors prefer to square off the defect in most cases as angular incisions produce straight scars that have a lower propensity to form trapdoor deformities compared with round or curvilinear scars. Unipedicle advancement flaps are effective for treating defects of the forehead, medial cheek, eyebrow, and helical rim; they are ideal for these aesthetic units due to the ability of the reconstructive surgeon to inconspicuously place incision lines within aesthetic boundaries. Cheek defects are frequently amenable to repair with unipedicle advancement flaps. Unipedicle flaps are ideal in this location because they take advantage of the

mobility and elasticity of the cheek skin. Cheek defects less than 2 cm can typically be closed primarily; however, cutaneous defects larger than 2 cm can necessitate local flap reconstruction for ideal aesthetic results. Advancement flaps may also be required for defects smaller than 2 cm adjacent to important aesthetic boundaries because primary closure can cause significant unwanted secondary movement and distortion. Unipedicle flaps of the cheek are best raised and placed in a lateral-to-medial vector to minimize adjacent tissue distortion of the nasofacial sulcus and lower eyelid. Tissue pull from repair can efface the natural concavity at the junction of the nose and cheek, creating the appearance of widened nasal bridge. Undesired secondary movement can be overcome by minimizing wound closure tension through a periosteal tacking suture between the dermis of the advancement flap and periosteum of the underlying bone of the pyriform aperture.

Defects that are within the upper half of the cheek near the junction of the cheek and nose along the natural nasofacial sulcus are amenable to unipedicle advancement flap reconstruction. Releasing incisions along the infraorbital crease and nasofacial sulcus allows for flap advancement and inconspicuous scars.

BILATERAL UNIPEDICLE ADVANCEMENT FLAPS

Bilateral flaps share the exact same characteristics, principles, and flap design of unilateral pedicle flaps. Bilateral flaps are paired flaps that advance toward one another into a defect (**Fig. 4**). The distinct advantage of bilateral flaps

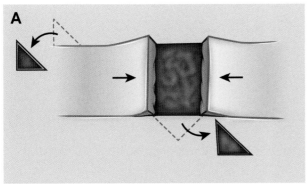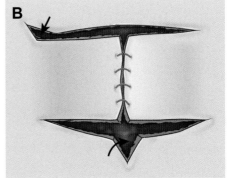

Fig. 4. Bilateral unipedicle advancement flap (H-plasty). (*A*) Paired isolated linear cutaneous flaps. Arrows demonstrate the bilateral advancement vectors over the central cutaneous defect. Burow triangle excisions remove standing cutaneous deformities. (*B*) Partial closure following bilateral flap advancement.

is the ability to distribute tension between the 2 opposing flaps, which lessens tissue distortion and improves flap perfusion. Bilateral flaps are particularly helpful for repair of larger midline structures, such as the lips, forehead, or chin.

Bilateral flaps commonly result in H- or T-shaped repair also known as H-plasty or T-plasty. Although mirrored flaps are an option, the 2 flap lengths do not have to be the same. Elasticity and redundancy of tissue from each donor site determine the appropriate length of each flap. Similar to single unipedicle flaps, advancement of bilateral flaps creates standing cutaneous deformities. Redundancy can sometimes be evenly distributed along the 2 flaps with the halving technique; excision of Burow triangles is often useful as well.

Some forehead defects are ideal for the use of bilateral advancement flaps. The forehead has relatively inelastic skin relative to other areas on the face, and, therefore, the use of 2 flaps can better distribute flap tension. Linear incisions for bilateral advancement flaps are easily hidden parallel to or in the horizontal forehead rhytids. An important consideration when using bilateral advancement flaps on the forehead is the placement of the vertical incision. Although horizontal incisions can be placed anywhere along the forehead and lie within a natural crease, vertical incisions are best placed within the central one-third of the forehead because of the natural dehiscence of the frontalis muscle that occurs near the midline.

T-PLASTY ADVANCEMENT FLAPS

The T-plasty is a modification of the bilateral unipedicle advancement flap. In contrast to bilateral advancement flaps where 2 parallel incisions are required, the T-plasty only uses one incision along the base of the cutaneous defect. Other names for T-plasty are A-to-T or O-to-T wound repair, named to represent the appearance of the cutaneous defect and eventual closure. T-plasty is created by one incision at the base of the cutaneous defect. These opposing sides are then advanced and slightly rotated to meet in the middle at the base of the cutaneous defect. This movement represents the horizontal limb of the T (**Figs. 5** and **6**). This horizontal movement leaves cutaneous redundancy at the distal end of the horizontal limb and in the tissue opposite the base of the defect along the vertical limb. To achieve an aesthetically pleasing result, the standing redundancy along the vertical limb is excised in triangular fashion. Excisions in this manner commonly take the "O" circular defect and turn it into an "A" to optimize reapproximation (see **Figs. 5** and **6**). Redundant tissue along the base of advancement can be removed using Burow triangles or the halving technique.

The T-plasty has 2 distinct advantages compared with other advancement flaps. First, the T-plasty minimizes the number of incisional scars present. The T-plasty only requires one incision to create both flaps compared with bilateral unipedicle advancement flaps requiring 2 parallel incisions. Second, the T-plasty uses 2 flaps to decrease wound tension as compared with unipedicle flaps. T-plasty reconstruction is optimal in defects where skin redundancy is limited or where additional stretching may compromise the vascular perfusion of the flap. Anatomic sites where the vertical and horizontal limb can be incorporated into natural creases or aesthetic boundary of the face are well suited for closure with T-plasty. Examples include the lip vermillion border (see **Fig. 6**; **Fig. 7**), hairline (**Fig. 8**), eyebrow (see **Fig. 5**; **Fig. 9**), preauricular, postauricular, and central forehead (see **Fig. 9**).

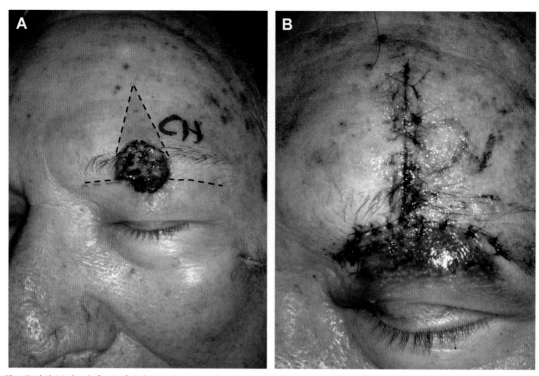

Fig. 5. (*A*) Mohs defect of right eyebrow and scalp measuring approximately 1.5 × 2 cm. A T-plasty bilateral uni-pedicle advancement flap was used to close the defect. The horizontal limb of the T-plasty was strategically placed along the aesthetic boundary of the left eyebrow. Anticipated excision marked with translucent triangle converts the oval "O" defect into an "A"-type defect. (*B*) Wound closed in a reverse T fashion.

Fig. 5 demonstrates an example of a Mohs defect of the left superior eyelid and forehead. Incisions are extended laterally at the base of the defect along the border of the eyebrow, creating the horizontal limb of the T (see **Fig. 5**A). The standing cutaneous deformity in this case is resolved using the halving suture technique.

A similar example can be seen following excision of an allograft placed at the time of Mohs resection of a forehead lesion (see **Fig. 9**). The square was turned into an "A" with triangular excision of tissue along the superior forehead (see **Fig. 9**A). Bilateral incisions were made along the base of the defect to inconspicuously rest within

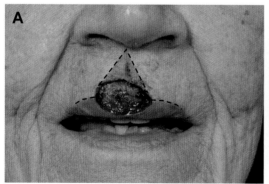

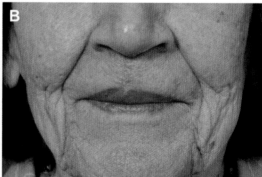

Fig. 6. (*A*) Mohs defect of upper lip measuring approximately 2.5 × 2 cm. (*A*) T-plasty bilateral unipedicle advancement flap design. The horizontal limb of the T-plasty was hidden in the vermillion border. Anticipated standing cutaneous defect marked with translucent triangle so the final vertical limb of the T-plasty falls within the philtrum. (*B*) Wound closed in a reverse T-type fashion.

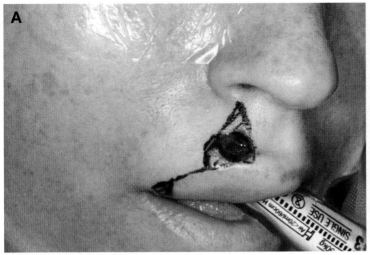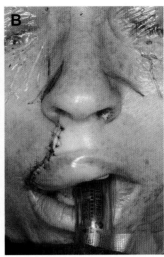

Fig. 7. (*A*) Mohs defect of the right upper lip just lateral to the philtrum column. Design for an A-T-plasty unipedicle advancement flap. Anticipated standing cutaneous deformity marked by horizontal lines for excision of Burow triangle. The "A" design places the incision lines along the left philtrum and vermillion border. (*B*) Wound closure.

the natural rhytids of the forehead (**Fig. 9**A). The standing cutaneous deformity was planned medially along the base of the flap to naturally coincide with the glabellar rhytid (see **Fig. 9**).

The upper and lower lips are common locations for cutaneous malignancies. The vermilion border of the lip provides an ideal location to hide the horizontal limb of T-plasty advancement flaps. **Figs. 5** and **6** demonstrate 2 cases where the modified A-to-T-plasty was used to inconspicuously hide the

incision lines within the vermillion border and philtrum for an optimal cosmetic outcome.

V-TO-Y AND Y-TO-V ADVANCEMENT FLAPS

The V-to-Y flap design is unique among advancement flaps in that it permits "pushing" of tissue into a defect. Other types of advancement flaps pull and create wound tension upon closure at the distal edge of a defect. The V-to-Y flap is advanced into the

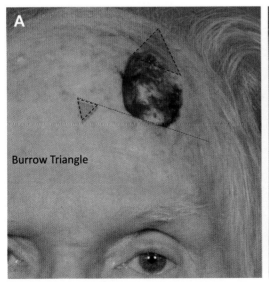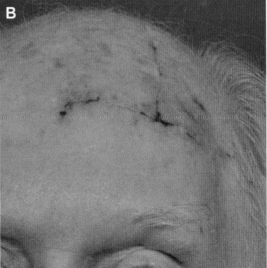

Fig. 8. (*A*) Large Mohs defect of the left superior scalp measuring approximately 3 × 4.5 cm. A T-plasty bilateral unipedicle advancement flap was used to close the defect. The anticipated standing cone excisions are marked with translucent triangles. (*B*) Wound closed in a reverse T-type fashion.

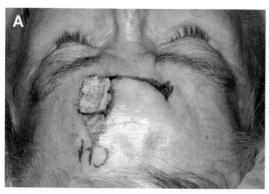 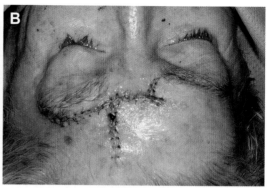

Fig. 9. (*A*) Planed excision of allograft placed at the time of Mohs resection of a forehead lesion. An A-T-plasty bilateral unipedicle advancement flap was used to close the defect. Incision lines were preplanned to naturally rest within upper brow and forehead. (*B*) Wound closed in a T-type fashion. A Burow triangle was placed medially in a glabellar rhytid line to remove the standing cutaneous deformity.

recipient site in a nearly tension-free fashion. The incision is made in a "V-" type fashion, and careful advancement of skin edges at the base of the V creates the vertical line of the Y (**Fig. 10**). The V-to-Y is a classic technique used to lengthen the columella with repair of cleft lip nasal deformities. Another V-to-Y application is correction of distortion along the vermillion border from scar contraction (**Fig. 11**). The V incision is created along the vermillion border with the base of the V along the contracted scar, creating a very broad based or widened "V." The common line of the Y is then closed to push the vermillion border back toward its desired location. The apex of the Y is then simply reapproximated along the repositioned vermilion border.

Medial cheek defects located at or below the ala are also amenable to closure with V-to-Y flaps. An ideal flap design minimizes tension on both the nasal ala and the lower eyelid. A "V"-type incision is created around the flap borders at the base or inferior extent of the cutaneous defect. Ideally, a limb of the V is placed within the nasolabial fold, allowing the flap vector to be parallel to the axis of the fold for ideal aesthetic results (**Figs. 12** and **13**). With proper placement, the common limb of the Y is closed to create a new nasolabial crease. By closing the inferior extent or vertical limb of the "Y," the tissue is "pushed forward" into the cutaneous defect, minimizing secondary tissue movement.

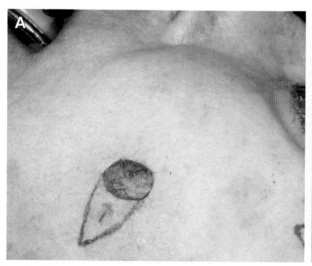 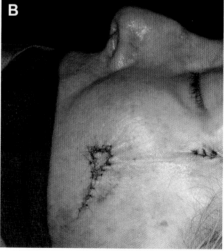

Fig. 10. (*A*) Cutaneous defect of the left cheek. V-Y advancement flap designed to mobilize the lateral cutaneous skin into the left cheek defect. The V-Y advancement flap "pushes" the lateral cheek medially. (*B*) Following closure of V-Y advancement flap.

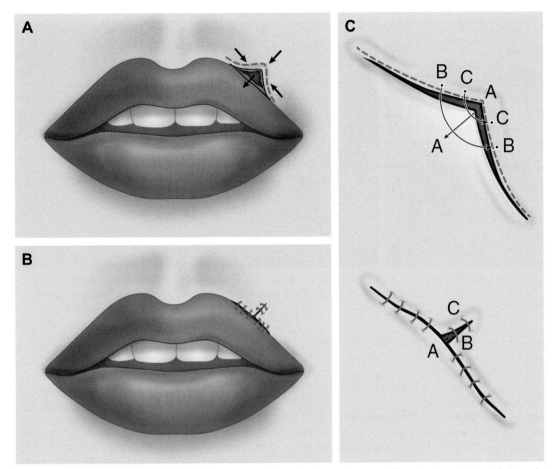

Fig. 11. V-to-Y advancement flap to correct a scar deformity along the vermillion border. (*A*) A wide-based V incision is created, marked by dotted lines, along the vermillion deformity. The *arrows* parallel to the vermillion border represent anticipated closure vector to convert the V into the main limb of the Y. The *arrows* perpendicular to the vermillion border represent anticipated vector of the flap closure, sliding the vermillion border back to its desired location. (*B*) Final closure of V-to-Y advancement flap, correcting the vermillion border shape. (*C*) Magnified view of the planned incision and closure. The "A" marks the planed advancement, while the "B" and "C" mark the planned closure. This closure "pushes" the distorted vermillion inferiorly.

The Y-to-V has a similar concept to the V-to-Y; however, the wound tension lines are opposite. In contrast to "pushing" tissue toward the defect seen with a V-to-Y, the Y-to-V is stretched or "pulled" into the common limb of the Y. An incision is made in a "Y"-type fashion, and the tissue from the top is advanced into the void created by the incision in the common limb of the Y. This advancement places maximum tension at the apex of the flap. Y-to-V advancement flaps are useful to relocate or reposition distorted facial structures into a more natural aesthetic line. Examples include medially displaced lateral canthus or vermillion border secondary to scar contracture. **Fig. 14** demonstrates a medially displaced oral commissure that can commonly occur after full-thickness lip reconstruction. The Y-to-V flap is carefully designed to help "pull" the oral commissure laterally to its more natural position.

CERVICOFACIAL FLAP

The cervicofacial advancement flap is a workhorse for large cheek defect repair that combines elements of both advancement and rotation. These flaps are well suited for defects of the cheek exceeding 3 to 4 cm and that cannot be readily closed with smaller flaps. Cervicofacial flaps are ideal for larger defects because these flaps not only take advantage of the ample laxity of the cheek but also recruit redundant skin from the neck. Advantages of cervicofacial flaps include mobilization of a large amount of tissue with incisions hidden along aesthetic boundaries such as the ear and hairline. Disadvantages include the amount of undermining required and risk of distal flap necrosis.

Cervicofacial rotation advancement flaps are designed to advance redundant cheek and

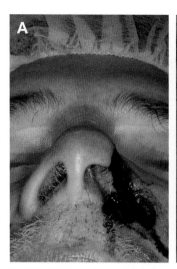
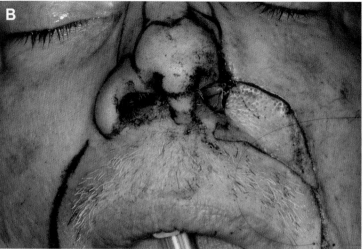

Fig. 12. (*A*) Mohs defect involving the left medial cheek and ala. (*B*) Closure of the defect with a V-to-Y advancement flap. The vertical limb of the Y was purposefully designed to rest in the nasolabial fold. The nasal portion of the defect was repaired secondarily with a paramedian forehead flap.

cervical skin into large cheek defects. Incisions lines for flap advancement typically run laterally from the defect and above the level of the lateral canthus in the temple to maintain superolateral tension on the lower eyelid upon closure. The incision then transitions into the preauricular crease, around the earlobe, along the posterior hairline, and into an inferior cervical crease (**Figs. 15 and 16**). For larger defects, the incision can be carried along the anterior border of the trapezius and/or down onto the chest to recruit more skin (see **Fig. 15**). For more medial defects, the incision can be hidden within the subciliary crease before transitioning into the lateral canthal and temporal region (**Fig. 17**). This incision allows further lateral-to-medial vector advancement. For more

superomedial movement, incision lines can be carried from the nasofacial groove and into the melolabial fold (see **Fig. 17**).

Cervicofacial flaps require carefully planned incision lines to recruit sufficiently redundant cheek and neck skin. Careful undermining in the subcutaneous plane protects the facial nerve that lies deep to the superficial muscular aponeurotic system (SMAS) and facial musculature. Anchoring the flap to sites such as periosteum near the medial canthus and temporalis fascia above the zygomatic arch minimizes undesirable wound tension on the lower eyelid. Plication of the SMAS can also decrease tension on the overlying skin.

Fig. 18 demonstrates a large Mohs defect measuring approximately 5 × 6 cm. Because of

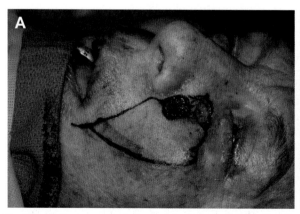
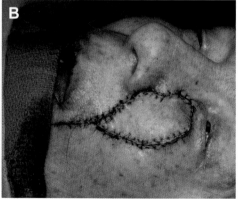

Fig. 13. (*A*) Two separate lesions of the left medial cheek and nasofacial sulcus. Planned V-to-Y advancement flap. (*B*) Following closure of V-to-Y advancement flap. The vertical limb of the "Y" lies within the melolabial fold; the medial limb of the "Y" lies along the nasolabial sulcus, and the advanced flap supports the lower eyelid.

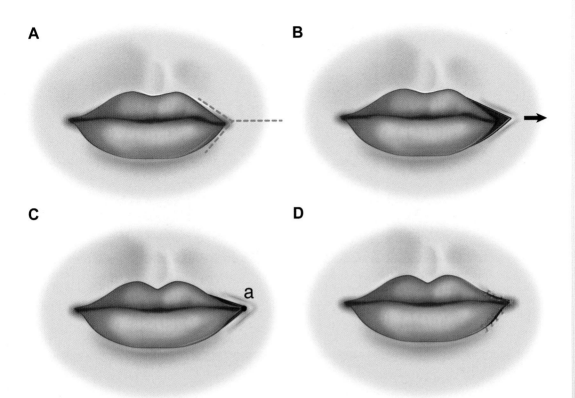

Fig. 14. Y-to-V advancement flap used to correct a medially contracted oral commissure. (*A*) The dashed lines represent the planned Y incision along the vermillion border and oral commissure. (*B, C*) The oral commissure is advanced laterally (arrow vector) to convert the Y into a V. The "a" demarks point of maximal tension. (*D*) After closure, the Y-to-V advancement flap "pulls" the oral commissure more laterally.

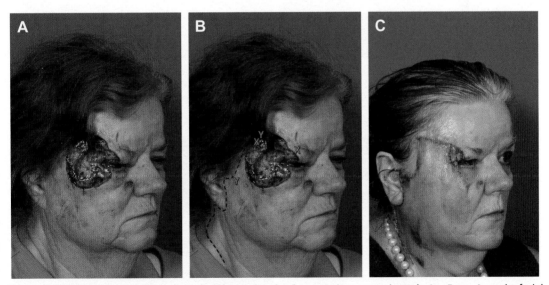

Fig. 15. (*A*) Mohs defect of the temporal and superior cheek measuring approximately 4 × 5 cm. A cervicofacial advancement flap is ideal for a defect of this size because of its ability to recruit redundant cervical skin. (*B*) Incision marked with dashed lines. Incision lines are inconspicuously hidden along the hairline, preauricular crease, and a natural neck crease. Because of the size of the defect, the incision line was carried down along the anterior border of the trapezius to allow additional mobility and skin recruitment. X and Y markings demonstrate the advancement, rotation, and anticipated attachment of the flap. (*C*) Following cervicofacial advancement flap closure.

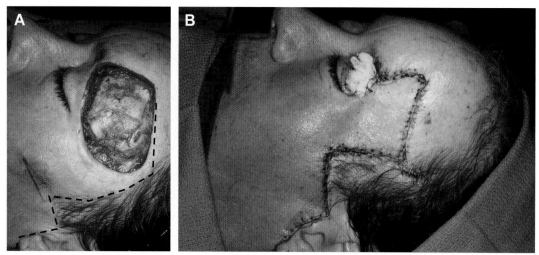

Fig. 16. (*A*) Large Mohs defect of the right superior brow and temporal skin. The dashed lines indicate planned incision lines for cervicofacial advancement flap. Incision lines were hidden along aesthetic boundaries. (*B*) Following cervicofacial advancement flap closure. Small skin graft with bolster was placed along the superior eyelid to minimize secondary movement of the eyelid.

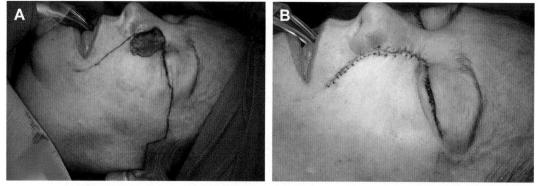

Fig. 17. (*A*) Mohs defect of the superior medial cheek. Planned incision lines are designed along the nasofacial, melolabial, and subciliary creases. Potential planned incision lines were drawn from the lateral canthus into the temporal region but were not required. (*B*) Following cervicofacial advancement flap closure.

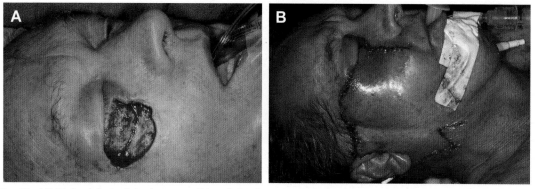

Fig. 18. (*A*) Mohs defect of the lower eyelid and cheek. A cervicofacial advancement flap was used to close the defect. Planned incision lines are carefully placed within the subciliary crease, temporal hairline, preauricular crease, and neck. (*B*) Following cervicofacial advancement flap closure. A Z-plasty was used inferiorly to eliminate the standing cone in the neck.

the size and location of the defect, a cervicofacial flap was selected for repair. The cervicofacial flap will allow for extensive recruitment and advancement of skin to cover the large defect. The planned closure vectors apply minimal tension along the lower lid, minimizing the risk of lower lid malposition. The flap incision lines were carried from the subciliary crease, laterally through the lateral canthus and temporal hairline, and inferiorly using the preauricular crease and cervical neck (see **Fig. 18**). A Z-plasty was used to close the inferior neck incision without excising additional skin.

SUMMARY

Advancement flaps are invaluable for solving complex facial reconstructive problems. When selecting and designing an advancement flap, the surgeon must account for primary and secondary movement to avoid distortion of structures, such as the lower eyelid, nasal ala, and lips. Ideally, incision lines are camouflaged by placing them along RSTLs and boundaries of facial subunits. Unipedicle and bipedicle (U- and H-plasty) advancement flaps are particularly useful for reconstruction of forehead, medial cheek, and brow defects. Lip and brow defects are often amenable to T-plasty closure. V-to-Y flaps have broad applications in the head and neck, allowing the surgeon to "push" tissue into a deficient area with minimal tension near the defect. Cervicofacial flaps are the workhorse for large cheek defects. Understanding how to design and execute all of these versatile flaps will allow for effective repair of a wide range of defects in the head and neck.

REFERENCES

1. Cutting C, Ballantyne D, Shaw W, et al. Critical closing pressure, local perfusion pressure, and the failing skin flap. Ann Plast Surg 1982;8(6):504–9.
2. Daniel R. The anatomy and hemodynamics of the cutaneous circulation and their influence on skin flap design. In: Grabb WC, Myers MB, editors. Skin flaps. Boston: Little, Brown and Company; 1975. p. 111–34.
3. Milton SH. Pedicled skin-flaps: the fallacy of the length: width ratio. Br J Surg 1970;57(7):502–8.
4. Tsur H, Daniller A, Strauch B. Neovascularization of skin flaps: route and timing. Plast Reconstr Surg 1980;66(1):85–90.
5. Cummings CW, Trachy RE. Measurement of alternative blood flow in the porcine panniculus carnosus myocutaneous flap. Arch Otolaryngol 1985;111(9): 598–600.
6. Folkman J. How is blood vessel growth regulated in normal and neoplastic tissue? G.H.A. Clowes Memorial Award lecture. Cancer Res 1986;46(2):467–73.

Flap Basics III
Interpolated Flaps

Lauren K. Reckley, MD[a],*, Jessica J. Peck, MD[b], Scottie B. Roofe, MD[c,d]

KEYWORDS

- Interpolated flaps • Paramedian forehead flap • Melolabial flap • Nasal ala • Nasal dorsum

KEY POINTS

- Interpolated flaps are designed from noncontiguous donor tissue, which is based on an axial or random blood supply with the pedicle passing under or, typically, over normal tissue.
- Interpolated flaps often require multistaged procedures with pedicle division typically performed at 3 weeks once neovascularization between the recipient and transposed tissue has occurred. Longer intervals between procedures are advised for patients with comorbidities that delay wound healing.
- Paramedian forehead flaps are an excellent option for reconstruction of the nasal dorsum with an axial blood supply based on the supratrochlear artery.
- The melolabial flap provides an aesthetic advantage to the reconstruction of the lateral nasal sidewall and ala due its preservation of the alar-facial sulcus and minimal distortion of the melolabial crease.

INTRODUCTION: INTERPOLATED FLAPS

Due to excellent reliability, vascularity, and skin color match, interpolated flaps are a valuable method for reconstruction of the midface following Mohs surgery. Interpolated flaps are designed from noncontiguous donor tissue, which is based on an axial or random blood supply. Therefore, the pedicle must pass under or, more commonly, over the intervening tissue. The overlying pedicle must typically be removed in a second stage after vascularity is established between the wound and the flap. Therefore, most interpolated flaps are performed in 2 stages. The first stage leaves a temporary bridge of vascularized tissue across normal adjacent skin and the second involves detachment of the flap pedicle after neovascularization from the recipient bed. It is this second stage requirement that is the greatest disadvantage of these flaps. Despite this, however, flaps such as the paramedian forehead and melolabial remain a popular technique when insufficient tissue or mobility in nearby skin prevents coverage of a surgical defect with primary closure or an adjacent flap.

Paramedian Forehead Flap

The paramedian forehead flap (PFF) serves as the workhorse flap for modern reconstruction of large, complex defects. Providing a superior match for nasal skin texture, color, and thickness, the ability of the PFF to reconstruct defects involving more than one layer has made it a classic choice for complex nasal reconstruction. However, the robust vascular supply, the ability to vary thickness of the design, and the ability to provide a large amount of tissue allow for reconstruction of

Disclosure: See last page of article.
[a] Otolaryngology-Head and Neck Surgery, Tripler Army Medical Center, Honolulu, HI, USA; [b] Facial Plastic and Microvascular Reconstructive Surgery, Otolaryngology-Head and Neck Surgery, Dwight Eisenhower Army Medical Center, Fort Gordon, GA, USA; [c] Uniformed Services University of the Health Sciences, Bethesda, MD, USA; [d] Otolaryngology-Head and Neck Surgery, Department of Surgery, Womack Army Medical Center, Fort Bragg, NC, USA
* Corresponding author.
E-mail address: lauren.k.reckley.mil@mail.mil

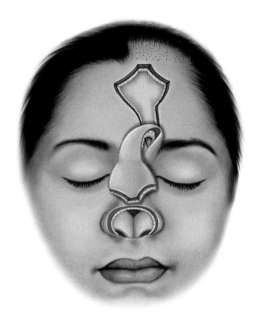

Fig. 1. Illustration of PFF for tip defect.

multiple areas of the midface. Defects of the medial canthal region, upper and lower eyelids, medial cheek, nasolabial region, and upper lip may all be reconstructed with a properly designed PFF.

History

The PFF has been used with a variety of modifications since at least 3000 BC. Initially, the primary design was based on the midline forehead involving the central forehead and glabellar skin, resulting in significant donor site deformity. However, in the late nineteenth and early part of the twentieth century, variations were introduced that altered the flap to the median position. Labat modified the median forehead flap to base it on a unilateral supratrochlear artery. Millard is credited with the shift to the paramedian design which excluded the central glabellar skin, subsequently eliminating a significant source of morbidity.[1]

Anatomy and Blood Supply

The PFF is clearly thicker than the original skin of the nose due to the unique composition of skin, subcutaneous tissue, frontalis muscle, and thin areolar tissue. Knowledge of the donor area anatomy is, therefore, essential because it allows thinning of the flap for better inset, as well as narrowing of the base of the flap for improved rotation without limiting the overall size of the flap. The primary blood supply of the PFF is the supratrochlear artery. This vessel runs in the submuscular

plane, passing deep to the orbicularis oculi muscle and ascending superficial to the corrugator supercilii muscle approximately 1 cm above the brow.[2] There are also important vascular anastomoses from branches of the angular and supraorbital arteries, as well as the medial forehead branch of the dorsal nasal artery.[2,3] The distal end of the flap is considered a random blood supply that allows for variation in design and preservation of vascularity well beyond the distal end of the axial vessel. It is this excellent vascularity that allows incorporation of cartilage or tissue grafts into the flap. These grafts can, in turn, serve as support or lining tissue in nasal reconstruction. **Fig. 1** is an illustration of a PFF used to reconstruct the nasal tip and **Fig. 2** illustrates the vascular supply of the flap. **Figs. 3** and **4** demonstrate intraoperative PFF reconstructive photos for nasal tip defects.

Design and Technique

The design of the PFF is based on the course of the supratrochlear vascular pedicle. For lateral nasal defects, the flap is generally based on the contralateral pedicle to avoid kinking of the vessels and for maximum rotation and length.[4] Doppler may be used to confirm the location of the vessel. However, cadaver studies show that the supratrochlear artery reliably exits the orbit

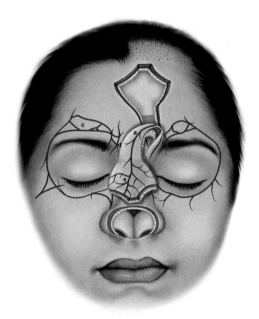

Fig. 2. Illustrated and labeled PFF anatomy. (a) Supratrochlear artery. (b) Supraorbital artery. (c) Supraorbital plexus. (d) Backfill through subdermal plexus. (e) Periosteal elevation captures the periosteal branch of supratrochlear artery.

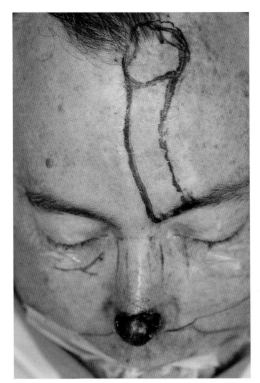

Fig. 3. Marked left PFF for nasal tip defect. Notice that the entire nasal subunit has been removed.

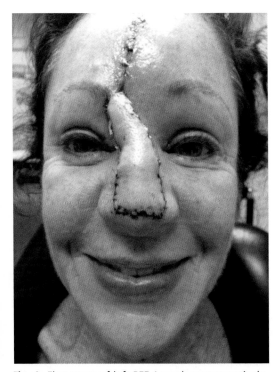

Fig. 4. First stage of left PFF 1 week postoperatively.

1.7 to 2.2 cm from the midline.[3] Taking this into account, the stalk of the flap may be designed to reliably include the supratrochlear pedicle without the use of Doppler, by making the vertical incisions at 1.5 and 2.5 cm from midline. The corrugator complex and frontalis muscles may also be incorporated into the base of the stalk, a technique that is advocated by some investigators to further ensure flap viability.[5]

The use of a foil or paper template is useful to match the defect to the proposed forehead flap. While confirming adequate length required to reach the defect in a tension-free manner, keep in mind the need to include a small amount of extra length to allow for flap thickness and swelling. The random nature of the distal portion of the flap lends itself to variety of designs without compromising blood supply to that area.[4] By extending the PFF superiorly into the hairline or by creating a flap that courses across the midline, the flap may be extended to reconstruct the lower nose and columella. Similarly, for full-thickness defects that involve the intranasal lining, the PFF can be folded over to close the intranasal defect as an alternative to full-thickness skin grafting or a mucosal flap.

Local anesthetic is injected along the periphery of the pedicle to aid in hemostasis while avoiding the supratrochlear vessels. The distal flap is then elevated in the subcutaneous plane from the underlying frontalis musculature, leaving 1 to 3 mm of subcutaneous fat on the underside of the flap. Maintaining the thinness of the flap distally avoids bulkiness and allows a more natural appearance of the flap after inset. As dissection proceeds proximally, the flap is then harvested in progressively deeper layers to preserve the supratrochlear vessels and nerves. After raising the portion for inset, dissection proceeds in the subgaleal plane to preserve the underlying periosteum.[4] Three centimeters above the supraorbital rim the periosteum is incised, and elevation continues in the subperiosteal layer to preserve the periosteal branch of the supratrochlear artery, which supplies additional perforators to the flap. This periosteal incorporation does not decrease the rotational freedom of the flap when using the contralateral forehead, nor does it deter flap length. It does, however, aid in supporting the base of the flap and preventing excessive pedicle torque.

Extending 7 mm above the supraorbital rim, the supraorbital plexus, composed of the supratrochlear, supraorbital, and dorsal nasal artery, provides additional perfusion to the PFF. In higher risk patients, such as smokers or those with poorly controlled diabetes, maintaining this plexus maximizes flap perfusion with a 3-vessel blood supply to the PFF. Conversely, extending the design below the orbital rim allows for maximal rotation.[2] The flap is then rotated and sutured into position.

To close the primary defect, wide undermining is performed. For wider defects, further laxity is achieved by performing galeotomies incised parallel to the skin margins. The wound is then closed in a layered fashion. Although most of the donor site may be closed primarily, often the distal aspect is too wide and under too much tension to close primarily. This portion of the donor site may be allowed to heal by secondary intention with excellent results and minimal scarring. Alternatively, a full-thickness skin graft may be harvested from the postauricular area, or the surgeon may consider a W-plasty closure along the frontal hairline with bilateral advancement flaps.[4]

If necessary, tissue expansion can be performed secondarily after nasal reconstruction to close the donor site or to allow for forehead scar revision.[1] Tissue expanders should be avoided before PFF harvest, however, due to the potential for the reconstructed area to contract after completion of nasal reconstruction.

Detachment

Once neovascularization between the recipient and the transposed tissue has occurred, the pedicle may be safely divided and inset. This has typically been performed at 3 weeks, with longer periods added for patients in whom impaired healing is expected, such as those with poorly controlled diabetes, vasculopathies, or a history of smoking. Klingenstrom and Nylen remarkably performed flaps on themselves to determine the optimal time for flap takedown and published their findings.[6] However, other studies have been performed to establish the appropriate time for takedown of forehead flaps using more objective techniques.[6,7] More than 3 decades ago, Gatti and colleagues[6] used fiberoptic perfusion fluorometry to measure tissue fluorescence, examining tissue in an animal model at various times after flap transposition and demonstrating that vascular ingrowth begins in the first few days. More recently, Woodard and Most[7] prospectively found evidence of vascular in-growth 1 week following transfer. In a later study, Surowitz and Most[8] demonstrated adequate vascular perfusion by 2 weeks in non-nicotine users using the same technology. Additionally, these investigators suggest that real-time imaging with this system can also be used to identify the origin and course of the supratrochlear artery preoperatively, as well as provide guidance for timing of flap transfer in high-risk patients.

The flap pedicle is taken down by incising the superior portion of the flap, in an inverted V.

Inferiorly, the flap is amputated near the margin of the defect and inset. If additional sculpting is required, further conservative thinning of the flap may be performed before closure. **Fig. 5** demonstrates a female patient years after multistaged right PFF for a dorsum defect after Mohs surgery.

Variations

Single-stage

To avoid the second-stage procedure associated with the traditional technique of forehead flaps, single-stage techniques have been described.[9,10] These include tunneling de-epithelialized tissue for transposition under existing intact skin to reconstruct a variety of defects. Avoidance of a second stage can be particularly advantageous in patients with significant comorbidities, or with those who are less likely to be compliant with follow-up. These flaps may be bulky and apparent under the bridging tissue between the donor site and the defect. However, this often resolves within a few months as the pedicle atrophies. Neurovascular injury secondary to compression is possible but unlikely with adequate undermining and avoidance of a narrow tunnel.[9]

Three-stage

Millard first described the 3-stage technique in 1974 using an intermediate procedure after flap transfer and before division of the pedicle with the intent of minimizing flap necrosis. During the intermediate phase, the flap was thinned and had the added benefit of some degree of aesthetic improvement over the traditional 2-stage technique. Some surgeons advocate that the 3-stage approach allows the use of skin grafts at the first stage for internal lining and placement of cartilage grafts at the second stage without putting them at risk because of tenuous vascularity. However, a review of 100 3-stage flaps by Stahl and colleagues[11] found no evidence to support a lower rate of necrosis or an enhanced aesthetic result.

Vascular delay

Vascular delay has been used for a variety of flaps in surgical reconstruction to improve survival but less frequently with forehead flaps. Vertical limbs of the flap are incised and elevated off of the loose areolar tissue at the deep surface. The flap is then sutured back into position. After 14 days, the superior margin is incised, and the flap is rotated to fill the distant defect. Four weeks later, the flap is inset and incised. Vascular delay improves flap perfusion through several transient effects. Early changes include vascular dilation caused by division of sympathetic nerves, causing initial release and then depletion of adrenergic factors

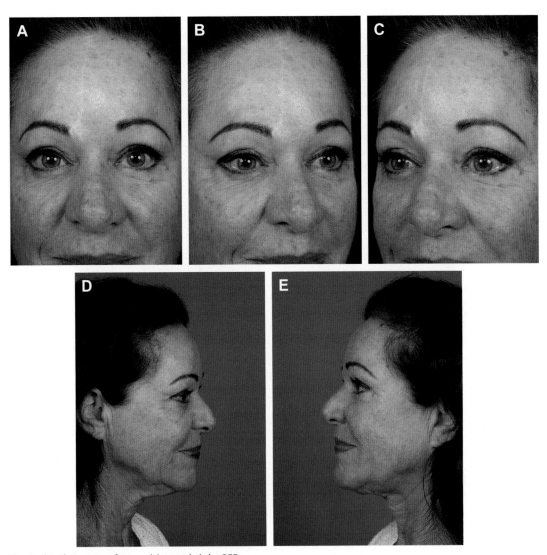

Fig. 5. (*A–E*) 2 years after multistaged right PFF.

from nerve endings.[12] A relative ischemia of the tissue and subsequent metabolic changes that contribute to increased flap survival. Later, prolonged alterations in tissue metabolism and neovascularization occur via both angiogenesis and vasculogenesis. This technique may be considered in smokers in whom vascular compromise can be expected.[13] However, most surgeons will simply prolong the time until takedown to 4 weeks or beyond in this subset of patients.

Other uses

The use of forehead flaps to provide internal lining, particularly in the case of large full-thickness nasal defects has been well described.[14] Paramedian flaps have also been described for use in reconstruction of periorbital defects. Similar to the concept of nasal reconstruction, these flaps with

their superior color match can also be contoured to match the variable skin thickness of the periorbital complex. Excellent coverage of the medial canthus, lacrimal drainage system, and medial upper eyelid has been achieved, particularly in defects that also involve the nose in that region.[15]

MELOLABIAL FLAP

The melolabial flap (also referred to as the nasolabial flap) is a versatile flap with multiple uses for midface reconstruction. It may be designed as a skin and subcutaneous tissue flap that is useful for partial-thickness nasal reconstruction or as a full-thickness flap of skin, subcutaneous tissue, and mucosa that is useful for reconstructing full-thickness defects of the lip. This flexibility in design, combined with the excellent skin color and texture match, makes it particularly useful for nasal reconstruction of the lower nasal sidewall, the ala, the columella, and the lateral internal lining.[16] The excellent vascularity allows incorporation of cartilage grafts to recreate structural support of the nose. Aesthetically, the most important advantage of the melolabial flap is that it does not violate the alar-facial sulcus, thereby minimizing distortion of the melolabial crease.[17] Similar to the PFF, it may be designed as a multistaged procedure. It may also be designed as a single-stage procedure for defects of the lower sidewall and ala.

History

The nasolabial flap was first described by Sushruta, an Indian surgeon, shortly after 700 BC. More than 300 surgical procedures were described, the most well-known of which covered reconstructive techniques following nasal amputation, performed at the time as a form of criminal punishment. During the 1800s, multiple alterations of the flap were described to reconstruct a variety of defects, including defects of the palate, tongue, and lips.[18]

Anatomy and Blood Supply

The ability to camouflage scarring in the nasolabial crease is an important advantage of using the melolabial flap for reconstruction. This crease begins slightly superior to the alar crease and extends to approximately 1 cm lateral to the oral commissure. The crease itself is created by a dense concentration of fibrous muscular attachments to the dermis. The blood supply is usually considered to be random, dependent on the subdermal plexus located between the reticular dermis and the superficial musculoaponeurotic system (SMAS) within the superficial adipose layer.[19] This plexus receives perfusion from branches of the distal facial and labial arteries perforating through the levator labii, as well as lesser contributions from the infraorbital artery. It is the rich anastomoses at the subdermal plexus that allow the flap to be based superiorly or inferiorly as the reconstruction requires.

Design

When used to reconstruct the lower nasal sidewall or ala, the melolabial flap is usually designed as a single-stage, superiorly based, flap. If the defect is greater than 50% of the aesthetic subunit, it is most advantageous to remove the skin and reconstruct the entire subunit with the melolabial flap. When reconstructing the ala, however, the surgeon should attempt to leave 1 mm of alar skin just anterior to the alar-facial sulcus, if still intact,

to preserve the normal concavity.[20] Superiorly, the excised nasal sidewall skin should reach the alar crease at an angle of less than 30° to prevent a dog-ear deformity at the point of rotation and to avoid torsion on the proximal melolabial blood supply. **Figs. 6–8** illustrate the typical superiorly based melolabial flap at different surgical stages.

The contralateral side conveniently serves as an appropriate template, keeping in mind to undersize the flap by approximately 20% to account for intrinsic elastic properties surrounding the defect, which will cause the enlargement from the initial excision.[19] However, when the defect is within 5 mm of the alar rim, it is advisable to design the flap to the exact size of the defect to prevent alar retraction. Whenever possible, the primary defect should be deepened to establish uniformity and symmetry with the contralateral side rather than overthinning the flap.[16]

The preferred pedicle width is generally 1.5 to 2 cm, with the medial border of the flap aligned with the melolabial crease.[16] Proximally, the pedicle skin incisions should narrow to facilitate closure of the donor site, whereas the subcutaneous portion is allowed to remain wide to maximize arterial perforators. The flap is elevated, defatted, and advanced medially, maintaining at least 3 mm of fat on the underside of the flap to optimize blood supply.[19] The flap is inset into the defect, proximally

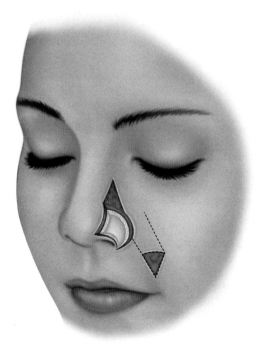

Fig. 6. Superiorly based illustration of melolabial flap for alar defect.

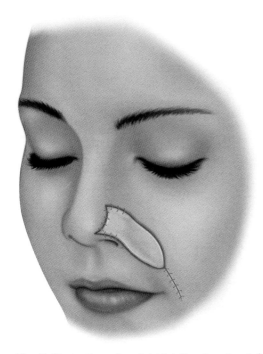

Fig. 7. Illustration of melolabial flap for alar defect after rotation and primary closure of donor site.

to distally. When the alar crease is reached, a buried permanent suture should be placed to anchor the flap, thus recreating the crease.

The donor site is closed primarily by undermining the cheek skin. The SMAS may also be plicated to aid in closure of larger donor site defects in a tension-free fashion.[17] However, due to tissue laxity lateral to the melolabial crease, particularly in the older patient, the closure of the donor site is usually uncomplicated.[16] For the best cosmetic result, the vectors for scar formation should be oriented within the melolabial crease and prevent distortion of the lower eyelid, upper lip, or oral commissure (**Fig. 9**). **Fig. 10** demonstrates a female patient after she has healed from completion of a right melolabial flap for right alar reconstruction.

Variations

The melolabial flap may be designed as an interpolated flap or as an island advancement flap based on a subcutaneous pedicle. The interpolated flap is elevated in the subcutaneous plane while preserving thickness of the pedicle base for flap survival.[16] The island pedicle is incised on the cutaneous borders while maintaining a vascularized subcutaneous and muscular pedicle at the central third of the flap.

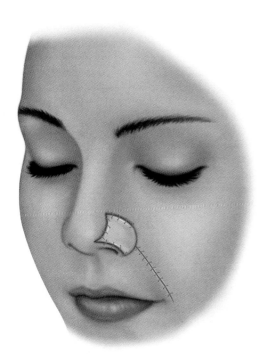

Fig. 8. Illustration of melolabial flap for alar defect after detachment.

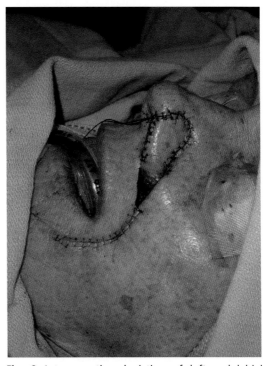

Fig. 9. Intraoperative depiction of left melolabial flap.

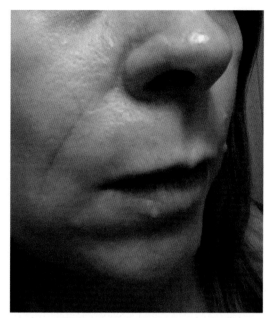

Fig. 10. Female patient 4 months after right alar reconstruction with melolabial flap.

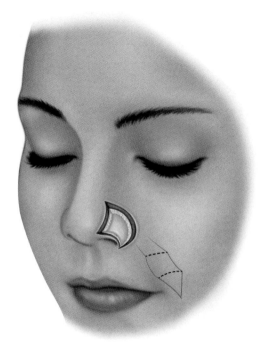

Fig. 11. Illustration of single-stage melolabial flap.

As with the PFF, when the melolabial flap is performed in 2 stages, detachment is typically performed after 3 weeks or longer in patients with comorbidities that impair healing or microvascularity. The distal aspect of the flap may be thinned initially to fit within the defect, while saving thinning of the proximal aspect for the second stage.

The melolabial flap may also be used to reconstruct the intranasal lining. By designing the melolabial flap to fold on itself, full-thickness alar defects can be repaired while avoiding additional difficult intranasal flaps.[21] Unfortunately, such reconstruction often results in excessive bulk, which can distort the alar-facial sulcus and crowd the airway.[22] Fig. 11 is an illustration of a single-stage melolabial flap reconstruction.

COMPLICATIONS

The most common complication following interpolated flaps is bleeding. Hematomas occur in 0.4%, whereas active bleeding requiring intervention occurs in 8.4% of cases.[23] Such bleeding may be prevented with meticulous hemostasis while raising the flap and, when it does occur, can be controlled without detrimental effects to the flap or patient.

Pincushioning occurs in up to 6.5% of cases.[24] Slightly undersizing the flap and avoiding curvilinear incisions aids in minimizing this complication. When

it does occur, however, patients may be treated with corticosteroids with reasonable improvement. Other common complications include nasal obstruction, thick scars, bulky flaps, and alar notching. It is also important to limit the incorporation of fibrofatty tissue into the defect and to not rely on fibrofatty tissue adding bulk to the ala. Preferably, a larger free cartilage graft is used to recreate bulk and provide structure to the nasal skeleton to prevent alar notching and collapse of the external nasal valve postoperatively.[24]

Overall, flap failure is uncommon, with complete flap failure limited to approximately 2%. Several risk factors have been evaluated for flap failure, including defect thickness, use of a cartilage graft, and presence of comorbidities. However, these factors did not affect outcome.[24] Not surprisingly, there is a greater risk of flap loss in active smokers.

SUMMARY

The reliability and ease of harvesting of interpolated flaps provide excellent functional and aesthetic results for reconstruction of large nasal defects. Their excellent skin color and texture match, along with the ability to contour to various thicknesses, allow superior long-term results. The complication rates are very low and, when they do occur, tend to be minimal. Patient selection is essential, and it is important to educate the patient about healing and the goals of each stage of the procedure to obtain the best result.

DISCLOSURE

Institution where the work was primarily performed: Tripler Army Medical Center, Hawaii, USA.

Source of Financial Support or Funding: None.

Financial Interests and Disclosures: None.

Financial Disclosure: (1) No financial and no material support for this research and work. (2) Authors have no financial interests in any companies or other entities that have an interest in the information in the contribution (eg, grants, advisory boards, employment, consultancies, contracts, honoraria, royalties, expert testimony, partnerships, or stock ownership in medically-related fields).

Conflict of Interest: None.

This article has not been presented at a meeting. The views expressed in this article are those of the authors and do not reflect the official policy or position of the Department of the Army, Department of Defense, or the US Government.

All authors met the criteria for authorship established by the International Committee of Medical Journal Editors, specifically: L.K. Reckley, J.J. Peck, and S.B. Roofe were responsible for substantial contributions to the conception, design, analysis, and drafting the work, revising the work, and reviewing the article. Additionally, all authors provided final approval of the version to be published and agreed to be accountable for all aspects of the work, including ensuring the accuracy and/or integrity of the work.

REFERENCES

1. Menick FJ. Aesthetic refinements in use of forehead for nasal reconstruction: the paramedian forehead flap. Clin Plast Surg 1990;17(4):607–22.
2. Reece EM, Schaverien M, Rohrich RJ. The paramedian forehead flap: a dynamic anatomical vascular study verifying safety and clinical implications. Plast Reconstr Surg 2008;121(6):1956–63.
3. Shumrick KA, Smith TL. The anatomic basis for the design of forehead flaps in nasal reconstruction. Arch Otolaryngol Head Neck Surg 1992;118(4):373–9.
4. Quatela VC, Sherris DA, Rounds MF. Esthetic refinements in forehead flap nasal reconstruction. Arch Otolaryngol Head Neck Surg 1995;121(10):1106.
5. Jellinek NJ, Nguyen TH, Albertini JG. Paramedian forehead flap: advances, procedural nuances, and variations in technique. Dermatol Surg 2014;40(Suppl 9):S30–42.
6. Gatti JE, LaRossa D, Brousseau DA, et al. Assessment of neovascularization and timing of flap division. Plast Reconstr Surg 1984;73(3):396–402.
7. Woodard CR, Most SP. Intraoperative angiography using laser-assisted indocyanine green imaging to map perfusion of forehead flaps. Arch Facial Plast Surg 2012;14(4):263–9.
8. Surowitz JB, Most SP. Use of laser-assisted indocyanine green angiography for early division of the forehead flap pedicle. JAMA Facial Plast Surg 2015;17(3):209–14.
9. Kishi K, Imanishi N, Shimizu Y, et al. Alternative 1-step nasal reconstruction technique. Arch Facial Plast Surg 2012;14(2):116–21.
10. Fudem GM, Montilla RD, Vaughn CJ. Single-stage forehead flap in nasal reconstruction. Ann Plast Surg 2010;64(5):645–8.
11. Stahl AS, Gubisch W, Haack S, et al. A cohort study of paramedian forehead flap in 2 stages (87 Flaps) and 3 stages (100 Flaps). Ann Plast Surg 2015;75(6):615–9.
12. Ghali S, Butler PE, Tepper OM, et al. Vascular delay revisited. Plast Reconstr Surg 2007;119(6):1735–44.
13. Kent DE, Defazio JM. Improving survival of the paramedian forehead flap in patients with excessive tobacco use: the vascular delay. Dermatol Surg 2011;37(9):1362–4.
14. Parikh S, Futran ND, Most SP. An alternative method for reconstruction of large intranasal lining defects: the Farina method revisited. Arch Facial Plast Surg 2010;12(5):311–4.
15. Price DL, Sherris DA, Bartley GB, et al. Forehead flap periorbital reconstruction. Arch Facial Plast Surg 2004;6(4):222–7.
16. Jewett BS. Interpolated forehead and melolabial flaps. Facial Plast Surg Clin North Am 2009;17:361–77.
17. Baker SR, Johnson TM, Nelson BR. The importance of maintaining the alar-facial sulcus in nasal reconstruction. Arch Otolaryngol Head Neck Surg 1995;121:617–22.
18. Schmidt BL, Dierks EJ. The nasolabial flap. Oral Maxillofacial Surg Clin N Am 2003;15(4):487–95.
19. Yellin SA, Nugent A. Melolabial flaps for nasal reconstruction. Facial Plast Surg Clin North Am 2011;19:123–39.
20. Drisco BP, Baker SR. Reconstruction of nasal alar defects. Arch Facial Plast Surg 2001;3:91–9.

21. Cook JJ. The reconstruction of the nasal ala with interpolated flaps from the cheek and forehead; design and execution modifications to improve surgical outcomes. Br J Dermatol 2014;171(2):29–33.

22. Weber SM, Wang TD. Options for internal lining in nasal reconstruction. Facial Plast Surg Clin North Am 2011;19:163–73.

23. Simmons A, Xu JC, Bordeaux JS. Improving the design and execution of interpolation flaps. Curr Dermatol Rep 2015;4:119–24.

24. Paddack AC, Frank RW, Spencer HJ, et al. Outcomes of paramedian forehead and nasolabial interpolation flaps in nasal reconstruction. Arch Otolaryngol Head Neck Surg 2012;138(4):367–71.

Skin and Composite Grafting Techniques in Facial Reconstruction for Skin Cancer

Michael J. Brenner, MD*, Jeffrey S. Moyer, MD

KEYWORDS

- Skin graft • Composite graft • Skin cancer • Mohs reconstruction • Facial reconstruction
- Melanoma • Local flap • Cartilage

KEY POINTS

- In Mohs reconstruction, full-thickness skin grafts are generally preferred over split-thickness grafts due to decreased contracture and improved color, contour, and texture.
- A variety of modifications to grafting technique can improve graft survival, restoration of normal contours, functional outcomes, and overall aesthetic results.
- Because grafts do not carry their own blood supply, optimizing recipient site conditions with a vascular bed is of paramount importance, particularly when performing composite grafts.
- Skin and composite grafts may be combined with other approaches to minimize distortion and optimize cosmetic subunits.

OVERVIEW OF SKIN ANATOMY IN RELATION TO GRAFTING

The skin is the body's largest organ, and it varies widely in thickness and character across the anatomic regions of the face. Successful grafting is predicated on a basic understanding of this functional anatomy. The skin's epidermis includes basal cell, prickle cell, granular cell, and keratin layers, and the epidermis attaches to the dermis via the basement membrane, which is the anatomic landmark that differentiates in situ or preinvasive lesions from invasive cutaneous malignancy. The dermis, in turn, affords skin most of it tensile strength. The dermis is penetrated by epidermal appendages, blood vessels, nerves, and cells. The richly vascularized and innervated pilosebaceous units include sebaceous glands, hair follicles, and arrector pili muscles that contain stem cells and have substantial regenerative potential.[1] The fibroblasts found in the dermis facilitate wound contraction during healing and produce collagen, elastin, and ground substance. Epithelialization of cutaneous defects occurs from wound edges and the basement membrane along hair follicles and adnexal structures. Blood supply derives from both a deep subdermal plexus and a superficial plexus that supplies the superficial dermal papillae.[2]

The skin serves a role as both graft and recipient in most cases of reconstruction. There are a variety of situations where skin grafts are indicated, and grafts are particularly useful for resurfacing superficial defects. Full-thickness skin grafts are also helpful in young patients who have tight skin and sizable defects that are not readily amenable

Disclosure Statement: The authors have nothing to disclose.
Division of Facial Plastic and Reconstructive Surgery, Department of Otolaryngology-Head and Neck Surgery, University of Michigan Medical Center, 1500 East Medical Center Drive SPC 5312, 1904 Taubman Center, Ann Arbor, MI 48109-5312, USA
* Corresponding author.
E-mail address: mbren@med.umich.edu

to adjacent tissue transfer. Although skin grafts often minimize the need for additional facial skin incisions, they are susceptible to developing a "patchlike" appearance due to mismatch of color, contour, or texture if not carefully planned. Because of such concerns, skin grafts are used judiciously, proving especially useful in cases that cannot be reconstructed with a local flap or where major distortion would ensue. With thoughtful application of the principles presented herein, many patients can benefit from these aesthetic approaches. As evidence-based approaches evolve in facial plastics,[3] grafting practices should become more consistent so as to achieve optimal outcomes.

Skin grafts may be harvested as full-thickness, split-thickness, or composite grafts with or without hair-bearing skin. The viability of the graft depends on the vascular supply to the recipient bed, thickness of the graft, appropriate compression of graft to recipient site, and patient factors, such as smoking, hypoxemia, diabetes, radiation, and history of prior surgery at the site.[4] Exposed bone,

tendon, and cartilage all decrease the probability of successful graft survival. Some irregularity at the junction of skin grafts and surrounding skin is common. When patients are routinely counseled preoperatively regarding the potential role for postoperative dermabrasion or other similar refinements, there is greater acceptance of procedures to achieve optimal match and camouflage of the reconstruction.

RECIPIENT BED PREPARATION

Several technical refinements may improve skin grafting outcomes. Meticulous attention to sterile technique is crucial, because infection greatly increases the likelihood of graft loss. Free grafts are particularly vulnerable to infection, because they do not carry their own blood supply. A variety of approaches may be used for bolstering, including conventional tie-down bolster, quilting sutures, and use of custom contoured compressive dressing. Nobecutane spray may also be used as a transparent antibacterial dressing that

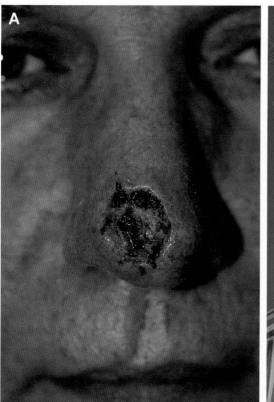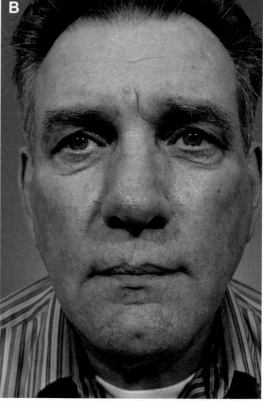

Fig. 1. (*A*) A 1.5-cm superficial defect of paramidline nasal tip after micrographic excision of carcinoma. (*B*) Defect repaired with full-thickness skin graft. Reconstruction with skin graft achieves favorable color and contour match, despite resurfacing only the resected portion of the nasal tip unit. Skin grafting avoided the alar distortion that would likely occur with local flap to a sizable defect at this location.

is gradually shed.[5] Regardless of dressing, the goal is to minimize shearing forces that may otherwise disrupt vascular connections forming between the graft and the recipient bed. Smoking cessation is also strongly encouraged as tobacco products significantly impair the survival of skin grafts.

In cases of exposed bone, the likelihood of skin graft survival can be improved by decorticating a thin layer of bone until punctuate bleeding is achieved. If using powered instrumentation, such as a diamond fraise burr, care must be taken to avoid inadvertently cauterizing the perforating nutrient vessels with heat/friction from the burr. Alternatively, holes can be drilled in the outer bone table to access the inner diploë. In cases of extensive bony loss, a muscle flap may be required before grafting. A similar approach may also be useful when grafting on ear cartilage without perichondrium by making windows in the native auricular cartilage. For deeper wounds, it is often helpful to delay skin grafting for roughly 2 weeks, until such time as granulation tissue has formed within the wound bed. The epithelium is then removed before grafting. To decrease bacterial load in granulating tissue, some authors advocate prophylactic use of antistaphylococcal antibiotic beginning 72 hours before skin grafting.

As in other approaches to facial reconstruction, the surgeon should consider facial aesthetic regions and surrounding anatomic landmarks. Marking out the borders of aesthetic units may help ensure preservation of natural facial contours and boundaries. Before skin grafting, defects may be conservatively enlarged to facilitate resurfacing of an entire aesthetic unit. The wound should be of uniform depth, and the edges should be freshened. In contrast to local flap reconstruction, where incisions are oriented 90°, in skin grafting it is often advantageous to maintain a gradual beveled contour transitioning between the skin graft and adjacent facial skin. Risk of trapdoor deformity can often be decreased by developing more acute (rather than rounded) angles in midface reconstruction.

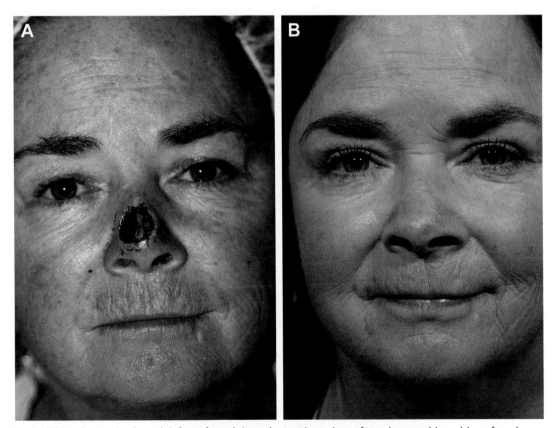

Fig. 2. (*A*) Moderate-sized nasal defect of nasal tip and supratip regions after micrographic excision of carcinoma, with underlying perichondrium preserved. (*B*) Defect repaired with full-thickness skin graft. Modifying the graft to have variable thickness was helpful in restoration of native contour, because the defect spanned tip and supratip nasal units.

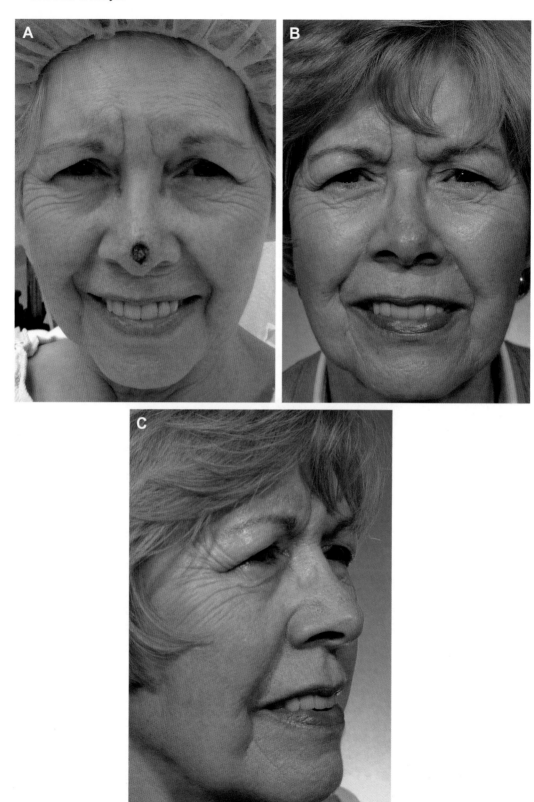

Fig. 3. (*A*) Nasal tip defect in a fair, thin-skinned patient, with preserved perichondrium and superficial muscu-loaponeurotic system in recipient bed. (*B*) Favorable color and contour match is noted after full-thickness skin graft reconstruction. (*C*) Natural profile could be achieved with graft because of favorable defect attributes.

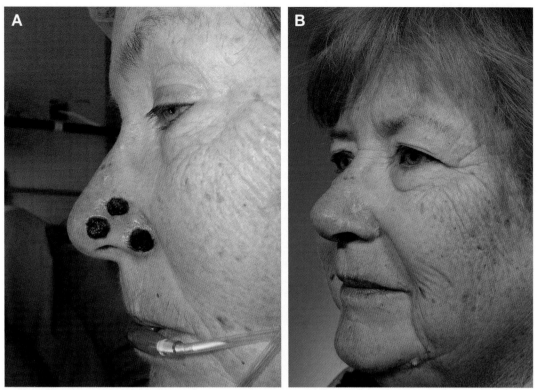

Fig. 4. (*A*) Multiple small nasal defects involving alar lobule, nasal tip, and nasal sidewall after micrographic excision. (*B*) Appearance after skin grafting. Skin grafting allowed for favorable camouflage while obviating 2-stage procedures and/or resurfacing of the entire alar lobule and surround areas.

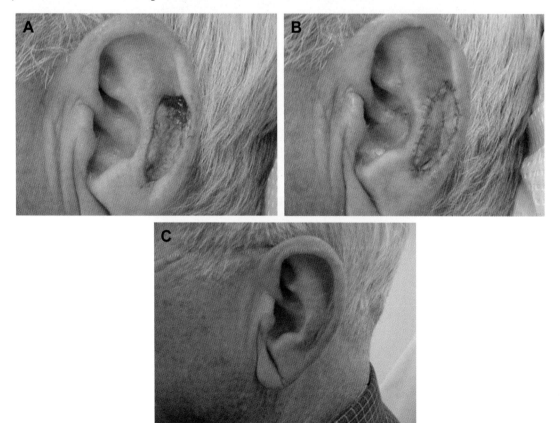

Fig. 5. (*A*) Defect of scapha of left ear, partially involving antihelical fold and helical rim. The wound was amenable to skin grafting because perichondrium was preserved. (*B*) Excellent take of skin graft is noted, made possible by the favorable vascular bed and bolster. (*C*) Long-term result.

FULL-THICKNESS SKIN GRAFTS TECHNIQUE

Full-thickness skin grafts consist of epidermis and full-thickness dermis, and they are harvested by incising down to subcutaneous fat. In instances where the graft donor site is thicker than the recipient site, judicious thinning to match thickness of skin in the recipient bed may be performed.[6] Conversely, in cases where the defect depth exceeds graft thickness, a small underlay vascular flap or small amount of adipose may be included to increase graft bulk, albeit with attendant decreased risk of take. Full-thickness grafts offer several advantages over split-thickness grafts, including decreased susceptibility to contraction, improved pigmentation and texture match, as well as additional thickness for deeper defects. Despite these advantages, full-thickness grafts nonetheless still contract 10% to 15% on average.[7] Patients are administered preoperative intravenous antibiotics, usually consisting of 2 g cefazolin or 900 mg clindamycin, if penicillin allergic. Patients receive local anesthesia (1%

lidocaine with 1:100,000 concentration of epinephrine) with or without intravenous sedation. The wound and donor sites are prepared sterilely with povidone-iodine. The 45° bevel of the saucerized defect is preserved to facilitate a smooth transition between graft and surrounding skin, thereby avoiding a step-off contour deformity. The template is made of the defect, and the graft is designed slightly larger to accommodate for graft contraction. Subcutaneous tissue is removed from the graft with curved iris scissors.

Because grafts survive initially by diffusion of nutrients (imbibition), the wound bed is optimized by removing eschar, nonvital tissue, or desiccated clot. Ideally, pinpoint bleeding is apparent along the defect, which is readily controlled with pressure and/or topical epinephrine. The graft is secured into position, often incorporating tacking or quilting sutures that help the graft adhere to the underlying tissue. Graft edges are secured with simple interrupted 5-0 chromic sutures. A variety of approaches

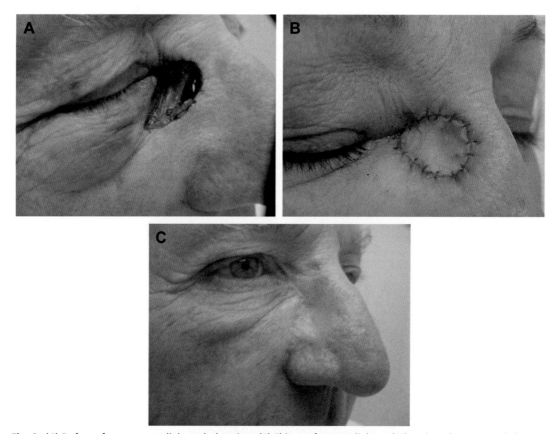

Fig. 6. (*A*) Defect of concave medial canthal region. (*B*) Skin graft to medial canthal region abuts on eyelid, nose, and cheek. (*C*) Favorable healing, without lower lid ectropion or other distortion. The skin graft resurfaces, rather than replaces, underlying topography; as a result, preexisting contours are preserved and graft is inconspicuous.

may be used to compress the graft flush to the underlying recipient bed. A bolster dressing may be made from nonadherent bandage with petroleum-based ointment. Alternatively, cotton balls covered with antibiotic ointment may be wrapped with petrolatum 3% bismuth tribromophenate (Xeroform). Larger bolsters are secured with silk sutures. For small irregular sites, such as the nasal tip or alar margin, it may be most effective to dress the wound and then provide compression with a thermoplast splint sculpted to the shape of the patient's nose. This custom bolster can then be secured to the surrounding skin with 5-0 Prolene sutures. Bolsters are left in place for 5 to 7 days. If the graft has adhered well to the recipient site, the patient is allowed to get the area wet and cleanse gently. With appropriate bolstering technique, complete graft loss is quite rare. In some cases, a graft may appear cyanotic due to a thin layer of blood deep to the graft or because of hyperemia.

Nasal defects are common sites for skin grafting. As shown in **Fig. 1**, skin grafts can achieve excellent aesthetic resurfacing of superficial defects. Skin grafts largely avert the risk of alar distortion that may occur when such defects are reconstructed with bilobe flap or other local flaps. Skin grafts can also provide favorable reconstruction of nasal tip/supratip, in cases where the underlying cartilage topography allows resurfacing with skin graft to restore nasal contours (**Fig. 2**). In reconstructing nasal tip defects, maintaining profile and avoiding depressed scars are critical; therefore, the surgeon must ensure appropriate graft thickness and adequate soft tissue volume in the recipient bed (**Fig. 3**). Granulation may be helpful in individuals with thick skin, in whom risk of depressed scar is anticipated. As **Fig. 4** demonstrates, even several small defects can be inconspicuously repaired with skin grafting, obviating a 2-staged flap reconstruction procedure while preserving aesthetic units.

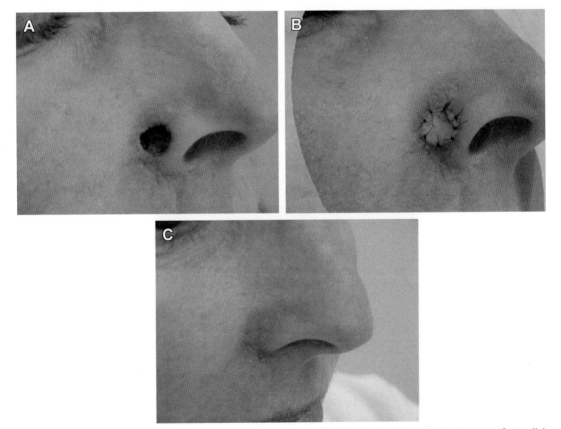

Fig. 7. (A) Defect of alar-facial sulcus, spanning alar lobule, and cheek subunits. A small subcutaneous fat pedicle from cheek was elevated before skin grafting to preserve structure and aesthetic contour. (B) Appearance of skin graft immediately postoperatively, showing natural contour. (C) Long-term result with favorable contour of alar-facial crease maintained.

Because skin grafts tend to assume the shape and contour of the underlying tissues, they are highly adaptable, allowing effective reconstruction to concave, convex, and planar surfaces. The ear is a common site for skin cancer, and it has many irregular contours. As a result, if often heals favorably with skin grafting, provided adequate perichondrium is preserved (**Fig. 5**). Skin grafts naturally conform to concave locations, such as the medial canthus (**Fig. 6**), alar-facial sulcus (**Fig. 7**), and supra-alar crease (**Fig. 8**). Tacking sutures are often helpful in preserving creases and junctions. Skin grafts also camouflage planar defects, such as the nasal sidewall (**Fig. 9**), and provide effective resurfacing for the fine skin found in the eyelids (**Fig. 10**) and the nasal infratip lobule.

Dermabrasion, if deemed helpful, is typically performed 6 weeks or more after the graft has healed. In some cases, injection of steroid deep to the graft may help in resolving early trapdoor deformity. Serial Z-plasties or other minor scar revision maneuvers are also occasionally performed to camouflage the transition between graft and surrounding skin. Dermabrasion helps to blend color, contour, and texture. Grafts may be dermabraded more than once if desired, but care must be taken to limit depth of dermabrasion to midpapillary dermis to avoid injury to melanocytes, because excessive depth can exacerbate hypopigmentation.[1] Vascular inosculation occurs over 24 to 48 hours, followed by capillary ingrowth. Development of pink color during 3 to 7 days signals neovascularization and successful graft take. Over the ensuing 1 to 2 months, pink color diminishes, but the graft may remain lighter than surrounding skin.

SPLIT-THICKNESS SKIN GRAFT TECHNIQUE

Split-thickness skin grafts include epidermis and limited dermis. They are thinner than full-thickness grafts and have capillary loops, making

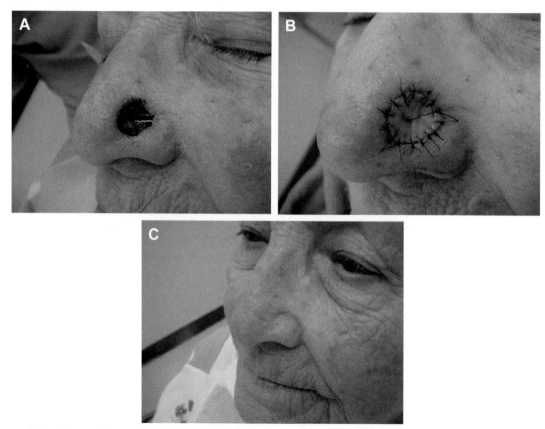

Fig. 8. (A) Defect of supra-alar crease, involving alar lobule and nasal sidewall. (B) Skin graft after inset, with tacking stitch at intended location of new supra-alar crease. Stitch both obliterates dead space and ensures preservation of natural crease. (C) Long-term result with favorable contour of alar-facial crease maintained. Note absence of "buttonlike" trap door deformity, often seen with local flaps that span a nasal crease. Preservation of contour favors a full-thickness skin graft for this location.

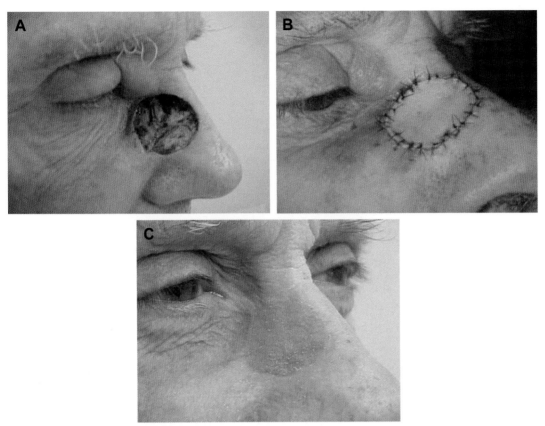

Fig. 9. (*A*) Defect of nasal sidewall and adjacent cheek. (*B*) Full-thickness graft to defect without local flap. (*C*) Long-term result, with satisfactory color and contour match. Improved camouflage may have been achieved by combining cheek flap with skin grafting (see **Fig. 15** for comparison).

them more conducive to imbibition of nutrients from the wound bed. Unfortunately, split-thickness grafts usually demonstrate poor color and texture match with surrounding skin. They are also more prone to contraction and depressed scars. The most common indication for split-thickness skin grafting is for extensive scalp defects, or as a temporary cover when monitoring a wound bed for potential cancer recurrence. When a melanoma resection is performed with pending margins, split-thickness grafting may be beneficial. In addition, split-thickness skin grafting is ideal for surveillance of aggressive malignancies for which definitive reconstruction is delayed. Split-thickness grafts may also be performed in staged fashion after achieving a vascularized bed of granulation using a dermal regeneration template or a latissimus free muscle flap.

The split-thickness skin grafts are usually harvested from the anterolateral thigh. An appropriate width blade is selected, and before using the dermatome, calibration is confirmed by setting the dial at 0.015 inch, which corresponds to most commercially available no. 15 scalpel blades. Split-thickness grafts are harvested with the dermatome set between 0.012 and 0.025 inches. After skin preparation, mineral oil is placed over the donor site. The dermatome is advanced while traction is maintained on the skin. Toothless forceps are used to prevent the graft from getting snared, and the dermatome is lifted away from the leg while still engaged. Split-thickness skin grafts are bolstered similar to full-thickness skin grafts to achieve effective compression. Wound care is also similar to that described for full-thickness grafts. Thicker split-thickness grafts, such as that shown in **Fig. 11**, can decrease the extent of graft contracture and allow for more natural skin texture and color and cosmetically sensitive areas.

COMPOSITE CHONDROCUTANEOUS GRAFTS

Composite grafts contain 2 or more tissue layers, most commonly including skin and cartilage.

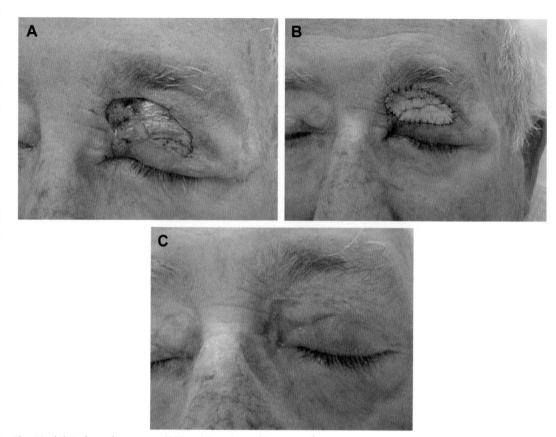

Fig. 10. (*A*) Defect of upper eyelid involving skin and subcutaneous fat, with preservation of orbicularis muscle. (*B*) Carefully thinned skin grafts to eyelid restore natural contour and texture while avoiding contracture. (*C*) Long term, there is favorable function, with no associated dry-eye or exposure keratitis.

These grafts are less reliable than single tissue free grafts due to the added distance required for diffusion of nutrients during the imbibition phase of healing that precedes neovascularization. This increased susceptibility to graft loss is a reflection of metabolic requirements.[8,9] Whereas early reports described graft loss approaching 50% with composite grafting, far higher survival rates can be achieved. Symonds and Crikelair[10] described use of composite auricular grafts for nasal reconstruction with an 89% graft survival rate. Composite grafts may be used to repair full-thickness defects of the nasal periphery, including alar margin, soft tissue facet, and nasal vestibule or columella. A typical nasal composite graft is shown in **Fig. 12**. The ear is a particularly attractive donor site because of its range of contours that can restore subtle nasal topography. If desired, the preauricular skin may be used with a composite graft to resurface larger nasal defects in which only limited cartilage is needed.[11]

Traditionally, the ideal nasal defect for composite grafting has been thought to be 1 cm or less.[12] For defects along the nostril margin, a composite graft may provide superior tissue match compared with other flaps that have bulky subcutaneous tissue. Composite auricular grafts harvested from the helical crus are particularly useful, because they provide thin skin that is tightly adherent to the underlying cartilage. The graft affords structural support and resembles fine nasal skin being reconstructed. Even with partial graft loss, there is often sufficient preservation of structure, such that with delayed healing there is acceptable contour restoration. An example of a composite graft with partial loss and secondary healing is shown in **Fig. 13**. Defects of the nostril margin are prone to notching, and composite grafts are particularly well suited to maintaining structural integrity while preserving a smooth, continuous nostril margin.[11] Weisberg and Becker[13] have reported use of auricular composite grafts with stabilizing struts that include extensions of cartilage placed beneath adjacent nasal skin in a tongue-and-groove fashion. Although convention has

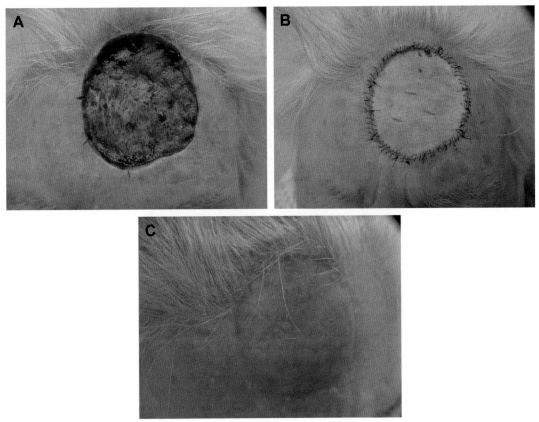

Fig. 11. (*A*) Large defect of forehead and anterior scalp with preservation of subcutaneous tissue and occipito-frontalis musculature. (*B*) Skin grafting to defect with a thick split-thickness skin graft to optimize color and contour. (*C*) Long-term results of skin grafting. Although large rotational flaps are often used in scalp and forehead, deep soft tissue allows for favorable match in this individual with fair complexion.

favored composite grafts of 1 cm or less (in order to decrease risk of graft failure), larger grafts will survive if placed in a vascular bed, and contact with viable tissue is maximized.[14–17] Reflecting a flap of granulation tissue and epithelium that has formed during secondary intention, healing also enhances the surface area of vascularized tissue in contact with the composite graft.[6]

COMPOSITE GRAFTING TECHNIQUE

The preferred patient for composite grafting is an individual without history of tobacco use who has a small to moderate defect involving the nostril margin or columella. Wound preparation is similar to that described for skin grafts, with heightened attention to preserving graft bed vascularity. Perioperative corticosteroids may enhance survival of composite grafts, and this steroid treatment is typically administered as a Medrol dose pack or with a higher dose regimen of 60 mg

prednisone with rapid taper, if no contraindication. Attempts to rescue compromised composite grafts with steroid have not been fruitful, however.[18,19] Cooling of composite grafts with ice application for 7 to 14 days will reduce metabolic requirements and has been found to improve graft survival in higher-risk patients, who have prior radiation, scar tissue, or advanced age.[20] There is improved survival rate if grafting is delayed until the defect has healed at least in part by secondary intention with granulation and is deepithelialized.

When harvesting the composite graft, it is preferable to design the graft larger than the defect, both to allow for contraction of the graft and to improve overlap between the graft and native tissue. Incorporating a flap of vascular soft tissue at the border will also enhance surface contact with the graft. After the donor site is closed, the graft is transferred and secured in place with a single layer of suture through skin and perichondrium, minimizing sutures

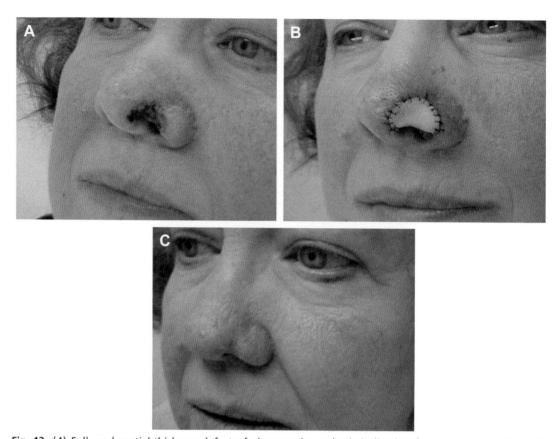

Fig. 12. (*A*) Full- and partial-thickness defect of alar margin, a classic indication for composite grafting. (*B*) Composite chondrocutaneous graft from auricle, with defect freshened and modified to allow for optimal inset maximizing contact with vascularized tissue. (*C*) Long-term favorable restoration of alar contour and patency.

passing through cartilage. Limiting sutures and graft trauma facilitates robust vessel ingrowth. A tongue-and-groove technique for composite grafting, in which the graft is situated between 2 layers of tissue in the recipient bed, improves surface contact area and graft viability. A dental roll or cotton ball bolster may be helpful in decreasing motion of the graft. Ice-saline compresses are applied for 72 hours, and successful grafts exhibit viable color during the first week. Although the primary concern is graft loss, other complications include partial graft resorption, contracture, and contour or pigmentary mismatch.

ADDITIONAL USEFUL COMPOSITE GRAFTS

Dermal underlay grafts may be particularly helpful for restoring contour and suppleness to atrophic skin. The original description of the dermal graft approach is a single-stage procedure at the time of initial reconstruction. In this approach, strips of dermis are placed at time of skin grafting for deeper defects.[21] The authors more commonly will perform such grafts in a delayed manner, several weeks or months postoperatively, if the initial skin graft failed to achieve adequate contour correction or soft tissue atrophy has occurred. Such grafts are often most effective when placed overlying a rigid structure, such as the osseocartilaginous nasal skeleton. Composite grafts containing other components may also be useful in selected applications. For example, skin and subcutaneous fat may be transferred from the earlobe or even the contralateral alar base. Stucker and Shaw[22] reported a 12-year experience using grafts of perichondrium and skin/subcutaneous tissue harvested from the cavum concha without cartilage. A postauricular skin flap may be used to reconstruct the donor site.[23] Tarsoconjunctival grafts are useful in posterior lamellar eyelid reconstruction. Transfer of skin, hair follicles, and fat from the scalp has been used for

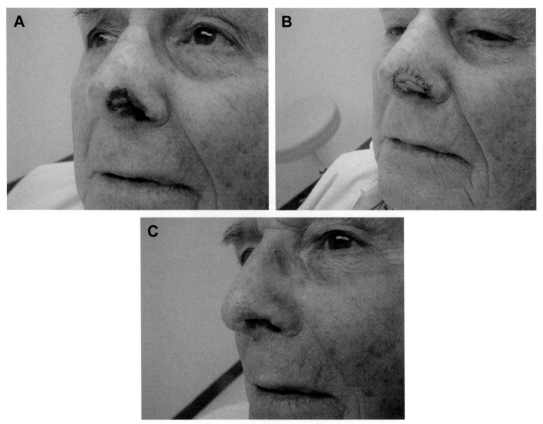

Fig. 13. (*A*) Defect of alar margin centered on soft tissue facet, involving nasal tip and alar lobule. (*B*) Composite graft restores topography of this region and provides structural support. (*C*) Long-term result. Despite partial graft loss, as is not uncommonly seen with composite grafts, there is favorable color match, satisfactory restoration of contour, and only subtle residual irregularity without external valve collapse.

eyebrow reconstruction, although microfollicular hair transfer is preferred.

COMBINING GRAFTS WITH OTHER RECONSTRUCTIONS

There are a variety of situations in which cutaneous defects of the face are best reconstructed using a combination of local flaps and skin grafting.[24] In some cases, the size of the defect precludes closure, and the need for grafting is self-evident. The scalp is prone to large skin cancers, and scalp tissue tends to be tough and relatively indistensable. After rotational flap and galeal-releasing incisions, skin grafts are used to complete wound closure. These skin grafts leave a zone of alopecia, but, as scalp tissue relaxes over time, the skin grafts can be removed with serial excisions for improved aesthetic results. In more nuanced cases, closure of the defect may be technically feasible, but a better outcome is achieved with grafting that restores normal structural and aesthetic attributes. Considerations of flap perfusion, aesthetic boundaries, and surrounding structures all inform surgical decision making.

Large facial defects often require combining cervicofacial advancement with full-thickness skin grafting to avoid distortion of facial structures (**Fig. 14**). When a cutaneous flap is under excessive tension, tissue perfusion pressure may fall below critical closing pressure, predisposing to ischemia. The surgeon should minimize risk of flap ischemia and also anticipate changes to surrounding anatomy that may arise from secondary tissue movement. Foresight in use of skin grafts can avoid undue tension on flaps, minimize ischemia, and decrease risk of tissue loss. Because flap necrosis leads to progressive deformity during secondary intention healing, careful planning is critical. The facial structures most susceptible to distortion include the eyelid, nostril margin, lip, and earlobe. Lower lid ectropion and retraction in the elderly patient are of particular

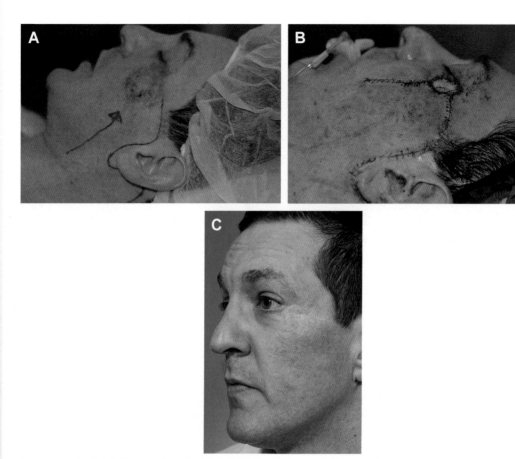

Fig. 14. Cervicofacial flap combined with full-thickness skin graft for a defect of cheek and eyelid after square procedure for lentigo maligna (melanoma in situ) with atypical junctional melanocytic hyperplasia. (*A*) Region to be excised is denoted by square, with planned cervicofacial flap designed along hairline. *Arrow* denotes direction of tissue advancement. (*B*) Reconstruction completed, with full-thickness skin graft placed to avoid ectropion of left inferolateral eyelid. (*C*) Long-term result, with favorable healing and preserved eyelid function.

concern, due to progressive canthal tendon laxity seen with advancing age. Distortion of hair-bearing structures, such as eyebrows and hairline, is also avoided.

Skin grafts have an important role in restoring and preserving aesthetic facial units. Cutaneous defects of the medial cheek commonly extend to the nose, spanning the aesthetic borders of the alar-facial or nasofacial sulcus. When defects cross these aesthetic facial regions, attempting to reconstruct the defect with a single cutaneous flap alone will often obscure or disrupt natural borders that separate these regions. Preserving the concave topography of the nose, cheek, and lips is necessary for satisfactory outcomes. Most commonly, a local flap is used to repair the cheek component of the defect, with a skin graft used to resurface the nasal sidewall defect (**Fig. 15**). The natural line of demarcation created when a skin graft abuts

on a local flap prevents blunting of obliteration of facial units.

A full-thickness skin graft can complement local flaps in other situations as well. For example, a subcutaneous tissue pedicle can be used to add bulk to a defect of the lateral alae that is subsequently grafted.[11] Similarly, reconstruction of the alar-facial sulcus may be achieved with a combination of a subcutaneous flap from the adjacent cheek fat and resurfacing with an overlying full-thickness skin graft.[25] Skin grafts are also extremely useful to cover the secondary defect that arises after transfer of a local flap. One example is use of a full-thickness skin graft to resurface a postauricular defect after skin has been transferred to resurface ear cartilage with too little perichondrium to allow reliable primary skin grafting (**Fig. 16**). Another common donor site for skin grafting is the bipedicled "bucket handle" intranasal vestibular skin flap. Grafts are

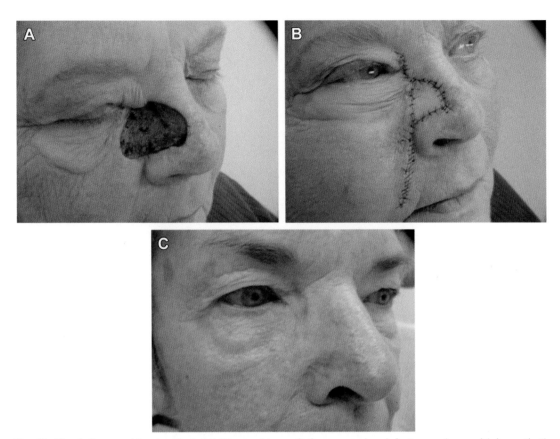

Fig. 15. Cheek flap combined with full-thickness skin graft for a complex defect spanning multiple aesthetic facial units. (*A*) Defect of lateral nose, cheek, and eyelid after micrographic surgery. (*B*) Reconstruction with cheek flap and full-thickness skin graft to preserve demarcation of nasal and cheek subunits. (*C*) Long-term result, with favorable aesthetic and functional outcome. Cosmetic result of combining cheek flap with skin graft is superior to that with skin graft alone, despite larger defect when compared with case shown in **Fig. 9.**

also used in scalp reconstruction after rotational advancement. Skin graft closure of secondary defects expedites wound healing and diminishes wound contraction. In a related approach, the frontalis-pericranial flap provides a vascular bed for exposed scalp that can be skin grafted.[26] Platelet-rich fibrin matrix also has an evolving role in promoting wound healing. Application of this approach to skin graft implants improved survival of free grafts in a porcine model.[27]

A key innovation in the use of composite grafts is in nasal reconstruction with paramedian forehead flap. Composite grafts may be used to reconstruct internal nasal lining and provide cartilaginous support, whereas a forehead flap provides covering for full-thickness defects extending along the alar margin. Another approach in nasal reconstruction involves combining full-thickness skin grafts with lateral crural strut grafts when there is loss of support after cancer excision from partial resection of alar fibrofatty tissue. Last, the composite grafts of

the internal nose may be used to correct or resist alar retraction, often placing a relatively larger cartilage graft relative to skin graft when rebuilding the nasal vestibule. These approaches are analogous to techniques used in rhinoplasty.[28] Skin grafting over free cartilage grafts can also be successful with adequate perfusion from surrounding tissues.[29]

SUMMARY

Skin grafts and composite grafts have extensive application in Mohs reconstruction, both as primary reconstruction and as adjuncts to local flaps procedures. Incorporating a skin or composite graft into a larger reconstruction will often improve functional or aesthetic outcome with minimal donor site morbidity. Skin grafts are particularly valuable in preventing late effects of secondary intention wound healing that may otherwise distort adjacent facial structures. These approaches can

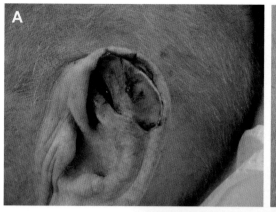
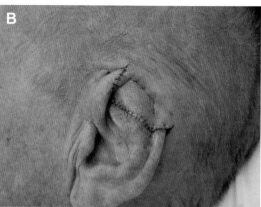
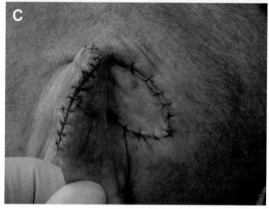

Fig. 16. Defect of left ear involving scapha, superior crus, triangular fossa, and helical rim. Because of removal of perichondrium during micrographic surgery, a flap was used to provide vascular covering for cartilage. (*A*) Defect of superior ear demonstrating exposed cartilage denuded of perichondrium. (*B*) Initial stage of reconstruction, involving a posteriorly based skin flap to ear. (*C*) Second stage, with detachment of skin flap and skin grafting to recipient donor site.

be used to achieve reconstruction in cases of inadequate tissue laxity as well as to improve aesthetic and functional results.

ACKNOWLEDGMENTS

The authors thank Robert Buzzell, MD, a Mohs micrographic surgery colleague for permission for inclusion of selected skin grafting examples in clinical examples.

REFERENCES

1. Brenner MJ, Perro CA. Recontouring, resurfacing, and scar revision in skin cancer reconstruction. Facial Plast Surg Clin North Am 2009;17(3):469–87.e3.
2. Frohm ML, Durham AB, Bichakjian CK, et al. Anatomy of skin. In: Baker SR, editor. Local flaps in facial reconstruction. 3rd edition. Philadelphia: Elsevier; 2014. p. 3–13.
3. Ishii LE, Tollefson TT. Evidence-based procedures in facial plastic and reconstructive surgery. Facial Plast Surg Clin North Am 2015;23(3):ix–xii.
4. Hom DB, Goding GS Jr. Skin flap physiology. In: Baker SR, editor. Local flaps in facial reconstruction. 3rd edition. Philadelphia: Elsevier; 2014. p. 14–29.
5. Brodovsky S, Dagan R, Ben-Bassatt M. Nobecutane spray as a temporary dressing of skin graft donor sites. J Dermatol Surg Oncol 1986;12(4):386–8.
6. Jewett BS. Skin and composite grafts. In: Baker SR, editor. Local flaps in facial reconstruction. 3rd edition. Philadelphia: Elsevier; 2014. p. 339–67.
7. Hill TG. Reconstruction of nasal defects using full-thickness skin grafts: a personal reappraisal. J Dermatol Surg Oncol 1983;9(12):995–1001.
8. Clairmont AA, Conley JJ. The uses and limitations of auricular composite grafts. J Otolaryngol 1978;7(3):249–55.
9. Konior RJ. Free composite grafts. Otolaryngol Clin North Am 1994;27(1):81–90.
10. Symonds FC, Crikelair GF. Auricular composite grafts in nasal reconstruction: a report of 36 cases. Plast Reconstr Surg 1966;37(5):433–7.
11. Jewett BS. Repair of small nasal defects. Facial Plast Surg Clin North Am 2005;13(2):283–99, vi.

12. Ballantyne DL Jr, Converse JM. Vascularization of composite auricular grafts transplanted to the chorio-allantois of the chick embryo. Transplant Bull 1958;5(4):373–7.

13. Weisberg NK, Becker DS. Repair of nasal ala defects with conchal bowl composite grafts. Dermatol Surg 2000;26(11):1047–51.

14. Avelar JM, Psillakis JM, Viterbo F. Use of large composite grafts in the reconstruction of deformities of the nose and ear. Br J Plast Surg 1984;37(1):55–60.

15. Becker OJ. Extended applications of free composite grafts. Trans Am Acad Ophthalmol Otolaryngol 1960;64:649–59.

16. Davenport G, Bernard FD. Improving the take of composite grafts. Plast Reconstr Surg Transplant Bull 1959;24:175–82.

17. Ruch MK. Utilization of composite free grafts. J Int Coll Surg 1958;30(2):274–5.

18. Aden KK, Biel MA. The evaluation of pharmacologic agents on composite graft survival. Arch Otolaryngol Head Neck Surg 1992;118(2):175–8.

19. Hartman DF, Goode RL. Pharmacologic enhancement of composite graft survival. Arch Otolaryngol Head Neck Surg 1987;113(7):720–3.

20. Conley JJ, Vonfraenkel PH. The principle of cooling as applied to the composite graft in the nose. Plast Reconstr Surg 1956;17(6):444–51.

21. Meyers S, Rohrer T, Grande D. Use of dermal grafts in reconstructing deep nasal defects and shaping the ala nasi. Dermatol Surg 2001;27(3):300–5.

22. Stucker FJ Jr, Shaw GY. The perichondrial cutaneous graft. A 12-year clinical experience. Arch Otolaryngol Head Neck Surg 1992;118(3):287–92.

23. Portuese W, Stucker F, Grafton W, et al. Perichondrial cutaneous graft. An alternative in composite skin grafting. Arch Otolaryngol Head Neck Surg 1989;115(6):705–9.

24. Moyer JS, Baker SR. The use of skin grafts with local flap. In: Baker SR, editor. Local flaps in facial reconstruction. Philadelphia: Elsevier; 2014. p. 368–84.

25. Lindsay KJ, Morton JD. Flap or graft: the best of both in nasal ala reconstruction. J Plast Reconstr Aesthet Surg 2015;68(10):1352–7.

26. Osorio M, Moubayed SP, Weiss E, et al. Management of a nonhealing forehead wound with a novel frontalis-pericranial flap and a full-thickness skin graft. Laryngoscope 2016;126(11):2456–8.

27. Reksodiputro M, Widodo D, Bashiruddin J, et al. PRFM enhance wound healing process in skin graft. Facial Plast Surg 2014;30(6):670–5.

28. Katira K, Guyuron B. Contemporary techniques for effective nasal lengthening. Facial Plast Surg Clin North Am 2015;23(1):81–91.

29. Zopf DA, Iams W, Kim JC, et al. Full-thickness skin graft overlying a separately harvested auricular cartilage graft for nasal alar reconstruction. JAMA Facial Plast Surg 2013;15(2):131–4.

Scalp and Forehead Defects in the Post-Mohs Surgery Patient

Michael D. Olson, MD*, Grant S. Hamilton III, MD

KEYWORDS

• Scalp • Forehead • Reconstruction • Mohs micrographic surgery • Skin cancer • Graft • Flap

KEY POINTS

- The loss of hair-bearing skin poses unique challenges in reconstruction.
- The scalp is less elastic than other areas of the head and neck, making reconstruction challenging.
- Forehead and scalp reconstruction after Mohs micrographic surgery is commonly encountered by head and neck reconstructive surgeons.
- Defects can be less than a centimeter or encompass most of the scalp, requiring a multitude of reconstructive techniques.
- Goals of forehead and scalp reconstruction are to maintain form and function while keeping patient facial aesthetics intact.
- For small to moderate lesions, local flaps are the mainstays of therapy, and for larger defects, microvascular free tissue transfer is becoming the backbone of therapy, especially for complex wounds.

INTRODUCTION

The scalp and forehead present specific and unique challenges to the head and neck surgeon when dealing with patients who have undergone Mohs micrographic surgery. For example, the scalp is thick, immobile, and hair bearing. In addition, the underlying skull challenges the surgeon to preserve and arrange tissue in an effort to prevent exposure of calvarial bone, a difficult problem in the best of circumstances. The forehead also presents significant challenges to the surgeon. Specifically, defects in this area may affect not only the patient's aesthetic result but also their function, with deficits in the patient's motor function leading to significant asymmetries. Several principles of reconstruction are used in this region, which include re-creation and preservation of the symmetry of the eyebrows, temporal and frontal.

hairlines, in addition to scar camouflage using the relaxed skin tension lines (RSTLs). Deformities in these 2 regions can range from almost complete scalp excision, requiring free-flap microvascular techniques for coverage, to small defects only requiring primary closure.

In order to best deal with these challenges and provide the patient with an optimal outcome, a comprehensive understanding of the anatomy, knowledge of a variety of reconstructive techniques coupled with the skills to execute, and careful wound analysis and planning are all surgical imperatives. In this review of forehead and scalp reconstruction, the authors aim to provide the reader with a thorough review and discussion of reconstruction options in an effort to outline strategies in dealing with defects in these complex areas.

Disclosure Statement: The authors have nothing relevant to disclose.
Otolaryngology, Mayo Clinic, 200 1st Street Southwest, Rochester, MN 55905, USA
* Corresponding author.
E-mail address: olson.michael@mayo.edu

Facial Plast Surg Clin N Am 25 (2017) 365–375
http://dx.doi.org/10.1016/j.fsc.2017.03.008
1064-7406/17/© 2017 Elsevier Inc. All rights reserved.

ANATOMY

The scalp and forehead comprise a large surface area in the head and neck, and therefore, abnormality in this area will be frequently encountered by the head and neck surgeon. Understanding the anatomy is the first step in deciding the best method of reconstruction.

From an anatomic perspective, the limits of the scalp and forehead are as follows: anteriorly the limit is the supraorbital rim, while the nuchal line establishes the posterior limit. The frontal process of the zygoma from the zygomatic arch to the prominence of the mastoid tip defines the lateral confines.

The scalp comprises 5 basic layers (**Fig. 1**): the skin (S), comprising the epidermis and dermis; the subcutaneous tissue (C), containing the subdermal vascular plexus; the galea aponeurosis (A); loose connective tissue (L); and finally, the periosteum (P). The acronym "SCALP" has been described in the literature and can be quite helpful and convenient in an effort to recall these layers on command.[1,2] The skin on the scalp, although not the thickest in the body, is the thickest skin in the head and neck region. Scalp thickness is the most robust in areas of thick hair growth; in patients with alopecia (from any cause), thickness decreases significantly. The outermost layers include the epidermis, dermis, and subcutaneous layer. Within these layers are the hair follicles, fat, and sweat glands. The galea (epicranial aponeurosis) is a tough, inelastic layer that connects the frontalis muscle anteriorly with the occipitalis muscle posteriorly (**Fig. 2**). Laterally, the galea is contiguous with, and ultimately becomes, the temporoparietal fascia. The galea has tight and loose components, and these are important to understand when designing flaps in the scalp. The tight areas comprise dense galeal tissue with no overlying muscle, such as the vertex of the scalp.

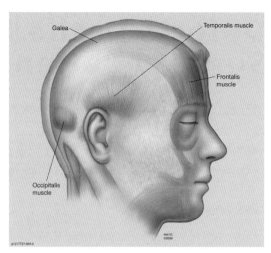

Fig. 2. Galea (epicranial aponeurosis) anatomy. (Used with permission of Mayo Foundation for Medical Education and Research. All rights reserved.)

These areas lack the ability to stretch, causing challenges in primary closure of large wounds. In contrast, the loose components of the galea include areas where the thickness of the tissue decreases, specifically in areas overlying muscle, such as the temporal regions and the occipital regions. Medium-sized defects in these areas are often easily managed with primary closure or small advancement flaps.

The scalp and forehead have an extensive blood supply (**Fig. 3**), giving the surgeon latitude in the design and ultimate survival of many different types of flaps in the scalp and forehead. The blood supply for these regions comes from both the internal and the external carotid artery systems. The internal carotid system gives branches that end in the

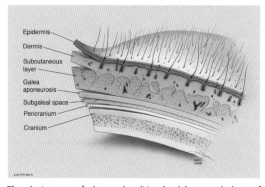

Fig. 1. Layers of the scalp. (Used with permission of Mayo Foundation for Medical Education and Research. All rights reserved.)

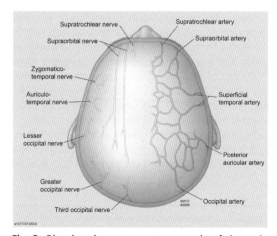

Fig. 3. Blood and nervous system supply of the scalp and forehead. (Used with permission of Mayo Foundation for Medical Education and Research. All rights reserved.)

supraorbital and supratrochlear arteries, the main blood supply to the forehead. The external carotid artery system provides most of the blood supply to the scalp via branches of the posterior auricular, occipital, and superficial temporal arteries.

The sensory and motor supply to the forehead and scalp are provided by a multitude of nerve branches. Anteriorly, the sensory component is primarily supplied by the first branch of the trigeminal nerve. Two main branches of this nerve include the supratrochlear and supraorbital nerves. The supratrochlear nerve exits the orbit and travels superiorly beneath the corrugator supercilii muscle to innervate the conjunctiva, upper eyelid, and medial forehead. The supraorbital nerve exits through the supraorbital foremen (or notch) as it travels superiorly in a more lateral course, continuing over the frontalis muscle to supply the central forehead. A deep branch of this nerve courses deep to the frontalis between the periosteum and galea, innervating the remainder of the anterior scalp and vertex. Posteriorly, the greater occipital nerve forms from branches of the first and second cervical nerves, where it then exits the posterior spine through the suboccipital triangle approximately 3 cm below the occipital protuberance and 1.5 cm lateral to the midline. The greater occipital nerve, lesser occipital nerve, and third occipital nerve are the primary sensory nerves to the posterior scalp. Finally, the lateral scalp and forehead sensory nerves include zygomaticotemporal nerve and the auriculotemporal nerve.

The motor innervation to the frontalis muscle in the forehead is supplied by the temporal branch of the facial nerve. It is critical to understand the complex anatomic relationships of this nerve as it courses through multiple tissue layers. Prevention of inadvertent harm to this nerve is paramount, because damage can lead to brow ptosis. The temporal branch is most at risk when elevating a flap near or over the zygomatic arch. This branch is small in size and is relatively close to the skin in this area, making iatrogenic damage possible. Once the nerve enters the forehead region, it travels under the frontalis muscle and innervates the muscle from below, making unintended transection much less likely in this area. Pitanguy line is a helpful way to accurately predict the location of the temporal branch.[3] Pitanguy line is drawn from 2 points: one point is made 0.5 cm inferior to the tragus and the other point is made 1.5 cm lateral to the supraorbital rim. The nerve crosses the zygomatic arch and travels along the deep surface of the temporoparietal fascia. It lies in a more superficial position in the temporal region. It then penetrates the temporoparietal fascia to innervate the frontalis muscle along its deep surface (**Fig. 4**).

Lymphatic drainage in the forehead and scalp occurs through lymphatic channels directly feeding the basins of the parotid, anterior and posterior auricular chains, and occipital regions. There are no lymph nodes present in the scalp or forehead, so attention to these downstream basins are important in the treatment of malignant tumors most common in this area.

RECONSTRUCTION GOALS

Before discussing the techniques of reconstruction, the goals of resection and reconstruction must be considered first. For the resection of forehead and scalp lesions, the first priority is the complete removal of the tumor. Complete removal of the lesion while sparing normal tissue is the underlying tenet of the Mohs micrographic technique. When considering reconstructive options, form and function are inextricably interrelated. For example, damage to the motor nerves of the forehead will result in brow ptosis leading to visual field defects and unwanted asymmetries.

The reconstructive ladder is a helpful principle when approaching the reconstruction of a scalp wound. This reconstructive paradigm organizes wound closure solutions in order from simplest to most complex. Categories of reconstructive techniques are outlined in the following section. Do the simplest thing that will make the patient happy.

SECONDARY INTENTION HEALING

There are indications where healing by secondary intention is advisable after Mohs micrographic tumor removal.[4] Patients who would otherwise not tolerate an extended general anesthetic or who would not tolerate a prolonged surgical procedure under local anesthesia would perhaps benefit from such an approach. Locations that are potentially amenable to healing by secondary intention include the vertex of the scalp in the bald patient and small lesions of the temple region. Ultimately, any region on the forehead or scalp can be closed using secondary intention, but there are some limitations to this method that need to be considered. First, the surgeon must consider the bed of tissue that is present after tumor removal. Exposed calvarium at the wound site will not readily form granulation tissue unless the outer table of the calvarial bone is removed to expose the diploic space, the vascular space between the 2 cortical sections of the skull.[5] Once exposed, the diploic space often allows for islands of granulation tissue to form. Of note, tissue that has been treated with radiation

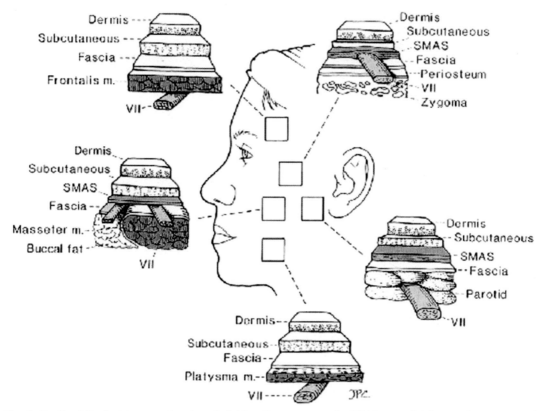

Fig. 4. Depth of the facial nerve at various facial locations. m., muscle; SMAS, superficial muscular aponeurotic system. (*From* May M, Schaitkin BM. Facial paralysis: rehabilitation techniques. New York: Thieme Publishers; 2003; with permission.)

therapy will often not readily form granulation tissue. This can lead to an extended period of healing and an increased risk of wound infection, including osteomyelitis, as a result of the prolonged healing process. Second, wounds on the scalp that heal by secondary intention will be devoid of hair, often an undesirable aesthetic complication. In addition, the expected wound contraction may distort nearby structures such as the eyebrows. Finally, the process of healing by secondary intention is often a long and laborious process by which the patient must be able to participate in wound care and maintenance on a daily basis. This can be a limiting factor in patients without significant social support and whose lesions are not readily visible, such as those located on the posterior scalp. Some patients, however, are too sick or want to avoid surgery, thus healing by secondary intention may be the best choice.

SKIN GRAFTING

Skin grafts were developed in India as far back as 2000 years ago.[6] Today, both full-thickness and split-thickness grafts are a commonly used method

of closure for a variety of wounds in the head and neck (**Fig. 5**). Full-thickness grafts, although not as commonly used as split-thickness skin grafts (STSG), are effectively used in scalp and forehead reconstruction. Grafts taken from the supraclavicular fossa and periauricular areas are common donor sites and are often used in head and neck reconstruction.[7] Full-thickness skin graft donor sites are typically closed primarily. This makes for uncomplicated postoperative wound care. It may be difficult, however, to obtain grafts large enough to cover the large and complex wounds encountered on the scalp after oncologic resection.

STSGs, which are typically 10 to 20 thousandths of an inch in thickness, are an appealing option in closure of scalp and forehead wounds in patients who would otherwise not be able to tolerate longer surgeries. Skin defects of 35 cm^2 or larger are technically straightforward and are not prone to marked wound contracture or significant postoperative pain.[7] Before considering placement of the graft, the surgeon must take into account the wound bed in which the graft is being placed. Exposed calvarial bone does not readily accept skin grafts due to the lack of vital tissue suitable

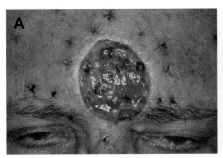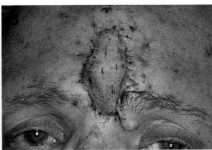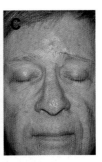

Fig. 5. (*A, B*) STSG placement on a large central forehead wound. (*C*) Results 9 months postoperatively.

for imbibition that can maintain the viability of the graft. Drilling away the outer cortex of the bone and exposing the diploic space can foster the formation of a suitable bed of granulation tissue. Rotation of a vascularized pericranial flap on top of the exposed bone can also support the STSG.[8]

For both full-thickness skin grafts and STSGs, there are specific factors that should be considered in an effort to increase graft survival. The first factor to assess is the status of the wound bed. Skin grafts need a well-vascularized bed to insure metabolic respiration. Devascularized tissue, such as exposed bone or cartilage without perichondrium, will not support these types of grafts. Systemic disease such as peripheral vascular disease related to arterial insufficiency or a history of radiation therapy localized to the scalp can also be limiting factors in the use of skin grafts. On the other hand, healthy tissues, such as dermis, fascia, fat, and muscle, all support skin grafts readily.

Infection is another contraindication to skin grafting in the Mohs patient. For patients with delayed reconstruction, wound infections are typically cleared with antibiotics before the skin graft is placed. This is especially true in the case of *Streptococcus pyogenes*. It is hypothesized that *S pyogenes* is a particular challenge for skin grafts secondary to the production of fibrinolysin, which releases the fibrin attachment of the graft to the underlying wound.[9] Hematoma can also be a factor for skin graft loss. Meticulous hemostasis must be performed during the operation to ensure excess blood does not separate the skin graft from the vascularized tissue below. However, aggressive use of the cautery will destroy the tissue needed to metabolically support the graft. In some cases, it may be advantageous to make an incision in the skin graft (pie crusting) as a way for accumulated blood to exit from beneath the graft. Finally, once the graft is secured to the underlying tissue, good contact between the graft and the wound must be accomplished in an effort to avoid any shear forces, which will prevent the inosculation needed to ensure survival. This is

typically done via a bolster dressing, and in some cases, wound vacuum therapy can be deployed.

In summary, for patients with forehead and scalp defects after Mohs surgery, the skin graft is a reliable option. They are an excellent option for patients with comorbidities that prevent extended or complex reconstruction and are a technically simple operation to use. Their disadvantages include the possibility of a poor aesthetic outcome, particularly on the scalp, due to a lack of skin follicles, and the need for a healthy vascularized bed to ensure graft survival.

PRIMARY WOUND CLOSURE

When considering primary closure of defects of the scalp and forehead, the size of the defect is typically the limiting factor in determining whether the wound edges can be successfully brought together. In the scalp, 3-cm-diameter defects can typically be repaired with primary closure.[10] This size, however, requires a significant amount of scalp undermining to be successful. The temporal and occipital areas of the scalp, given their relatively loose tension, will make primary closure of defects in this area more successful than in comparison to lesions in the vertex of the scalp, where tension is higher. Dissecting bluntly under the galea, often with just finger dissection, will relax the underlying subgaleal connections, allowing for primary closure without significant skin tension at the wound site. In addition to undermining the skin around the wound, galeal relaxing incisions are often used to further reduce skin tension. It is important that these incisions are limited to just the galea and are not carried too far into the subcutaneous tissue, where the blood supply of the skin is located. They should be oriented parallel to the final wound closure.

On the forehead, primary wound closure of circular defects requires the excision of healthy skin on either side of the defect to avoid standing cutaneous deformities. As a general guideline, the proportions of a fusiform excision without the propensity for a standing cone deformity are 3:1. Horizontal incisions are recommended for closure of forehead defects to use the RSTLs of the forehead for optimal scar camouflage. However, a carefully closed vertical incision will heal well with proper wound eversion. When closing wounds on the forehead that are near the eyebrows, make certain that the tension on the closure does not distort the eyebrow. A well-camouflaged scar will be of little benefit in the setting of significant eyebrow asymmetry.

DERMAL ALTERNATIVES AND TISSUE EXPANSION

Dermal alternatives, such as Alloderm (LifeCell Corporation, Branchburg, NJ, USA), an allogenic acellular matrix, and Integra (Integra LifeSciences Corporation, Plainsboro, NJ, USA), a matrix of bovine collagen and chondroitin-6-sulfate, have been used as a bridge to delayed skin grafting. This gives the underlying tissue adequate time to set up a healthy bed of granulation tissue that can be covered at a later date. For patients with large scalp-wound defects, these techniques represent an alternative the microvascular free-flap reconstruction. Richardson and colleagues[11] described a series of 10 patients who were treated with Integra and subsequently treated with an STSG 2 weeks later. These patients had large defects that would otherwise have required free-flap reconstruction. Disadvantages of dermal substitutes include the additional procedures required and the extended wound care associated with a 2-stage procedure. However, in the setting of a large full-thickness defect in patients who may not tolerate an extended surgical procedure, this option is an attractive alternative to microvascular reconstruction.

Tissue expansion is also an alternative option for large defects that would otherwise require a sizable reconstructive effort. Its primary advantage is the ability to mobilize tissue adjacent to the wound, such as the hair-bearing areas of the scalp. The expanders are placed in the subgaleal layer and slowly expanded over time. Disadvantages of internal tissue expansion include the extended period of expansion that large wounds require for coverage. In some cases, up to 8 months of expansion have been reported.[12] In addition, inflation of the implant is typically done 2 to 3 times per week, making the process labor intensive for both the patient and the surgeon. Expanders may also become infected or extrude, and patients should be counseled about these possible complications. Finally, for oncologic resection, internal tissue expanders are infrequently deployed as the priority of the tumor removal outweighs the benefits of the tissue expansion.

External expanding devices to assist in the primary closure of larger scalp defects have been developed in an effort to provide constant mechanical pressure to the wound, bringing the skin edges in close proximity while reducing the tension on the primary skin closure (**Figs. 6** and **7**). Advantages of this system are the ability to close larger defects without the use of multiple incisions, rotation flaps, and the avoidance of free tissue transfer in otherwise unsuitable candidates. The device is typically left in place for 1 to 2 weeks to allow for proper expansion of the surrounding scalp skin while reducing tension on the primary closure. Disadvantages of this type of system include the need for frequent intraoffice advancement of the device (typically every 48–72 hours) and discomfort of the advancement process. In addition, patients with thinned skin from prior radiation therapy are more likely to develop complications due to the underlying weakness of the skin and its inability to tolerate the mechanical stress placed upon it.[13,14]

LOCAL FLAPS

Local flaps are a mainstay for reconstruction in a variety of head and neck wounds. In the scalp and forehead, and particularly the forehead, wounds generated by Mohs excision will often be amenable to a simple transposition, advancement, or rotation flap.

In the forehead, cutaneous and musculocutaneous flaps are excellent options for those wounds that are not easily closed by primary closure. For cutaneous flaps, undermining of the flap is done in the subcutaneous plane, preserving the subdermal plexus located in the fat. This is more challenging than the musculocutaneous flaps because more bleeding is typically encountered, and one must dissect around important

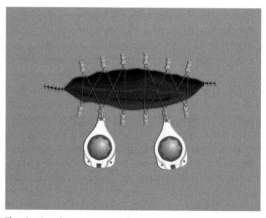

Fig. 6. Continuous external tissue expander (Dermaclose; Wound Care Technologies). (*Courtesy of* Wound Care Technologies, Inc, Chanhassen, MN; with permission.)

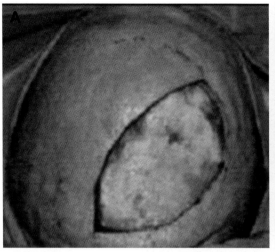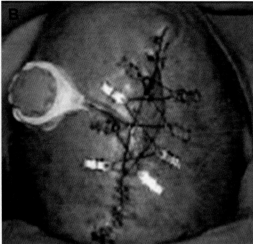

Fig. 7. Before and after application of external tissue expander. (*From* O'Reilly AG, Schmitt WR, Roenigk RK, et al. Closure of scalp and forehead defects using external tissue expander. Arch Facial Plast Surg 2012;14(6):419–22; with permission.)

neurovascular bundles. Once the skin flap is raised and inset, there are typically few functional limitations, and recovery is rapid without sensory or motor deficits. Musculocutaneous flaps are typically used for larger defects of the forehead. They are dissected beneath the frontalis muscle and are lifted in an avascular plane under the fascia. Once the musculocutaneous flap is raised, mobilization of the flap may be more difficult due to the unyielding bone, which often causes excessive tension at closure.

For forehead reconstruction, advancement flaps are one of the most commonly used flaps for patients who have undergone excision of their tumor with Mohs techniques (**Fig. 8**). The benefits of advancement flaps include the use of adjacent tissue, the ability to maintain the contour of the forehead, and well-camouflaged incisions in the RSTLs. Advancement flaps usually provide enough skin for reconstruction. Multiple different flaps designs are possible, including unilateral and bilateral advancement flaps. In addition, O-T and A-T flaps are also commonly used (**Fig. 9**). The disadvantages of this type of flap are related to the moderate amount of undermining, which needs to occur in large defects, as well as the multiple incisions required to execute the outcome. Note the orientation of the line of maximal tension in the flap in **Fig. 8**. This flap was designed to minimize distortion of the brow.

Transposition flaps, although a commonly used flap in other areas of head and neck reconstruction, are not often used in forehead reconstruction. These flaps often need to be oriented in ways that violate the RSTLs, making scars less than ideal in many situations. If used, the rhomboid flap and the 30° flap are often used.

Rotation flaps, such as the O-Z closure, are also commonly used flaps because their benefits include the ability to cover larger areas in comparison to the advancement flap or transposition flap (**Fig. 10**). They are usually designed as larger flaps with the incision lines being slightly diagonal to the horizontal RSTLs, which often produce less than appealing scar positioning. They are often better suited to defects on the scalp where the RSTLs are of minimal concern.

In the scalp, local flaps are a mainstay of treatment and for small- to medium-sized defects. As in the forehead, common flaps include transposition, advancement, and rotational flaps (**Figs. 11** and **12**). Given the hair in the scalp, one must be aware of any flap that rearranges hair follicle orientation. Make sure that patients have an understanding of how this will impact their appearance. Multiple flap designs for the scalp have been described in the literature. Some examples include pinwheel flaps, double opposing advancement flaps, O-to-T, and Y-to-T flaps[15–17] (**Fig. 13**). Given the lack of RSTLs in the scalp, incisions can be arranged in such a way as to maximize the blood supply to the flap. After the incision is made, elevation is performed in the subgaleal plane, and a large area of surrounding tissues is freed to allow for a tension-free closure. Once the flap has been rotated into place and secured, it is often the case that a standing cutaneous deformity is created. Many of these will resolve with patience and time. If needed, a small surgical revision can be performed at a later date.

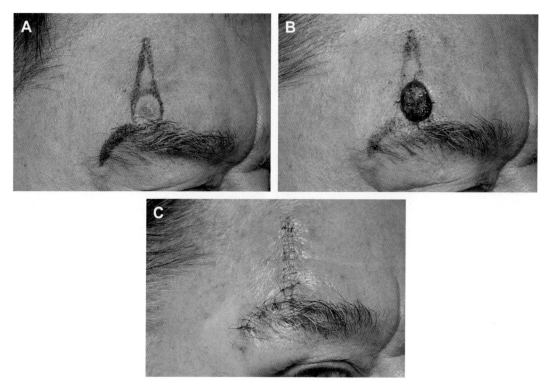

Fig. 8. O-to-L advancement flap reconstruction of a basal cell carcinoma (1.7 cm × 1.0 cm).

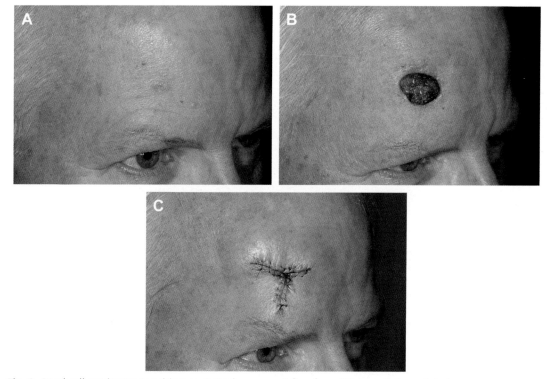

Fig. 9. Basal cell carcinoma requiring an O-T advancement flap for a 2.0 cm × 1.5 cm defect.

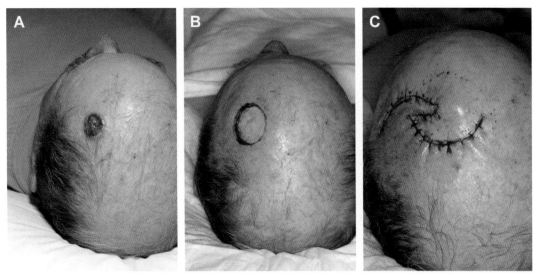

Fig. 10. O-to-Z flap reconstruction for a 2 cm × 2 cm squamous cell carcinoma of the frontal scalp. Note the length of the incisions relative to the size of the original defect. This is a consequence of the inelasticity of the scalp.

Multiple rotation flaps and pinwheel flaps are a useful and frequently used strategy in closure of moderate to large defects, especially on the vertex of the scalp. Using the multiple incisions allows for the recruitment of tissue from areas of the scalp with more tissue laxity, such as the occiput and temporal areas, allowing for a more tension-free closure. If using a pinwheel flap with 4 arms, make certain to show an example of this to the patient before surgery, because the resulting closure and scar may resemble a swastika, which would most likely be objectionable. Pinwheel flaps with 3 limbs should be considered.

Last, pericranial (galeal) and temporoparietal fascial flaps have also been used in scalp and forehead reconstruction. Both flaps are thin and vascularized and can be rotated to cover exposed bone or provide a vascularized bed for skin grafts. For the temporoparietal flap, take care to preserve the superficial temporal vessels when making the skin incision. They may be inadvertently injured due to their close proximity to the skin.

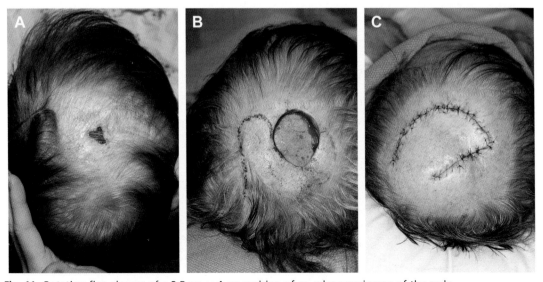

Fig. 11. Rotation flap closure of a 3.5 cm × 4 cm excision of an adenocarcinoma of the scalp.

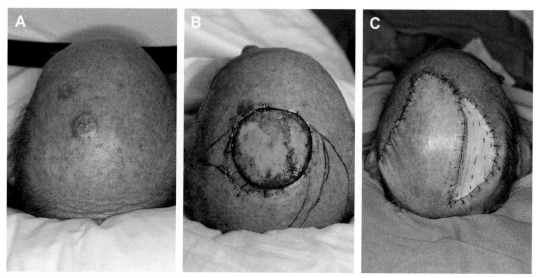

Fig. 12. Leiomyosarcoma of the scalp (7 cm × 7 cm) with rotation flap reconstruction and placement of a large full-thickness skin graft from the abdomen.

MICROSURGICAL RECONSTRUCTION

Microvascular reconstruction of large cranial excisions has become a reliable technique that is now considered by many to be the method of choice in the closure of these large wounds. These flaps are often deployed after failure of more traditional reconstruction and in difficult cases such as chronically infected wounds, wounds that have had prior radiation therapy, and exposed neurocranial structures or reconstructive hardware.[18]

The most common free flaps in this area include the latissimus dorsi, anterolateral thigh (ALT), and radial forearm. In particular, the latissimus dorsi free flap has distinct advantages, which include the ability to conform uniformly to the calvarium, the ability to cover a large portion of the scalp, and the uniformly thin muscle, making it ideal for scalp reconstruction (**Fig. 14**). Disadvantages include the lack of skin, requiring skin grafting or secondary intention epithelialization, and the related alopecia. Alternatively, the ALT and radial forearm flaps are harvested with skin in place, but with the ALT flap in particular, a large amount of subdermal fat often makes appropriate contouring a challenge.

Once considered an excessively long and challenging surgery, especially for elderly patients,

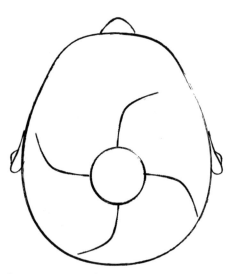
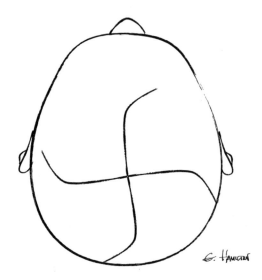

Fig. 13. Four-armed pinwheel flap.

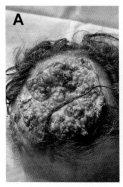 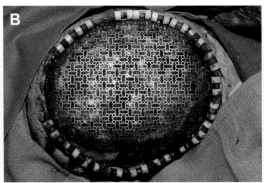 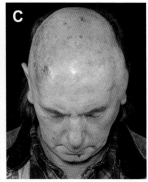

Fig. 14. (*A*) Large (13 cm × 9 cm × 5 cm) squamous cell carcinoma on the vertex of the scalp. (*B*) After surgical excision and titanium mesh cranioplasty. (*C*) One year after latissimus dorsi free flap with STSG reconstruction.

experienced surgeons are now routinely placing these flaps with minimal morbidity and reliable results.[19] For oncologic patients with large scalp wounds and the need for postoperative radiation therapy, free-flap reconstruction should be the method of choice to reduce the chance of post-treatment wound complications.[10]

SUMMARY

Scalp and forehead reconstruction after Mohs micrographic surgery encompasses a broad range of techniques, from primary closure to microvascular free-flap reconstruction. An excellent understanding of the underlying anatomy and range of reconstructive options will prepare the head and neck surgeon for the variety of defects seen in these areas.

REFERENCES

1. Seitz IA, Gottlieb LJ. Reconstruction of scalp and forehead defects. Clin Plast Surg 2009;36:355–77.
2. TerKonda RP, Sykes JM. Concepts in scalp and forehead reconstruction. Otolaryngol Clin North Am 1997;30:519–39.
3. Pitanguy I, Ramos AS. The frontal branch of the facial nerve: the importance of its variations in face lifting. Plast Reconstr Surg 1966;38:352–6.
4. Lam TK, Lowe C, Johnson R, et al. Secondary intention healing and purse-string closures. Dermatol Surg 2015;41(Suppl 10):S178–86.
5. Dingman RO, Argenta LC. The surgical repair of traumatic defects of the scalp. Clin Plast Surg 1982;9:131–44.
6. Ratner D. Skin grafting. From here to there. Dermatol Clin 1998;16:75–90.
7. Quilichini J, Benjoar MD, Hivelin M, et al. Split-thickness skin graft harvested from the scalp for the coverage of extensive temple or forehead defects in elderly patients. Arch Facial Plast Surg 2012;14:137–9.
8. Molnar JA, DeFranzo AJ, Marks MW. Single-stage approach to skin grafting the exposed skull. Plast Reconstr Surg 2000;105:174–7.
9. Perry AW, Sutkin HS, Gottlieb LJ, et al. Skin graft survival–the bacterial answer. Ann Plast Surg 1989;22:479–83.
10. Desai SC, Sand JP, Sharon JD, et al. Scalp reconstruction: an algorithmic approach and systematic review. JAMA Facial Plast Surg 2015;17:56–66.
11. Richardson MA, Lange JP, Jordan JR. Reconstruction of full-thickness scalp defects using a dermal regeneration template. JAMA Facial Plast Surg 2016;18:62–7.
12. Mangubat EA. Scalp repair using tissue expanders. Facial Plast Surg Clin North Am 2013;21:487–96.
13. Laurence VG, Martin JB, Wirth GA. External tissue expanders as adjunct therapy in closing difficult wounds. J Plast Reconstr Aesthet Surg 2012;65:e297–9.
14. O'Reilly AG, Schmitt WR, Roenigk RK, et al. Closure of scalp and forehead defects using external tissue expander. Arch Facial Plast Surg 2012;14:419–22.
15. Moulton-Barrett R, Vanderschelden B. Double-opposing unilobar rotation flaps in the reconstruction of moderate-to-large defects of the scalp. J Craniofac Surg 2015;26:e523–5.
16. Ransom ER, Jacono AA. Double-opposing rotation-advancement flaps for closure of forehead defects. Arch Facial Plast Surg 2012;14:342–5.
17. Simsek T, Eroglu L. Versatility of the pinwheel flap to reconstruct circular defects in the temporal and scalp region. J Plast Surg Hand Surg 2013;47:97–101.
18. Hierner R, van Loon J, Goffin J, et al. Free latissimus dorsi flap transfer for subtotal scalp and cranium defect reconstruction: report of 7 cases. Microsurgery 2007;27:425–8.
19. Simunovic F, Eisenhardt SU, Penna V, et al. Microsurgical reconstruction of oncological scalp defects in the elderly. J Plast Reconstr Aesthet Surg 2016;69:912–9.

Defect of the Eyelids

Guanning Nina Lu, MD[a], Ron W. Pelton, MD, PhD[b],
Clinton D. Humphrey, MD[a], John David Kriet, MD[a],*

KEYWORDS

- Eyelid reconstruction • Post-MOHS reconstruction • Eyelid flaps • Eyelid defects • Eyelid anatomy

KEY POINTS

- The primary goals of eyelid reconstruction are restoration of eyelid function, corneal protection, and recreating the natural appearance and symmetry of the eyelids.
- The anterior and posterior lamella and the tarsoligamentous sling are considered discrete subunits of the eyelid and their distinction can guide reconstructive options.
- Disruptions of the lacrimal system should be repaired to prevent epiphora.
- Whenever possible, vertical surgical tension near the lid margin should be converted to horizontal tension in the eyelids to minimize vertical tension, lid retraction, and cicatricial ectropion.
- A variety of options exist for eyelid reconstruction and familiarity with many different methods will give the reconstructive surgeon the ability to analyze an eyelid defect and choose an optimal method for repair.

INTRODUCTION

The eyelids are an important aesthetic unit of the face. They have multiple functions, most notably serving as the primary protectant of the globe. Surgically restoring the natural form and function of the eye can be complex and challenging. Defects of the upper and lower eyelids frequently result from cancer ablation but also arise from trauma, burns, congenital defects, and autoimmune disease. The eyelids are composite structures with an anterior lamella comprising skin and orbicularis oculi muscle, the middle lamella comprising the orbital septum and lower lid retractors, and a posterior lamella comprising tarsus and conjunctiva. This article discusses the anterior and posterior lamellae as discrete units during repair. Eyelid reconstruction involves replacing one or both lamella, depending on the size and anatomic position of the defect, as well as other structures such as the lacrimal drainage system. Thus, reconstruction can be approached in a variety of ways and familiarity with a diversity of methods will yield the best reconstructive outcome.

CONTENT

Physiology of the Eyelid and Lacrimal System

The primary functions of the eyelids include the protection and maintenance of the orbital contents, light regulation, and facial expression. They also serve as an important aesthetic focal point of the face. Intact eyelid closure establishes an air-tear barrier over the cornea. Eyelids rest on the surface of the globe and wick tears across as they glide over the corneal surface. The bulbar conjunctiva on the surface of the globe is continuous with the palpebral conjunctiva lining the inner surface of eyelids by means of a redundant fornix. Conjunctival relationships must be maintained or restored during reconstruction to preserve blink efficiency for corneal wetting and normal tear flow. Corneal drying and irritation leads to exposure keratopathy that, if prolonged, can result in corneal scarring and infection.

The lacrimal system is closely associated with the medial canthus of the eyelid and allows for proper outflow of tears into the nasal passage. Physical disruption of the lacrimal system can

[a] Otolaryngology-Head and Neck Surgery, University of Kansas Medical Center, 3901 Rainbow Boulevard, MS 3010, Kansas City, KS 66160, USA; [b] Oculofacial Cosmetic and Reconstructive Surgery, 2770 North Union Boulevard, Suite 100, Colorado Springs, CO 80909, USA
* Corresponding author.
E-mail address: dkriet@kumc.edu

Facial Plast Surg Clin N Am 25 (2017) 377–392
http://dx.doi.org/10.1016/j.fsc.2017.03.009

cause epiphora, blurred vision, and severe patient annoyance. Lacrimal punctal eversion (aka punctal ectropion) after lower lid reconstruction can also result in improper tear drainage.

Surgical Anatomy of the Eyelids

The eyelids are essentially bilamellar structures comprising the anterior and posterior lamella and supported by the tarsoligamentous sling a branch of the oculomotor nerve

- The anterior lamella comprises skin and orbicularis oculi muscle.
- The posterior lamella comprises the tarsal plate and conjunctiva.

The upper eyelid layers vary depending on their distance from the palpebral fissure or eyelid crease. The eyelid crease is formed by the cutaneous insertion of the aponeurosis of levator palpebrae superioris muscle (**Fig. 1**):

- Below lid crease: epidermis, orbicularis oculi, levator aponeurosis, tarsus, and conjunctiva.
- Above lid crease: epidermis, orbicularis oculi, orbital septum (inserts onto the levator aponeurosis before attaching to the tarsal plate), orbital fat, levator aponeurosis, Müller muscle, and conjunctiva.

In the lower eyelid, the capsulopalpebral fascia (aka lower lid retractors) is similar and analogous to the levator aponeurosis of the upper lid. This is a fascial extension of the inferior rectus muscle sheath and causes downward movement of the lower lid via the ophthalmic nerve (cranial nerve 3). Additionally, the inferior tarsal muscle is analogous to Müller's muscle and causes downward movement of the lid via sympathetic input.

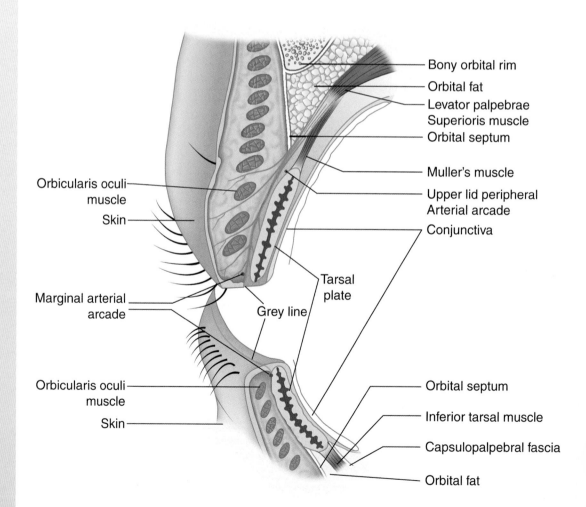

Fig. 1. Cross-sectional view of upper and lower eyelids.

The medial and lateral canthal tendons attach to the tarsal plates and provide anterior-posterior stability to the eyelids as the tarsoligamentous sling. The medial canthus attaches to the anterior and posterior lacrimal crest. The lateral canthus attaches posterior to the lateral orbital rim at Whitnall's tubercle. The levator aponeurosis and capsulopalpebral fascia attach to the superior and inferior tarsal plates, respectively, and provide vertical stability.

The orbicularis oculi muscle, innervated by the facial nerve, is subdivided into the pretarsal, preseptal, and orbital segments based on its location overlying the tarsus, septum, and orbital rim, respectively. The gray line of the eyelid margin represents the pretarsal orbicularis insertion. The pretarsal and preseptal orbicularis muscles surround the lacrimal system and facilitate the movement of tears from the canaliculi to the tear sac. The lacrimal puncta are located at the medial edge of the upper and lower eyelid. They open into the lacrimal canaliculi, which are encased in orbicularis oculi muscle as discussed previously. Lacrimal canaliculi coalesce into the lacrimal sac, which is located posterior to palpable anterior limb of medial canthal tendon (**Fig. 2**). The orbicularis oculi muscle inserts on the lateral wall of the lacrimal sac, which aids in dilation of the sac for tear drainage. The lacrimal sac continues into the nasolacrimal duct, which drains into the inferior nasal meatus.[1]

The ophthalmic branch of the internal carotid is the major vascular contribution to the eyelids, supplying the superior and inferior tarsal arcades in the eyelids, as well as the supraorbital and supratrochlear arteries of the superior orbit. The facial and maxillary artery branches of the external carotid systems contribute to the medial and lateral canthus. The upper lid has a marginal lid arterial arcade, located 2 to 3 mm from the eyelid margin, and a peripheral arcade, located at the border of the levator aponeurosis and Müller's muscle. The lower lid only has a marginal arcade, located 4 mm below the eyelid margin (see **Fig. 1**). Vascular compromise exists if the arterial arcades are disrupted both medially and laterally. The venous supply to the lids is ample and complex. The angular and superficial temporal veins receive the superficial eyelid venous drainage and the muscular tributaries of the ophthalmic vein receive the deep venous drainage.

Reconstructive Principles

A detailed knowledge of the components and anatomy of the eyelid serve as a framework for

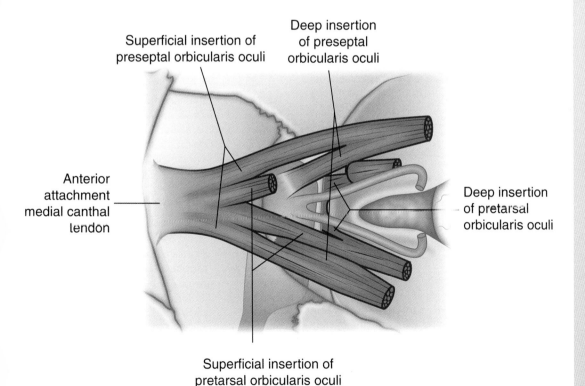

Superficial insertion of preseptal orbicularis oculi

Deep insertion of preseptal orbicularis oculi

Anterior attachment medial canthal tendon

Deep insertion of pretarsal orbicularis oculi

Superficial insertion of pretarsal orbicularis oculi

Fig. 2. Orbicularis oculi relationship to lacrimal system at medial canthus.

reconstruction based on the underlying structures involved. Surgical objectives rely on the principles of restoring the basic function and appearance of the eye (**Box 1**).

In other areas of facial reconstruction, closure is oriented parallel to relaxed skin tension lines (RSTLs) to minimize the appearance of scars. In the periocular areas, use of RSTLs provides satisfactory outcomes at the glabella, medial canthus, lateral canthus, and eyebrows. However, at the eyelid margin, closure parallel to the RSTLs can create vertical surgical tension and cicatricial ectropion. Thus, wound closure along the eyelid margin should be oriented perpendicular to RSTLs to convert vertical tension to horizontal tension. In certain cases, dermatochalasis (redundant skin) may permit horizontally oriented ellipses in the lid crease.

Partial-thickness eyelid defects can first be subdivided into anterior lamellar or posterior lamellar defects. In isolated anterior lamellar defects, horizontally oriented local flaps are preferred over free skin grafts or secondary healing.[2,3] Local flaps provide excellent adjacent skin texture and color match and less tissue contraction. The rich vascular supply of the eyelid provides a unique environment for what might otherwise be considered a tenuous flap. One exception to healing via secondary intention exists in small (<1 cm) medial canthal defects centered between the upper and lower eyelids because of the concave nature of this area.

In full-thickness defects, reconstruction should be considered for each lamella separately with an intact blood supply for at least one. Typically, a local flap will be used to reconstruct one lamella and a graft use to reconstruct the other lamella. Full-thickness defects are categorized based on the percentage of lid involvement.

Box 1
Surgical objectives

- Restore a nonkeratinizing mucosal epithelium to the inside of the eyelid to protect and wet the cornea.

- Provide a rotationally stable eyelid margin to protect the cornea from skin, hairs, and lashes.

- Ensure eyelid apposition to the globe to facilitate formation of corneal tear film.

- Use flexible and firm connective tissue frame to provide support and shape for the eyelid.

- Restore protractor and levator muscle function to close and open the eyelid.

- Achieve symmetry with the contralateral eyelid.

Upper lid reconstruction poses more challenges than lower lid reconstruction because of several factors. The upper lid levator function must be preserved in contrast to reconstructions in the relatively stationary lower lid. Likewise, the narrower lower lid tarsus (4-5 mm) versus the upper lid tarsus (11–12 mm) provides less tarsal tissue for cross-lid transfer. The upper lid is wider and its adjacent forehead and temporal skin are thicker and less mobile than the cheek and zygomatic tissue adjacent to the lower lid. Fortunately, most eyelid cancers, and thus defects, are found on the lower eyelid.

Grafts for Partial-Thickness Reconstruction

A variety of grafts can be used to reconstruct partial-thickness lid defects. Anterior lamellar defects can be reconstructed with a full-thickness skin graft from an ipsilateral or contralateral blepharoplasty incision to provide the best color and contour match (**Fig. 3**). Skin grafts are usually reserved for cases not amenable to local flaps because of defect size or patient comorbidities that preclude a complex reconstruction. Skin graft repairs obviate additional incisions or scars near the defect but tend to have a patch appearance with skin texture and color mismatch. The tendency of elderly patients to have thinner skin results in a better color and texture match when compared with similar grafts in younger patients (**Fig. 4**).

Posterior lamellar defects can be managed with a variety of grafts: upper lid tarsoconjunctiva, buccal mucosa with or without additional cartilage grafting, hard palate mucoperiosteum, nasal septal mucoperichondrium with or without cartilage, and auricular cartilage. Typically, posterior lamellar grafts are used in conjunction with a local skin flap to repair a full-thickness defect because isolated posterior lamellar defects are exceedingly rare.

Local Cutaneous Flaps for Partial-Thickness Reconstruction

A variety of local flaps exist for anterior lamellar defects. Rhomboid transposition flaps are a useful adjacent skin flap for periocular defects and provide particularly good results for medial and lateral canthal defects (**Fig. 5**).[4,5] Final closure for these flaps must follow the principles of horizontal tension distribution at the lid margins and vertical tension at the lateral and medial canthal regions to avoid canthal height distortion. Unipedicle-shaped and bipedicle rectangle-shaped advancement flaps are preferred for eyelid defects of the medial upper and lower lid for small to moderate

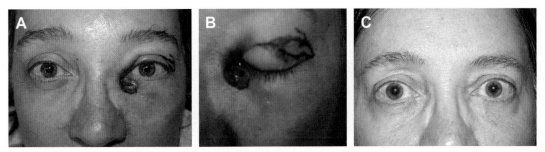

Fig. 3. Medial canthal full-thickness skin graft repair. (*A*) Medial lower eyelid and inner canthus defect. (*B*) Full-thickness skin graft harvested from ipsilateral lateral blepharoplasty site. (*C*) Six months postoperatively with good symmetry, texture, and color-match.

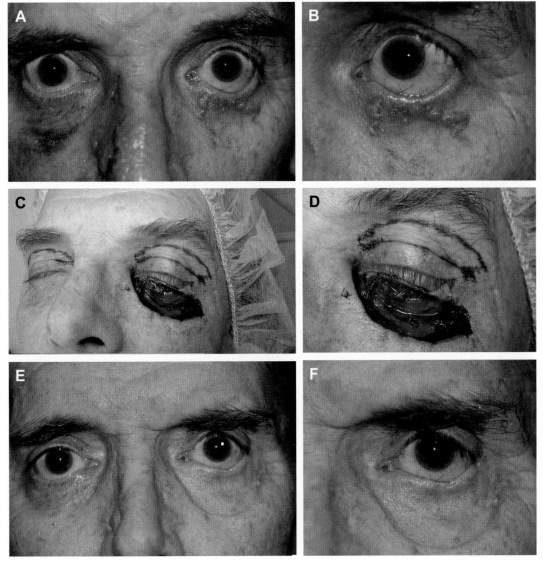

Fig. 4. Lower eyelid full-thickness skin graft repair. (*A, B*) Original lesion along the left lower eyelid. (*C, D*) Bilateral full-thickness skin grafts were harvested from upper blepharoplasty incisions to repair large anterior lamellar defect of the left lower eyelid. (*E, F*) Six month postoperative appearance.

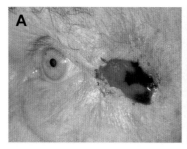
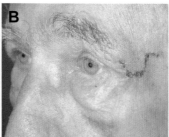
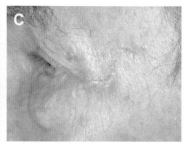

Fig. 5. Left lateral canthus rhomboid flap repair. (*A*) Defect of left lateral canthus. (*B*) Rhomboid flap closure of lateral canthal defect. (*C*) Six month postoperative scar appearance.

sized defects (**Fig. 6**). Other advancement and transposition flaps are used solely or in combination for a variety of unilamellar defects (**Fig. 7**). Lateral tarsal strip procedures to tighten the lateral canthal tendon are used in conjunction to prevent lower eyelid ectropion or malposition.[6]

Full-Thickness Defect Classification

A variety of reconstruction options exist for marginal full-thickness defects and have been traditionally classified based on defect size (**Table 1**). Each type of repair is applicable over a defect size range, reflecting the contribution of patient factors such as eyelid laxity, skin condition, and prior surgery. The same size defect in an older patient with skin and eyelid margin laxity may be closed primarily, whereas in a young patient with tight eyelids or scarring from prior surgery a local flap may be required.

PRIMARY CLOSURE

Full-thickness eyelid defects less than one-third of the eyelid will permit primary closure with reasonable tension. Additional laxity may be gained with concomitant lateral canthotomy and cantholysis (LCC) at the expense of inferior displacement of the reconstructed eyelid. Primary closure has been described in defects up to 50% in size with LCC in addition to baseline tissue laxity (**Fig. 8**).[7] Exact vertical alignment is the most crucial aspect of primary closure. Primary closure recreates the eyelid margin and preserves lashes in a single-stage procedure while restoring anatomically corresponding tissue layers. Complications include notching of the eyelid margin, trichiasis, eyelid retraction, blepharoptosis, pyogenic granuloma, and corneal exposure.

LOCAL FLAP RECONSTRUCTION

Several orbicularis musculocutaneous flaps exist for midsized defects of the upper and lower eyelids (defects 1/3-2/3 of the eyelid). These flaps differ in their incisions and design but all involve dissection in the suborbicularis plane, LCC, lateral incision extension, and need for additional posterior lamella repair.

The Tenzel semicircular advancement flap, initially described in 1978, is the most well-established orbicularis musculocutaneous flap and the basis for many current variations

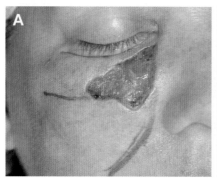
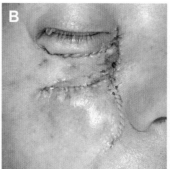
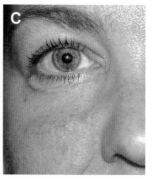

Fig. 6. Horizontal advancement flap repair (*A*) Defect of left medial cheek and lower eyelid junction. (*B*) Unipedicle rectangular shaped advancement flap combined with rotational flap of cheek skin for closure. (*C*) 6 month postoperative scar appearance.

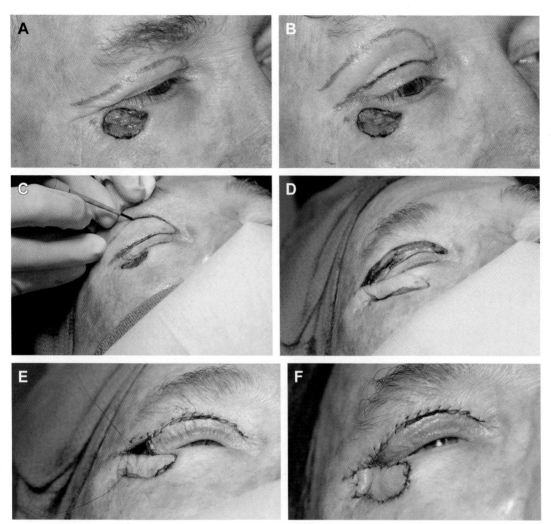

Fig. 7. Rectangular transposition flap repair. (*A–D*) Rectangular transposition flap designed from right upper lid to lower lateral eyelid defect. (*E, F*) Donor site closed along blepharoplasty incision and defect connected with flap base.

Table 1
Full-thickness defect reconstruction classification

Defect Size	Repair
<25%	Direct
25%–50%	Direct with lateral canthotomy and cantholysis
33%–66%	Semicircular flap with periosteal flap
25%–75%	Tarsoconjunctival graft and skin-muscle flap
50%–100%	Cutler-Beard flap (upper lid) Hughes tarsoconjunctival flap with full-thickness skin graft (lower lid)

(**Fig. 9**).[8] It is well-suited to close eyelid defects involving one-third to two-thirds of the upper and lower eyelids if adequate lateral canthal skin laxity is present. The broad-based design allows for robust blood supply to the flap even in patients with prior radiation or burn injury. The musculocutaneous flap is raised widely off of the orbital rim in the suborbicularis plane, continued along the subcutaneous plane beyond the orbital rim to avoid zygomatic nerve injury, and rotated for primary closure of the defect. The cantholysis incision is extended in a gentle semicircular pattern either superiorly or inferiorly depending on the eyelid reconstructed. Lateral canthal height can be reestablished with suture fixation to the superolateral orbital rim periosteum or lateral orbital rim periosteal flap secured to the musculocutaneous flap.

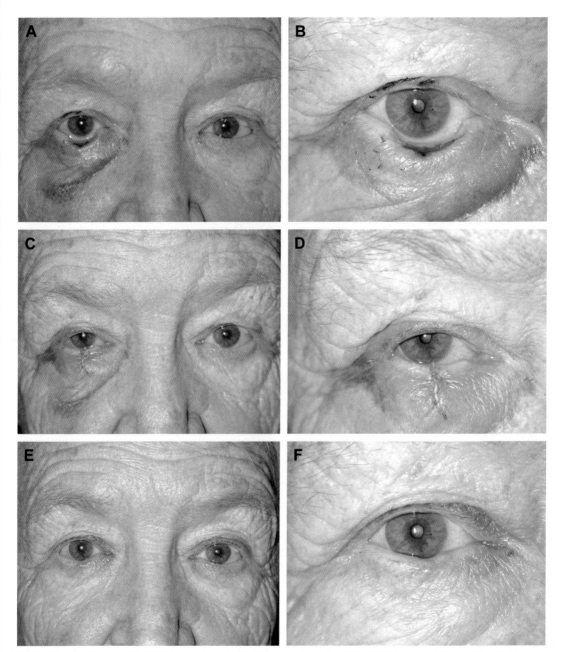

Fig. 8. Primary closure of full-thickness defect. (*A*, *B*) Approximately 50% full-thickness defect of the right lower eyelid with baseline eyelid laxity. (*C*, *D*) Primary closure of full-thickness after wedge excision. (*E*, *F*) 6 month postoperative appearance.

The lateral orbital rim periosteal flap allows for concurrent posterior lamellar repair, whereas suture fixation does not. For larger defects, tarsus bolstering with cartilage, mucosa, and mucoperichondrial grafts may be necessary. Conjunctival advancement from the inferolateral fornix may be necessary unless grafting is concomitantly performed. Complications of the Tenzel flap include eyelid notching, ectropion, lateral canthal webbing, trap-door deformity, and symblepharon formation.

In 2015, Alvaro Toribio[9] described a lateral tarsoconjunctival flap via subciliary approach and lateral periosteal flap (**Fig. 10**). This technique involves subciliary and canthotomy incisions away from the defect site and dissection down to the

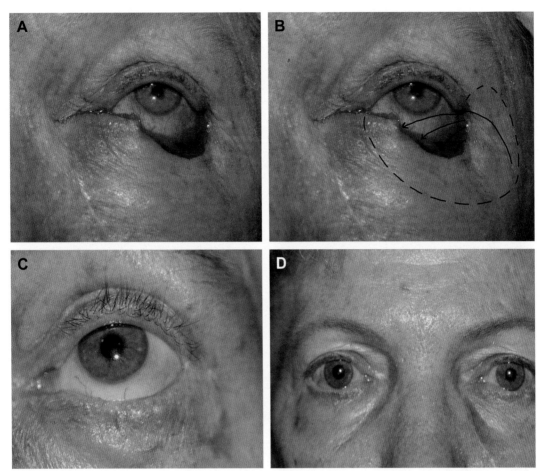

Fig. 9. Tenzel flap repair. (*A*) Defect involving approximately two-thirds of the left lower eyelid. (*B*). Dotted line represents area of undermining in the suborbicularis plane. Solid black line represents extension of incision into lateral canthal skin. Arrows represent advancement of Tenzel flap to close defect. (*C*). Postoperative close-up view. (*D*) Satisfactory symmetry to right eye achieved postoperatively.

preseptal level, preserving the pretarsal orbicularis. The tarsoconjunctival flap with a pedicle base of the orbicularis muscle can then be medially displaced. A lateral orbital rim periosteal flap is created and secured to the tarsoconjunctival flap to repair the newly created lateral defect. This technique effectively mobilizes the posterior lamella medially, prevents anterior lamellar distortion, and avoids vertical incisions. Short-term follow-up (ranging 5–31 months) in 9 subjects did not result in any complications.

CROSS LID FLAPS: LOWER EYELID DEFECTS

The Hughes tarsoconjunctival flap was first described by William Hughes in 1937 for lower eyelid reconstruction of defects involving 66% to 100% of the lower eyelid.[10] The posterior lamellar defect is replaced by autogenous conjunctiva-lined tarsus from the upper lid. The anterior lamellar defect is reconstructed with either a full-thickness skin graft or a local advancement flap (**Fig. 11**). Unfortunately, this 2-staged procedure causes visual obstruction until the flap is divided and inset for 2 to 4 weeks after reconstruction, although division as early as 7 days has been described.[11] The upper eyelid conjunctival incision is made 4 to 5 mm from the eyelid margin to leave a portion of the tarsus for upper eyelid stability. An incision is made through the tarsus only and dissection continued superiorly, posterior to the levator aponeurosis along the anterior surface of the tarsus. At the level of Muller's muscle, dissection transitions subconjunctivally to travel posterior to Muller's muscle and leave it intact; including Muller's muscle will result in upper eyelid retraction. The superior tarsal border of the flap is approximated to the presurgical

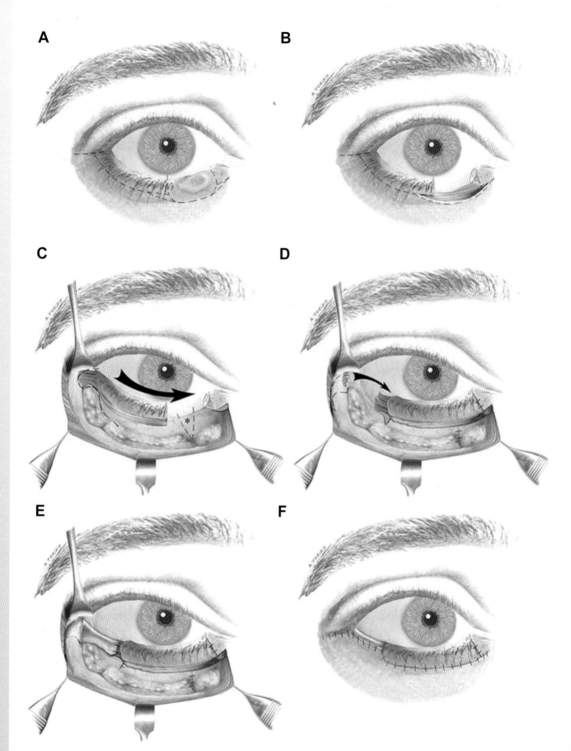

Fig. 10. Double lateral flap for eyelid repair. (*A*) Incision lines (dotted) are drawn. (*B*) Subciliary and canthotomy incisions are made and advancement triangles created beside the lesion. (*C*). Dissection carried along the preseptal level through the subciliary incision, preserving the pretarsal orbicularis. The lateral canthal tendon, lateral attachment of the orbital septum, capsulopalpebral fascia, and conjunctiva are sectioned. The newly created tarsoconjunctival flap is medially displaced (*arrow*). A small wedge of conjunctiva is removed from below the medial defect (*asterisk*). (*D*) To cover the newly created lateral defect, a second flap is created from the periosteum of the outer surface of the zygomatic bone and advanced medially (*arrow*). (*E*) The periosteal flap is stitched to the remainder of the canthal ligament from the tarsoconjunctival flap. (*F*) The commissure is reconstructed and incisions closed. Frost suture may be used but is not necessary. (*From* Alvaro Toribio J. Double lateral flap: a new technique for lower eyelid reconstruction alternative to the Tenzel procedure. Aesthetic Plast Surg 2015;39(6):936;Figure 1; with permission.)

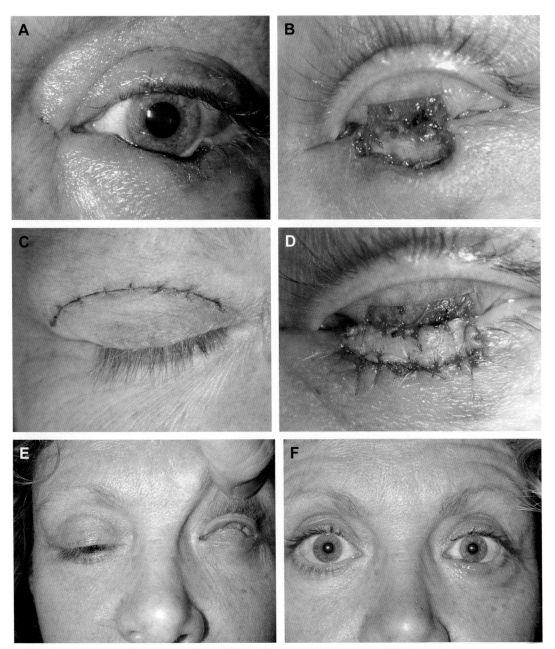

Fig. 11. Hughes tarsoconjunctival flap. (*A*) 50% to 60% full-thickness defect of the left lower eyelid. (*B*) The upper eyelid tarsoconjunctival flap secured to lower eyelid to replace posterior lamella. (*C, D*) A contralateral full-thickness skin graft from the upper blepharoplasty incision is harvested and secured to repair the anterior lamella. (*E*) Healed flap at 3 weeks before division. (*F*) Postoperative appearance.

lower eyelid margin. The flap is released 2 to 4 weeks after initial reconstruction.

In the recent literature, there has been debate of performing traditional Hughes flaps versus tarsal autografts with additional anterior lamellar reconstruction.[12,13] A retrospective case series by Hawes and colleagues[14] in 2011 compared 70 subjects who underwent full-thickness lower eyelid defect repair using free autogenous tarsoconjunctival grafting versus a standard Hughes tarsoconjunctival flap. The free tarsoconjunctival graft group was a younger population than the

Hughes flap group (63 vs 73 years) and the defect sizes were smaller (52% vs 72%) in the tarsoconjunctival group. Overall, free tarsoconjunctival graft subjects were less likely to require revision surgery for eyelid margin erythema. The investigators advocate using tarsoconjunctival graft repair in patients with defects 50% to 75% of the horizontal eyelid margin and continued use of Hughes flaps for those with greater than 75% defects.

CROSS LID FLAPS: UPPER EYELID DEFECTS

First described in 1955, the Cutler-Beard flap is a lid-sharing reconstruction method used for upper eyelid reconstruction (**Fig. 12**).[15,16] Unlike the relatively static position of the lower lid, upper lid reconstruction poses additional challenges in restoring the dynamic blink and range of movement required for corneal integrity. The Cutler-Beard incision starts 5 mm below the eyelid margin to ensure the lower lid tarsal blood supply remains undisturbed. A skin-muscle-conjunctiva flap from lower eyelid is tunneled underneath the undisturbed lower lid tarsus bridge to connect with the upper eyelid defect. Additional contralateral tarsal or cartilage grafting is used to reconstruct the upper lid tarsus. Similar to the Hughes tarsoconjunctival flap, there is visual obstruction of the eye for about 2 to 4 weeks after surgery. A study of 18 subjects undergoing Cutler Beard flaps performed by Kopecky and colleagues[17] in 2015 did not result in any lower lid damage but revealed a 23% upper eyelid entropion rate.

First introduced in 1994, the reverse modified Hughes procedure has been presented as an alternative to the Cutler-Beard procedure for large upper eyelid defects.[18] A tarsoconjunctival flap from the lower eyelid is used to reconstruct the posterior lamella of the upper eyelid and a skin graft or advancement flaps to reconstruct the anterior lamella.[19] Compared with the Cutler-Beard, the lower eyelid tarsus is able to be mobilized in this procedure and advocates cite decreased risk of cicatricial entropion. Additionally, the superior lid orbicularis muscle can be mobilized inferiorly in a bipedicled fashion and secured over the tarsoconjunctival flap to aid in eyelid closure and prevent cicatricial change. Flap division occurs between 2 to 4 weeks postoperatively.[19]

In recent literature, some surgeons have advocated against use of cross-lid flaps for upper eyelid reconstruction. In 2004, Scuderi and colleagues[20] described upper eyelid reconstruction based on a nasal chondromucosal flap for large, full-thickness upper eyelid defects. In their series

of 15 subjects, flaps were viable without total or partial necrosis. Subjects reported satisfactory cosmetic outcomes, adequate levator function, and no incidences of nasal valve distortion. Another group from Turkey described 8 subjects who underwent upper eyelid reconstruction via an orbicularis oculi musculocutaneous island advancement flap.[21] Remaining upper eyelid skin adjacent to the eyelid defect was advanced with a submuscular tissue pedicle attachment to reconstruct the anterior lamella. In their series, no major complications were noted and levator function was within normal limits.

COMPLEX DEFECT CLOSURE

Occasionally, a post-Mohs defect will encompass the eyelid as well as an adjacent area, such as the cheek or the nasal dorsum. These defects involve a large area of tissue that is not amenable to the previously mentioned reconstruction techniques alone and require the use of additional regional flaps.

In the lower eyelid, the Mustarde cheek rotation flap has proven to be a reliable technique for repairing large defects. The cheek flap incision runs laterally from the level of the lower eyelid and lateral canthus to the superior aspect of the auricle and down the preauricular skin crease. The incision may be extended behind the ear as needed, depending on the defect. The cheek flap is undermined in the subcutaneous facelift plane to the lower border of the mandible and rotated medially to cover the defect. The remaining donor defect may be repaired primarily or with a full-thickness skin graft as seen in **Fig. 13** below.

In the upper eyelid, nose, and medial canthus, the paramedian forehead flap allows for transfer of a large portion of donor tissue for large, complex defects. The forehead flap is an axial-patterned, transposition flap based on the supratrochlear artery. In the case in **Fig. 14**, the defect over the nasal dorsum and medial canthus was repaired with a forehead flap and a modified Hughes tarsoconjunctival flap was used to reconstruct the lower lid defect.

CANTHAL RECONSTRUCTION

Proper reattachment of the medial and lateral canthi is critical for eyelid conformity to the globe and corneal protection. Medial canthal fixation is directed toward the posterior lacrimal crest located posterior to the lacrimal sac. Reattachment to the anterior reflection of the medial canthal tendon will cause the lid to be pulled away from the

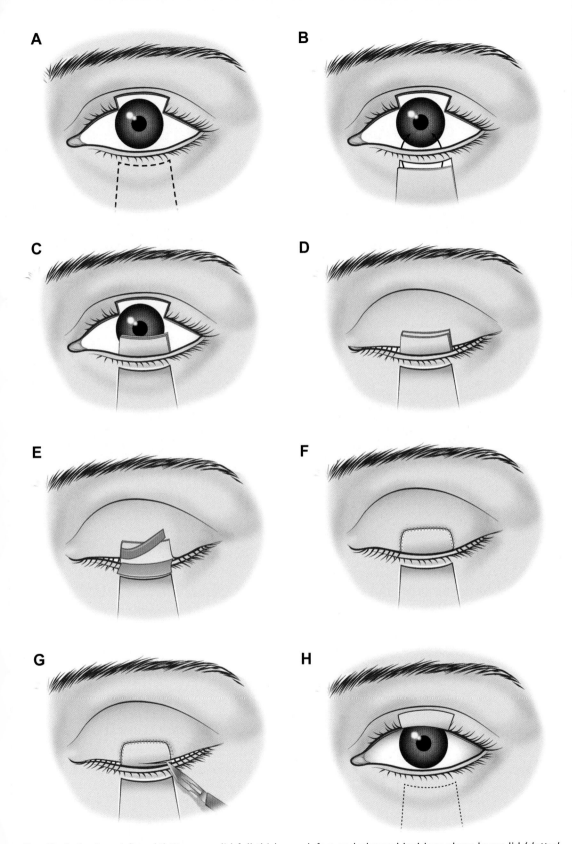

Fig. 12. Cutler beard flap. (*A*) Upper eyelid full thickness defect and planned incisions along lower lid (*dotted line*). (*B, C*) Skin-muscle-conjunctiva flap raised from lower lid and tunneled underneath intact lower eyelid tarsus. (*D*) Conjunctiva separated from lower lid flap and secured along defect to replace posterior lamella. (*E*) Additional grafting (eg, contralateral tarsus, cartilage, perichondrium) may be placed between the reconstructed posterior and anterior lamellae. (*F*) Skin and orbicularis is secured to the upper eyelid and left attached for 2-4 weeks. (*G, H*) Pedicle is divided and remaining flap replaced along the lower lid.

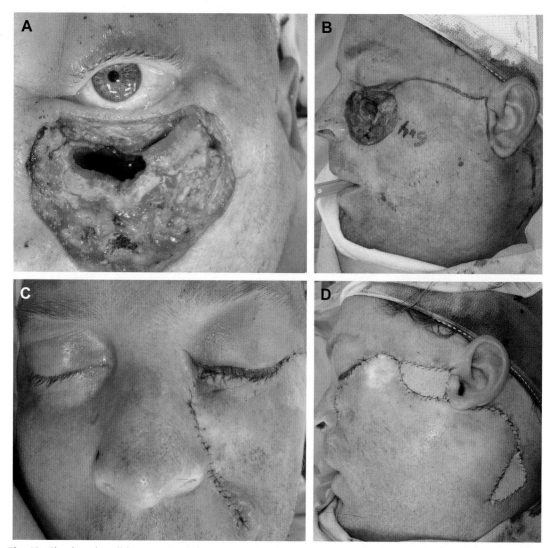

Fig. 13. Cheek and eyelid composite defect repair. (*A*) Large defect of the left lower eyelid and cheek soft tissue, as well as a small, bony defect of the midorbital rim and anterior wall of the maxillary sinus. (*B, C*) Mustarde flap was designed extending from the lateral canthus laterally to the preauricular crease then inferiorly and posterior to the postauricular soft tissue. (*D*) Full-thickness skin grafts were used to repair the preauricular and cervical defects created after rotational flap inset.

globe. Fixation to a periosteal flap, miniplates, or a transnasal wire may be necessary with increasing tissue loss. Lateral canthal fixation is directed toward the posterior aspect of the lateral orbital rim to Whitnall's tubercle. Placement inside of the lateral orbital rim assures the lid remains flush with the globe and prevents lower lid sag and downward retraction at the lateral canthal area. Fixation may occur directly to the periosteum, to a periosteal flap, or to a drill hole placed at the lateral orbital tubercle, depending on the degree of tissue loss.

CANALICULAR AND LACRIMAL RECONSTRUCTION

Medial eyelid and medial canthus defects will frequently disrupt the puncta and canaliculi of the lacrimal drainage system. In cases in which there is partial loss of the canaliculi or puncta, silicone intubation of the remaining intact lacrimal system can be performed at the time of eyelid repair and typically left for 6 months. In cases of complete loss of the canaliculi, a conjunctivodacryocystorhinostomy with Jones tube placement

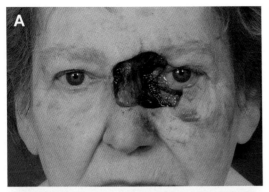

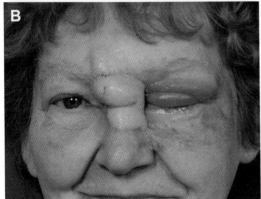

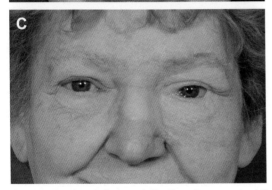

Fig. 14. Forehead flap and Hughes flap repair. (*A*) Large defect extending from the nasal dorsum to involve the entire medial canthus and 50% of the left lower eyelid. (*B*) Forehead flap was used to cover the nasal dorsum and medial canthus and Hughes flap was used to repair the lower eyelid. (*C*) The pedicle was divided at 3 weeks with satisfactory functional and cosmetic outcome at 10 months postoperative.

may be necessary. Jones tube functionality depends on a normal-shaped canthal angle and is best placed after healing occurs.

SUMMARY

Eyelid reconstruction is surgically challenging given the complex natural form and function of the eye. The anterior lamella, posterior lamella,

and tarsoligamentous sling should be considered as discrete subunits of the eyelid and their distinction can guide reconstructive options. Additionally, care should be taken to restore the lacrimal system function associated with the primary defect or arising during reconstruction. A variety of options exist for eyelid reconstruction and familiarity with many different methods will give the reconstructive surgeon a better ability to analyze an eyelid defect and choose an optimal method for repair. Further studies in the nature of flap revascularization and survival will be important in further refining current techniques.

REFERENCES

1. Anderson RL. Medial canthal tendon branches out. Arch Ophthalmol 1977;95(11):2051–2.
2. Lowry JC, Bartley GB, Garrity JA. The role of second-intention healing in periocular reconstruction. Ophthal Plast Reconstr Surg 1997;13(3):174–88.
3. Shankar J, Nair RG, Sullivan SC. Management of peri-ocular skin tumours by laissez-faire technique: analysis of functional and cosmetic results. Eye (Lond) 2002;16(1):50–3.
4. Shotton FT. Optimal closure of medial canthal surgical defects with rhomboid flaps: "rules of thumb" for flap and rhomboid defect orientations. Ophthalmic Surg 1983;14(1):46–52.
5. Shotton F. Rhombic flap for medial canthal reconstruction. Ophthalmic Surg 1973;14:46.
6. Anderson RL, Gordy DD. The tarsal strip procedure. Arch Ophthalmol 1979;97(11):2192–6.
7. Anderson RL, Ceilley RI. A multispecialty approach to the excision and reconstruction of eyelid tumors. Ophthalmology 1978;85(11):1150–63.
8. Tenzel RR, Stewart WB. Eyelid reconstruction by the semicircle flap technique. Ophthalmology 1978; 85(11):1164–9.
9. Alvaro Toribio J. Double lateral flap: a new technique for lower eyelid reconstruction alternative to the Tenzel procedure. Aesthetic Plast Surg 2015; 39(6):935–41.
10. Herde J, Krause A, Rau V. Results of the Hughes operation. Ophthalmologe 2001;98(5):472–6 [in German].
11. Leibovitch I, Selva D. Modified Hughes flap: division at 7 days. Ophthalmology 2004;111(12):2164–7.
12. Toft PB. Reconstruction of large upper eyelid defects with a free tarsal plate graft and a myocutaneous pedicle flap plus a free skin graft. Orbit 2016; 35(1):1–5.
13. Skippen B, Hamilton A, Evans S, et al. One-stage alternatives to the Hughes procedure for reconstruction of large lower eyelid defects: surgical techniques and outcomes. Ophthal Plast Reconstr Surg 2016;32(2):145–9.

14. Hawes MJ, Grove AS Jr, Hink EM. Comparison of free tarsoconjunctival grafts and Hughes tarsoconjunctival grafts for lower eyelid reconstruction. Ophthal Plast Reconstr Surg 2011;27(3):219–23.

15. Cutler NL, Beard C. A method for partial and total upper lid reconstruction. Am J Ophthalmol 1955; 39(1):1–7.

16. Fischer T, Noever G, Langer M, et al. Experience in upper eyelid reconstruction with the Cutler-Beard technique. Ann Plast Surg 2001;47(3):338–42.

17. Kopecky A, Koch KR, Bucher F, et al. Results of Cutler-Beard procedure for reconstruction of extensive full thickness upper eyelid defects following tumor resection. Ophthalmologe 2016;113(4):309–13 [in German].

18. Mauriello JA Jr, Antonacci R. Single tarsoconjunctival flap (lower eyelid) for upper eyelid reconstruction ("reverse" modified Hughes procedure). Ophthalmic Surg 1994;25(6):374–8.

19. Sa HS, Woo KI, Kim YD. Reverse modified Hughes procedure for uppereyelid reconstruction. Ophthal Plast Reconstr Surg 2010;26(3):155–60.

20. Scuderi N, Ribuffo D, Chiummariello S. Total and subtotal upper eyelid reconstruction with the nasal chondromucosal flap: a 10-year experience. Plast Reconstr Surg 2005;115(5):1259–65.

21. Demir Z, Yuce S, Karamursel S, et al. Orbicularis oculi myocutaneous advancement flap for upper eyelid reconstruction. Plast Reconstr Surg 2008; 121(2):443–50.

Repair of Auricular Defects

Deborah Watson, MD[a], Avram Hecht, MD, MPH[b],*

KEYWORDS

- Auricle • Auricular • Reconstruction • Reconstructive • Defect

KEY POINTS

- Repairing defects of the auricle requires an understanding of the complex underlying framework, the structural properties of the cartilages, and typical healing tendencies of the surrounding tissues.
- The auricle is divided into various subunits: central (anterior auricle, posterior auricle) and peripheral (superior, mid, inferior).
- The optimal reconstructive approach for any given auricular defect will depend on its specific location and the quality of the surrounding available tissues.

The human auricle is an important component of facial aesthetics with functional, cultural, and physiologic significance. Not only is it a sound gathering structure but we rely on it practically for modes of cultural expression and support for eyewear. Asymmetry or deformity of the ear is obvious, even by the untrained eye. The auricle is composed of multiple subunits with numerous convexities, concavities, varying skin thickness and a complex underlying cartilaginous framework (**Fig. 1**). Accordingly, reconstructing a functional and aesthetically pleasing auricle is challenging. As a general principle, size, projection, tissue matching, and contour are all important considerations with the understanding that the goal is to create a likeness that incorporates as many of the features of a normal auricle as possible.

When considering any individual reconstruction, not limited to the auricle, it is vital to evaluate all possible options. The paradigm of the reconstructive ladder[1] involves considering reconstructive methods starting with the simplest and progressing to the most complex. For any given site of reconstruction, the chosen method should represent an optimal balance of factors, such as aesthetic result, restoration of function, recovery time, operative time, and donor site morbidity. The simplest method for reconstruction at any site is to close the defect primarily. However, in many instances this can lead to an unfavorable aesthetic outcome and is not always possible given the size or location. Secondary intention is a very useful method; however, it can also have negative cosmetic or functional results. Both primary closure and secondary intention are great options for many small defects; however, the additional time allocation for healing and wound care must be taken into consideration if the wound is to heal by secondary intention. Skin grafts and local flaps are excellent options in certain settings and can be easily undertaken. Composite grafts and free distal flaps have significantly more

Disclosure Statement: The authors have no relevant commercial or financial disclosures.
a Division of Otolaryngology–Head & Neck Surgery, Department of Surgery, University of California, San Diego, 3350 La Jolla Village Drive, 112-C, San Diego, CA 92161, USA; b Division of Otolaryngology–Head & Neck Surgery, Department of Surgery, University of California, San Diego, 200 West Arbor Drive, #8895, San Diego, CA 92103, USA
* Corresponding author.
E-mail address: ahecht@ucsd.edu

A   B

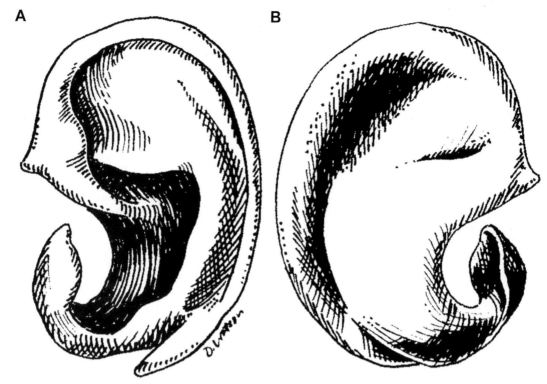

Fig. 1. The underlying cartilaginous framework of the auricle. (*A*) Anterior. (*B*) Posterior.

involvement and require more surgical expertise and comfort with these options; however, sometimes these latter choices are necessary.

With respect to repair of auricular defects, primary closure and secondary intention are the least complex options and work well for many small defects. Although secondary intention may initially be one of the simplest approaches, longer healing times and the ability of the patient to perform the necessary wound care should be considered, particularly if the patient is elderly or has difficulty lifting his or her hands to the affected area. If the cartilaginous framework is intact, free skin grafts may be used to cover larger defects. For anterior defects, full-thickness grafts are generally preferred, though split thickness grafts may suffice in patients with thin skin. Both the lateral neck and preauricular skin are convenient donor sites and typically offer good color match; however, the postauricular skin tends to be a good match as well and favorably hides the donor wound. If the vascular supply in the wound is not sufficient enough to support a free dermal graft, then local random flaps are preferred and tend to do well given the rich blood supply within the dermal plexus of skin surrounding the auricle. Large

defects with missing cartilaginous framework often require the use of local flaps and composite grafts to provide structural support and coverage with vascularized tissue. Although the focus of this article is the repair of postsurgical defects, it is important to know that microvascular surgery has been used successfully in the acute trauma setting for reimplantation.[2–4]

Preoperative planning is essential for the reconstruction of auricular defect. It is important to determine the specific anatomic subunits involved because each subunit has unique characteristics. The structural integrity, skin thickness, contour, and visibility of the subunit involved, and the availability of healthy surrounding tissues will determine which reconstructive option will give an optimal result.

For purposes of analysis, the auricle is divided into central and peripheral zones. The peripheral auricle is divided into 2 main subunits: the helix (which is further subdivided into thirds) and the lobule. The central zone of the auricle is divided into anterior and posterior regions. The anterior central zone is divided into subunits, including the concha, helical root, and antihelix. The posterior central zone does not have further subdivisions. **Table 1** summarizes

Table 1 Analytical zones for auricular reconstruction		
Central		
Anterior	**Posterior**	**Peripheral**
Concha Helical root Antihelix	Entire posterior surface	Helix (upper, mid, lower) Lobule

the analytical zones of the auricle. **Table 2** summarizes some of the highlighted reconstructive options for each of these areas.

TOTAL OR NEAR TOTAL AURICULAR DEFECTS

One of the most challenging types of facial reconstructive surgery is recreating the entire auricle. When a patient is left with a total or near total auricular defect, a prosthesis should be considered. By using a mold created from the contours of the contralateral ear, a prosthesis can be fashioned that provides an excellent cosmetic result. The lack of further local tissue disruption or rearrangement is particularly helpful when

tumor surveillance is needed. Prostheses can be attached to osseointegrated implants in the mastoid region if necessary.[5,6]

When total auricular reconstruction is required, a staged approach is necessary[7,8] with the use of autologous tissue. At the initial stage, rib cartilage should be harvested and the new cartilage framework sculpted (**Fig. 2**). Harvesting cartilage from the contralateral 6th to 8th ribs is optimal; leaving a superior margin of the 6th rib cartilage in place will help to prevent chest deformity. The contralateral ear is used as a template to determine the appropriate amount of cartilage to harvest. The use of 3-dimensional (3D) modeling techniques based from the contralateral ear has been shown to be useful in reconstructive efforts, and this relatively new technology is becoming increasingly accessible.[9] The components of the new cartilaginous framework are sutured together and then implanted in a postauricular subcutaneous pocket. At a subsequent staged procedure, the lobule is transposed (**Fig. 3**). The auricle is elevated from the head at the next staged procedure, and a skin graft is placed postauricularly to define the posterior margin of the auricle (**Fig. 4**). The tragus may be created using a graft from the contralateral ear (**Fig. 5**).

Table 2 Reconstructive summary for auricular defects by size and analytical zone		
Location	**Small Defects**	**Large Defects**
Total		Microtia-type repair Temporoparietal fascia flap with autologous cartilage or synthetic implant Prosthesis
Peripheral		
Helix, upper 1/3	Secondary intention Full-thickness skin graft	Helical advancement Pre- or postauricular transposition flap Staged retroauricular tube flap
Helix, mid 1/3	Secondary intention Full-thickness skin graft	Helical advancement Wedge excision Staged retroauricular advancement flap Composite wedge graft from contralateral ear
Helix, lower 1/3	Secondary intention Full-thickness skin graft	Helical advancement Composite wedge graft from contralateral ear
Lobule	Primary closure	Bilobed flap
Central		
Anterior (concha, helical root, antihelix)	Secondary intention Full-thickness skin graft	Retroauricular pull-through flap (concha, antihelix) Preauricular pedicle flap (helical root) +/− cartilaginous struts
Posterior	Secondary intention Primary closure	Full-thickness skin graft Split thickness skin graft

396

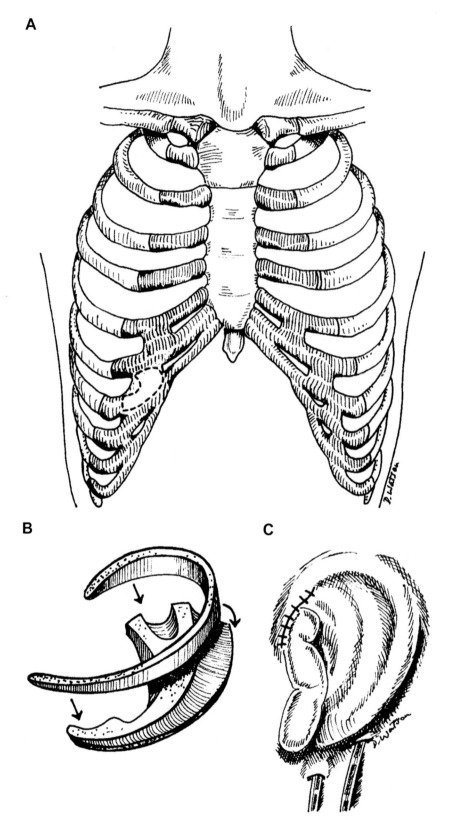

Fig. 2. Harvest of rib cartilage and implantation. (*A*) Cartilage can be taken from the confluence of the 6th to 8th ribs on the contralateral side. (*B*) Harvested cartilage is sculpted and sutured together to create the new auricular framework. (*C*) Placement of the assembled new framework is inserted into a subdermal pocket over the mastoid with suction drains in place.

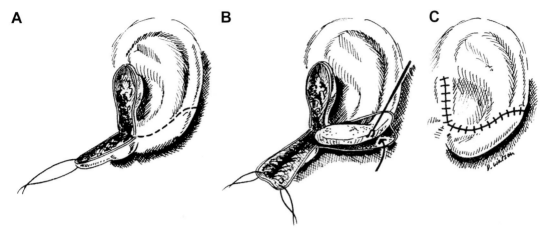

Fig. 3. Lobular transposition. (*A*) The auricular-lobular remnant is elevated to create an inferiorly based flap. (*B*) The inferior portion of the cartilage is exposed before the lobular remnant is rotated inferiorly to cover the cartilage. (*C*) The donor area, which is closed primarily, will become the tragus.

Another option for augmenting repair of near total defects is the use of the temporoparietal fascia flap, based from the superficial temporal vessels (**Fig. 6**).[10,11] This flap can be used to provide a significant amount of vascularized tissue that is robust enough to support both the autologous costal cartilage graft and overlying skin graft, and it may be helpful in the postradiated or other complex field.[12]

PERIPHERAL AURICULAR DEFECTS
Helix

The eye is easily drawn to abnormalities in the peripheral contours of the auricle; therefore, maintenance of natural contours is a primary consideration in reconstruction of helical defects. For analysis and planning, the helix is divided into superior, middle, and inferior subunits. Small cutaneous defects of the upper third of the helix with intact cartilage and perichondrium can frequently be left to heal by secondary intention or can be covered with full-thickness skin grafts. For superiorly-located defects, the helical advancement flap uses the abundance of anterior donor tissue available (**Fig. 7**). For smaller defects with intact cartilage, local skin can be advanced alone. For larger cartilaginous defects of the upper third of the helix, a chondrocutaneous flap can be mobilized.[13,14] Defects of the superior helix can also be repaired with preauricular or postauricular transposition flaps (**Fig. 8**). A staged retroauricular tube flap can be used to reconstruct large full-thickness defects of the superior and middle helix (**Fig. 9**).[15,16]

Two-stage reconstructions are frequently necessary for defects of the middle third of the helix given the limitations of local donor tissues. Double helical advancement flaps can be used in this area with flaps mobilized both superiorly and inferiorly, although this has the potential to distort the shape of the auricle if overcorrected. Small wedge excisions of the middle third of the helix can be closed primarily (**Fig. 10**). However, if the defect is too large or if the repair is poorly planned, then the resultant auricle can become cup-shaped and noticeably asymmetric. Although the size of the auricle is reduced with a wedge excision, the lateral position of the auricle on the head makes this reduction minimally noticeable from a head-on view. To reduce the likelihood of cupping and visible asymmetry, a stellate pattern is used with the wedge excision. Composite grafts from the contralateral ear can be used to reconstruct the mid-helix (**Fig. 11**) with a wedge, allowing for good cosmesis of the donor site. A staged postauricular advancement flap (**Fig. 12**) is used to provide a healthy amount of donor tissue with good color match to cover a large defect of the middle third of the lateral auricle and tends to hide the donor site well.[17]

Small superficial defects of the inferior helix can frequently heal well by secondary intention or with full-thickness skin grafts. However, the inferior helix has a more favorable donor skin supply than the middle helix, given the laxity of the lobe, which can be mobilized for reconstruction. Composite grafts from the contralateral ear and helical advancements are used for larger defects. **Fig. 13** demonstrates a defect of the inferior helix with

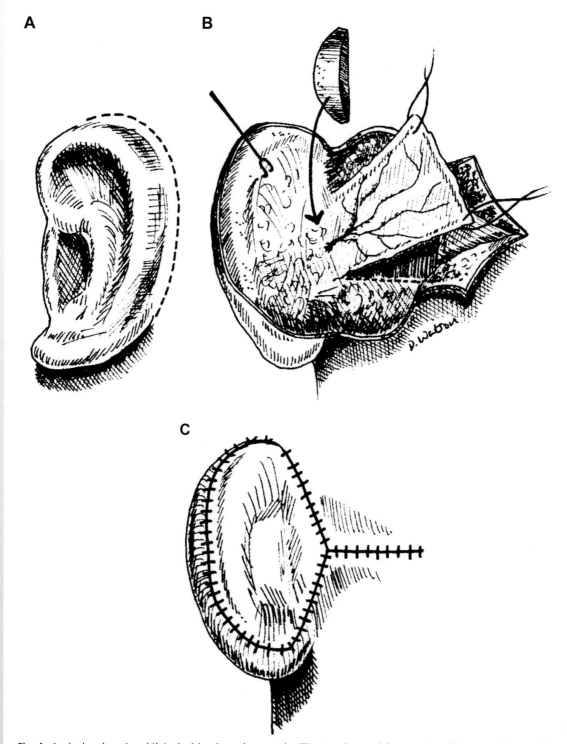

Fig. 4. Auricular elevation. (*A*) An incision is made several millimeters beyond the margins of the underlying auricular framework. (*B*) The auricular framework is elevated. A wedge of harvested cartilage can be used to create the auriculomastoid angle. The cartilage wedge can be covered with a small temporoparietal fascial flap. (*C*) A skin graft can be used to cover the posterior surface of the temporoparietal fascial flap and cartilage wedge.

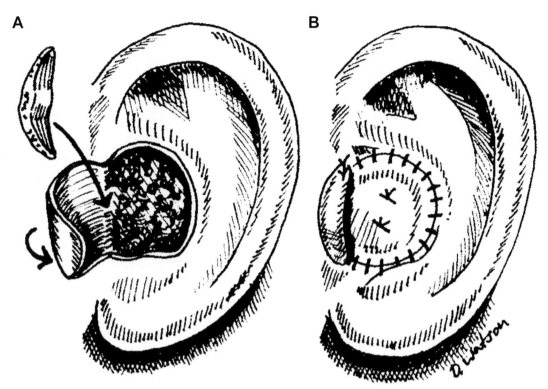

Fig. 5. Creation of the tragus. (*A*) The skin of the neoconcha can be used to create an anteriorly based flap, under which a crescent-shaped cartilage graft is placed and sutured in place to create the neotragus. (*B*) The conchal defect is usually covered with a full-thickness skin graft.

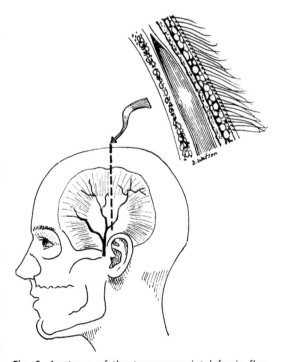

Fig. 6. Anatomy of the temporoparietal fascia flap. The temporoparietal fascia is supplied by the superficial temporal vessels and is found just below the subdermal adipose tissue of the scalp.

reconstruction using helical advancement flap with posterior wedge and anterior dart excisions that facilitate an undistorted closure.

Lobule

The lobule can often be closed primarily due to its inherent laxity (**Fig. 14**) and lack of underlying cartilaginous framework. Accordingly, skin grafts should be avoided on the lobule because they are at risk for significant contraction given no underlying support framework. Total or subtotal defects of the lobule can be repaired with a bilobed flap which can be used to create an excellent likeness of a native lobule (**Fig. 15**).

CENTRAL DEFECTS
Anterior

Small lesions of the antihelix, helical root, and concha can heal well with either secondary intention or full-thickness skin grafts. Assuming the peripheral cartilaginous framework is intact, central defects typically require little more than skin coverage alone and have minimal noticeable loss

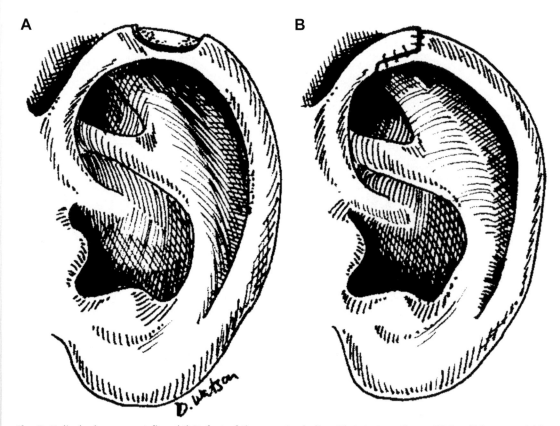

Fig. 7. Helical advancement flap. (*A*) Defect of the superior helix with intact cartilage. (*B*) Parallel tangential incisions are made along the rim of the helix anterior to the defect, and this anteriorly based peninsular-shaped flap is elevated and advanced to cover the defect posteriorly.

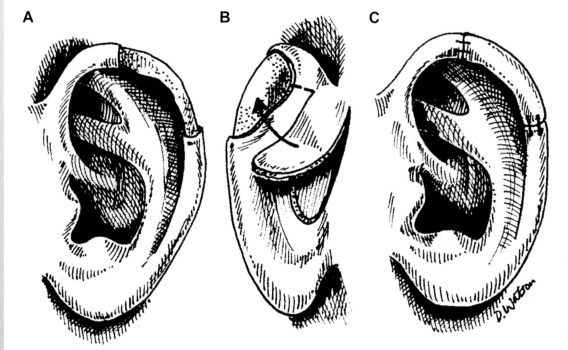

Fig. 8. Postauricular transposition flap. (*A*) The superior third of the helix with a large defect. (*B*) Elevation of a superiorly based flap from the postauricular sulcus. The dotted line represents an area to be incised, allowing for inset of the flap without a pedicle. (*C*) Appearance of final reconstruction.

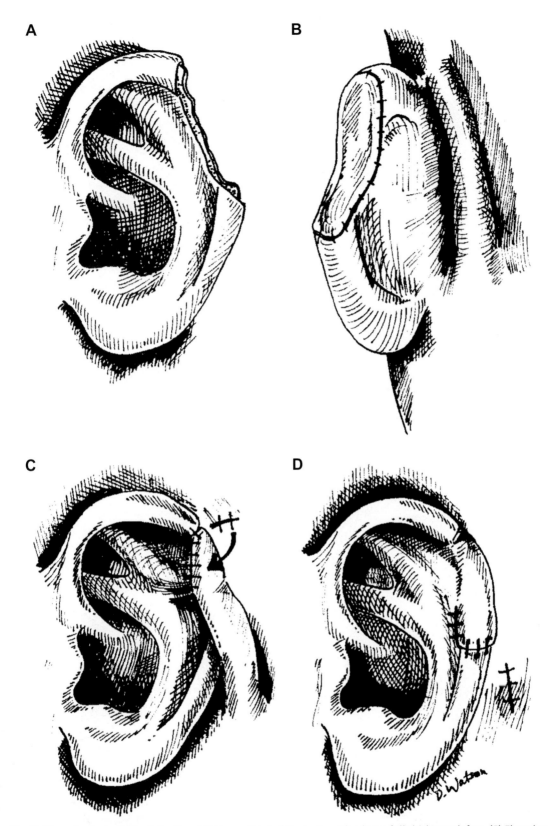

Fig. 9. Staged retroauricular tube flap. (*A*) Upper third of the helix with a large full-thickness defect. (*B*) Elevation of a full-thickness bipedicled flap in the mastoid skin with each end of the pedicle intact. The flap is sutured to create a tube. Primary closure of the underlying donor site. Placement of a skin graft to cover the defect during the delay. (*C*) After a 2-week delay, the superior aspect of the tube is separated and advanced to cover the defect. (*D*) After another 2-week delay, the inferior aspect is separated and inset to restore contour to the helix.

A   B

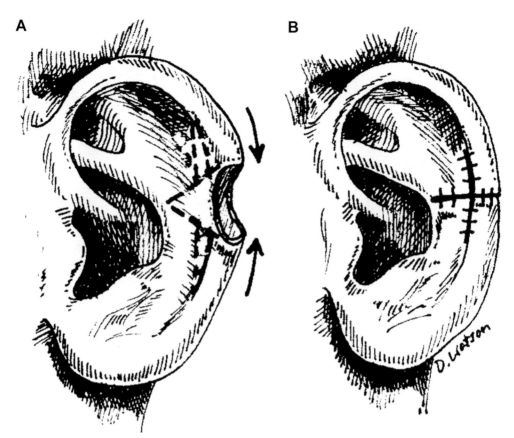

Fig. 10. Wedge excision. (*A*) Wedge planned according to defect, with stellate excision to prevent cupping. (*B*) Appearance of final reconstruction.

A   B

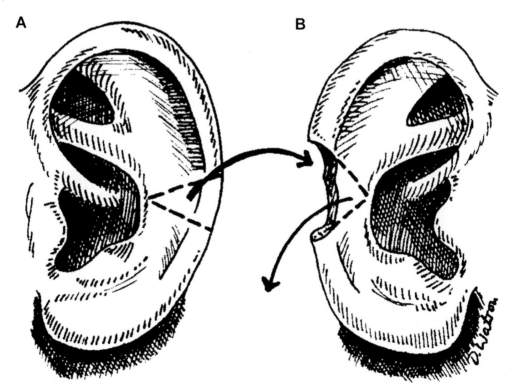

Fig. 11. Composite wedge graft. (*A*) A full-thickness wedge is taken from a similar location on the contralateral ear to reconstruct the defect (*B*). Note that to achieve symmetry between the ears, the harvested wedge should be approximately half the size of the defect.

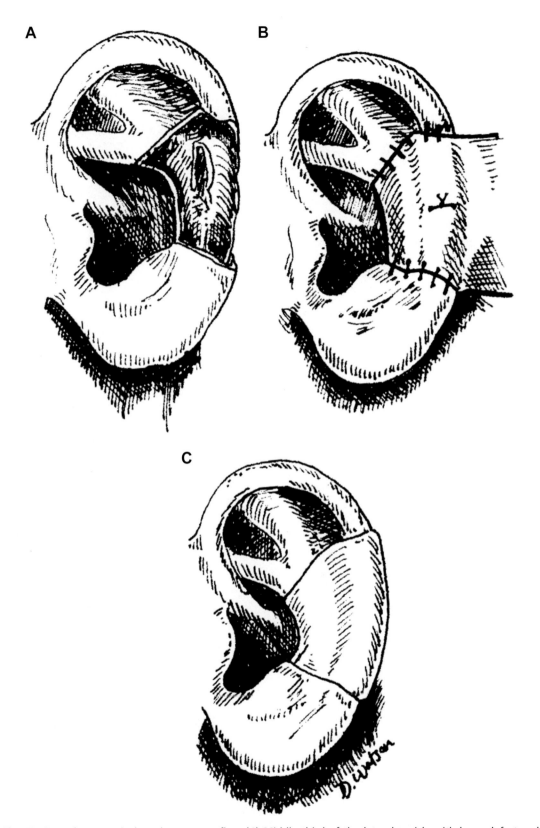

Fig. 12. Staged retroauricular advancement flap. (*A*) Middle third of the lateral auricle with large defect and exposed cartilage. (*B*) A posteriorly based flap (skin from the posterior auricle, sulcus, mastoid can be included) is planned. Elevation and advancement to cover the defect. Basting sutures may be necessary to conform the flap to the underlying framework. (*C*) The flap is allowed to mature for 2 to 3 weeks before dividing the pedicle and using it to repair the posterior portion of the defect. If the resultant cutaneous mastoid defect is large, a skin graft may be necessary for coverage.

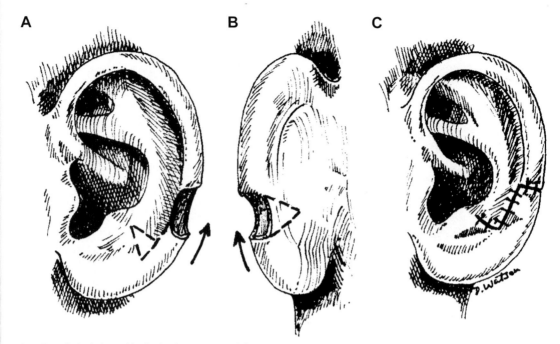

Fig. 13. Inferiorly based helical advancement. (*A*) Tangential rim is incised with a central dart to reduce cupping. (*B*) A posterior wedge may be excised to facilitate closure. (*C*) Appearance of final reconstruction.

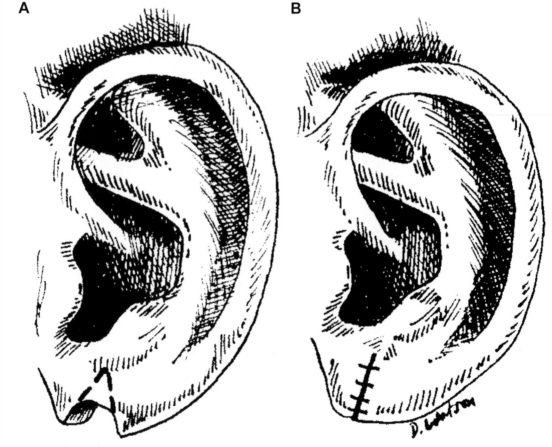

Fig. 14. Primary closure of small lobular defect. (*A*) The defected is extended to form a wedge to facilitate primary closure (*B*).

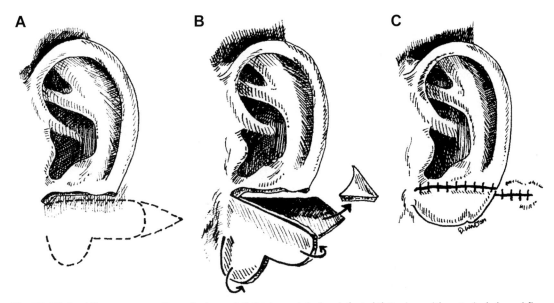

Fig. 15. Bilobed flap reconstruction of a large full-thickness lobular defect. (*A*) Design with anteriorly based flap, short limb oriented inferiorly. To facilitate closure, an additional triangle may be removed posteriorly. (*B*) The distal portion of the horizontal limb is folded posteriorly with the inferior limb being rotated underneath to recreate the most inferior aspect of lobule (*C*).

of contour, even if cartilage is missing. Additionally, if cartilage is left exposed without overlying perichondrium, it should be removed to allow the vascular supply of the posterior perichondrium or soft tissues to assist with wound healing. Alternatively, if a large surface area of cartilage is exposed and the wound is to be left to granulate or a graft is to be placed, numerous perforations should be made into the cartilage using a 4 mm biopsy punch before placement of a full-thickness graft. This will allow the posterior vascularized tissues to assist with the wound healing anteriorly. As shown in **Fig. 16**, a large defect of the concha and antihelix can be repaired with a postauricular pull-through transposition flap.[18] Similarly, it can be repaired with a postauricular pull-through island flap that is either random or axial.[19–21] If the central cartilaginous defect is very large, or the peripheral cartilage framework is compromised, then autologous cartilaginous struts harvested from the contralateral auricle, septum, or rib can be placed to prevent contracture. A superiorly based preauricular transposition flap can be used to close large defects of the helical root (**Fig. 17**).

Posterior

As previously mentioned, the posterior auricle and retroauricular skin is well hidden from view and can be used for donor tissue for other areas.

Additionally, as long as it is clinically appropriate, nearly half the surface area of the posterior auricle can be left to heal by secondary intention, assuming intact perichondrium or the cartilage has been removed and the postauricular sulcus is not involved. Although small lesions near the sulcus may be closed primarily, larger defects should be covered with full-thickness or split-thickness skin graft to prevent further contracture. Contraction of wounds involving the sulcus can result in an acute auriculomastoid angle that creates noticeable asymmetry.

SUMMARY

The auricle and periauricular areas present a uniquely challenging anatomic landscape with which the postresection reconstructive surgeon works. Weighing the various options for reconstruction will most likely result in a favorable outcome. This determination is largely influenced by the specific anatomic location of the defect and the characteristics of the surrounding tissues. The reconstructive surgeon should be familiar with and respect the limitations of the unique topographic and structural properties of each subunit. As a guiding principle, the approach chosen to repair any auricular defect should be that which most simply balances aesthetic outcome, donor site morbidity, and recovery time.

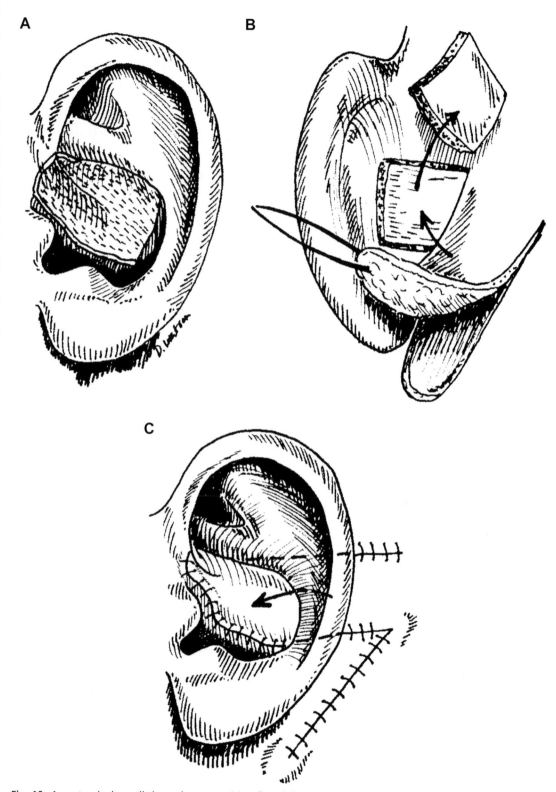

Fig. 16. A postauricular pull-through transposition flap. (*A*) A large defect of the concha. (*B*) Elevation of a superiorly based postauricular axial flap. The postauricular window is removed, allowing access to the anterior defect. (*C*) The flap gets pulled through and transposed to repair the anterior defect, and the donor site is closed primarily.

A   B

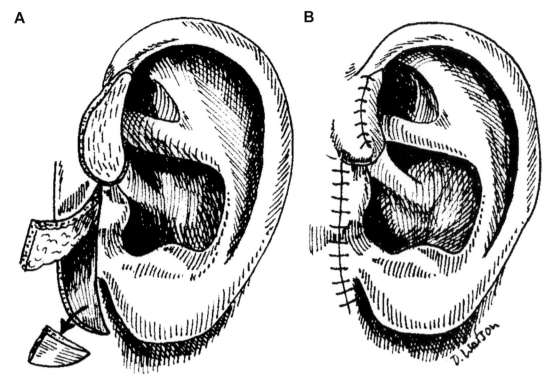

Fig. 17. Preauricular transposition flap to reconstruct the helical root. (*A*) The distal tip of the preauricular flap is tapered so that primary closure of the donor site may be achieved. (*B*) The scar from the donor site easily camouflages in the preauricular crease.

REFERENCES

1. Sieczka EM, Weber RV. Climbing the reconstructive ladder in the head and neck. Mo Med 2006;103: 265–9.
2. Senchenkov A, Jacobson SR. Microvascular salvage of a thrombosed total ear implant. Microsurgery 2013;33(5):396–400.
3. Sadove RC. Successful replantation of a totally amputated ear. Ann Plast Surg 1990;24:366–70.
4. Schonauer F, Blair JW, Moloney DM, et al. Three cases of successful microvascular ear replantation after bite avulsion injury. Scand J Plast Reconstr Surg Hand Surg 2004;38:177–82.
5. Mevio E, Facca L, Mullace M, et al. Osseointegrated implants in patients with auricular defects: a case series study. Acta Otorhinolaryngol Ital 2015;35(3): 186–90.
6. Westin T, Tjellstrom A, Hammerlid E, et al. Long-term study of quality and safety of osseointegration for the retention of auricular prostheses. Otolaryngol Head Neck Surg 1999;121:133–43.
7. Frenzel H. The rib cartilage concept in microtia. Facial Plast Surg 2015;31(6):587–99.
8. Brent B. Technical advances in ear reconstruction with autogenous rib cartilage grafts: personal experience with 1200 cases. Plast Reconstr Surg 1999;104:319–34 [discussion: 335–8].
9. Zhu P, Chen S. Clinical outcomes following ear reconstruction with adjuvant 3D template model. Acta Otolaryngol 2016;136(12):1236–41.
10. Cheney ML, Varvares MA, Nadol JB Jr. The temporoparietal fascial flap in head and neck reconstruction. Arch Otolaryngol Head Neck Surg 1993;119: 618–23.
11. Park SS, Wang TD. Temporoparietal fascial flap in auricular reconstruction. Facial Plast Surg 1995;11: 330–7.
12. Brent B, Byrd HS. Secondary ear reconstruction with cartilage grafts covered by axial, random, and free flaps of temporoparietal fascia. Plast Reconstr Surg 1983;72:141–52.
13. Stella C, Adam MF, Edward L. Helical Rim Reconstruction: Antia-Buch Flap. Eplasty 2015; 15:ic55.
14. Low DW. Modified chondrocutaneous advancement flap for ear reconstruction. Plast Reconstr Surg 1998;102:174–7.
15. Ellabban M, Maamoun MI, Elsharkawi M. The bipedicle post-auricular tube flap for reconstruction of partial ear defects. Br J Plast Surg 2003;56(6): 593–8.

16. Dujon DG, Bowditch M. The thin tube pedicle: a valuable technique in auricular reconstruction after trauma. Br J Plast Surg 1995;48:35–8.

17. Johnson TM, Fader DJ. The staged retroauricular to auricular direct pedicle (interpolation) flap for helical ear reconstruction. J Am Acad Dermatol 1997;37: 975–8.

18. Wood-Smith D, Ascherman JA, Albom MJ. Reconstruction of acquired ear defects with transauricular flaps. Plast Reconstr Surg 1995;95:173–5.

19. Adler N, Ad-El D, Azaria R. Reconstruction of nonhelical auricular defects with local flaps. Dermatol Surg 2008;34(4):501–7.

20. Turan A, Turkaslan T, Kul Z, et al. Reconstruction of the anterior surface of the ear using a postauricular pull-through neurovascular island flap. Ann Plast Surg 2006;56:609–13.

21. Masson JK. A simple island flap for reconstruction of concha-helix defects. Br J Plast Surg 1972;25: 399–403.

Reconstruction of Cutaneous Nasal Defects

Gregory S. Dibelius, MD*, Dean M. Toriumi, MD

KEYWORDS

- Mohs reconstruction • Nasal reconstruction • Skin grafts • Bilobe flaps • Forehead flaps

KEY POINTS

- The paranasal region permits several flap designs based on the well-established pattern of anastomoses between the major vessels of the central face.
- Defect characteristics, such as size and location, as well as the principles of subunit reconstruction as outlined by Burget and Menick guide the surgeon in choosing the most appropriate type of reconstruction.
- Full-thickness skin grafts have a valuable place in the management of cutaneous defects of the nose, including the lower third, if applied correctly in appropriate patients.
- The nasal ala has unique structural properties that make reconstruction a challenge for even experienced surgeons.
- Dermabrasion, steroid injections, and staged debulking or scar revision procedures can be valuable tools in the postoperative period and can greatly improve results.

INTRODUCTION

Mohs micrographic surgery has become the standard of care for the treatment of cutaneous malignancies because of its high treatment efficacy with maximal preservation of normal tissue. Successful management includes both a sound oncologic operation as well as meticulous reconstruction.

The nose is the most common subsite of cutaneous malignancies in the head and neck, the vast majority (90%) of which are basal cell carcinomas. Of the remaining cancers, squamous cell carcinomas and melanomas are the most common.[1] The nose is a distinctive facial feature with a complex 3-dimensional shape, a skin envelope that varies in thickness across nasal subunits, and an important functional role as an entry point to the airway. Thus, defects of the nose present unique reconstructive challenges.

The surgeon must weigh multiple options across the spectrum of the reconstructive ladder and choose the most appropriate technique for both the defect and patient. Form and function must be respected to the greatest extent possible.

Surgical planning is frequently defined by the aesthetic subunit principle proposed by Burget and Menick,[2,3] which emphasizes the reconstruction of topographic subunits rather than defects. This especially applies to defects that comprise a significant portion (>50%) of a nasal subunit, where reconstruction within the subunit could result in less favorable outcomes. In this approach, incisions are designed to lie within the junctions between subunits (these include the nasal dorsum, sidewalls, tip, alar lobules, and soft tissue facets) and, thus, remain hidden by the natural demarcations perceived by the human eye. A necessary component of this technique is the resection of

Disclosure: The authors have nothing to disclose.
Department of Otolaryngology–Head & Neck Surgery, Eye and Ear Infirmary, University of Illinois–Chicago, 1855 W Taylor St Chicago Room. 2.42 Chicago, IL 60612, USA
* Corresponding author.
E-mail address: gdibel2@uic.edu

Facial Plast Surg Clin N Am 25 (2017) 409–426
http://dx.doi.org/10.1016/j.fsc.2017.03.011

normal skin. The surgeon must balance these principles with a defect-only approach to reconstruction, which emphasizes the preservation of native tissue and has also been applied successfully in many circumstances.[4]

The reconstructive ladder for post-Mohs cutaneous defects consists of healing by secondary intention; skin grafting; recruitment of local tissue; and the 2 interpolated workhorse flaps, the forehead flap and the melolabial flap. Cutaneous defects may be accompanied by defects of the nasal framework and/or the internal nasal lining that will need to be reconstructed simultaneously. Preserving or rebuilding structural support should be a primary goal in nasal reconstructive surgery.

SECONDARY INTENT AND PRIMARY CLOSURE

Allowing cutaneous wounds to heal by secondary intent is the simplest method of reconstruction. This technique is most effective for very small (<5 mm) defects on the concave surfaces of the nose. Along with skin grafting, healing by secondary intent may serve a role when aggressive tumor characteristics warrant surveillance of the wound rather than immediate reconstruction. Small defects in the medial canthal area, the anatomy of which is easily distorted by local tissue rearrangement, are best suited to this technique.[5] In aesthetically prominent regions of the nose, the relatively large amount of contracture can lead to poor scarring as well as alar notching or retraction. These distorting forces increase with increasing size and depth of the defect. The concavities of the alar groove, alar-facial sulcus, and naso-facial sulcus may occasionally tolerate scars from small, very superficial defects allowed to heal by secondary intention; however, these important contours can be irrevocably lost if webbing occurs across a defect that is too large or too deep. The scars themselves are less favorable, often healing with a smooth, shiny surface that is visually distracting. Overall this technique is limited and is reserved for very carefully selected patients.

Primary closure of cutaneous defects can be effective for small wounds typically less than 1 cm, although the technique is fundamentally limited by the poor mobility and stiffness of the nasal skin. Consequently, primary closure is more feasible in elderly patients who have additional skin laxity. Additionally, fusiform excisions with primary closure result in linear scars, which can have poor cosmesis depending on their location relative to the nasal subunits and relaxed skin

tension lines. In the distal third, cephalocaudad vectors of tension may result in a cosmetically unfavorable distortion of the normal alar contour. This option is most effective on the nasal dorsum and sidewalls. It is appropriate in select patients but has limited applicability.

SKIN GRAFTING

Skin grafting serves an important role in nasal cutaneous reconstruction, but whether it is aesthetically comparable with local skin flaps is a matter of debate.[6–9] In general skin grafts are a viable option for defects less than 2 cm in size. Full-thickness skin grafts are preferred as split-thickness grafts tend to have excessive contraction and poor recipient site match. Initial skin graft survival depends on stable contact with a vascularized defect bed, and the use of bolster dressings is required. A common criticism of skin grafting for nasal reconstruction is that it can result in discrepancies in thickness and color that may provide a poor match to the recipient site. This criticism is in contrast to local repair techniques, which are conversely more affected by centripetal forces of contraction that lead to pincushion deformities. The common donor sites for full-thickness skin grafts used in nasal reconstruction include preauricular, supraclavicular, forehead, and postauricular full-thickness skin.

When contemplating skin graft resurfacing of a cutaneous nasal defect, thickness of the nasal skin is an essential consideration that is both highly patient and defect specific. Defects in the upper two-thirds of the nose are particularly amenable to skin grafting because of the flat-to-concave contours of these regions and the relative thinness of the nasal skin. In the lower third, increased skin thickness and convexity of the nasal tip contours make successful utilization of full-thickness skin grafts a more challenging problem. Ethnicity also has a profound influence on skin thickness and sebaceous quality. Where a large discrepancy between graft and donor site exists, the tendency is to heal with an obvious depression at the reconstructed site. Careful patient selection and operative technique can help ameliorate these difficulties and allow for successful reconstruction of these areas with skin grafts.

The authors' experience with full-thickness skin graft reconstruction of cutaneous nasal defects challenges the notion that local flaps are superior to skin grafts. The senior author (DMT) conducted a retrospective study of 103 nasal cutaneous reconstructions comparing 39 patients with full-thickness skin graft reconstruction with 64 patients undergoing local reconstruction.[6] Outcomes were assessed on visual analog scales by independent observers blinded to reconstructive technique. By this method, skin grafts were found to have equivalent cosmetic outcomes and required significantly fewer postoperative triamcinolone injections than the local flap group. In contrast, rates of postoperative dermabrasion were not statistically different. This technique represents a good option for single-stage reconstruction with potentially fewer postoperative interventions. The keys to the successful use of skin grafting likely include the use of preauricular skin as a donor site and certain patient characteristics, such as thin, less sebaceous skin and Fitzpatrick I or II skin type. Additionally, thickness discrepancies in the nasal tip were managed with the inclusion of cartilage grafts in the defect deep to the skin graft with preservation of a layer of vascularized tissue in between. Using these techniques, defects of the dorsum, sidewalls, tip, and ala were all reconstructed successfully. The thoughtful application of full-thickness skin grafting in appropriate patients can be an important tool for reconstructing

cutaneous nasal defects, including defects of the lower third (**Fig. 1**).

LOCAL FLAPS
Bilobed Flap

There have been countless local flap designs described throughout the literature for the purpose of cutaneous nasal reconstruction; however, the bilobed double transposition flap is the most well established and widely used. These flaps can be used effectively for defects of the sidewalls, dorsum, and lower third less than 1.5 cm in diameter and a safe distance (>5 mm) from the alar margin.[10,11] Thin nasal skin is preferable for this type of reconstruction, as thick sebaceous skin is more prone to pincushion deformities.

The flap is designed as a random-pattern double transposition flap rotated over an arc of 90° to 180° that recruits full-thickness cephalic skin into a more caudally positioned defect. Skin is, thus, rotated into the defect from an area of relative laxity. The double flap design allows greater dispersion of tension compared with a single transposition flap, such as a rhombic or note

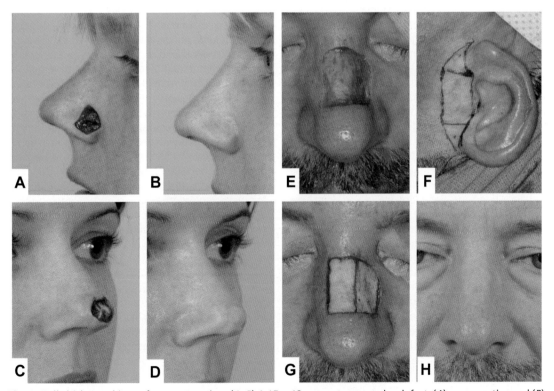

Fig. 1. Full-thickness skin graft reconstruction. (*A, B*) A 15 × 12-mm cutaneous alar defect. (*A*) preoperative and (*B*) postoperative appearance at 4 months. (*C, D*) A 20 × 20-mm cutaneous tip defect (*C*) preoperative and (*D*) postoperative at 8 months. (*E*) A 26 × 20-mm cutaneous defect of dorsum and sidewall. (*F*) Preauricular donor graft site marked. (*G*) Bilaterally harvested grafts used to perform subunit reconstruction. (*H*) Postoperative at 6 months.

flap. The original description of this flap described tissue transposition over two 90° arcs.[12] This description has subsequently been modified, most significantly by Zitelli,[13] who demonstrated the utility of limiting the arc of rotation to a total arc length of 90° to 100° with individual arcs of 45° between the two flaps. Burget and Menick[3] described the flap as a musculocutaneous flap incorporating the underlying muscle layer further increasing the flaps blood supply and survivability. The authors think the incorporation of the muscle layer significantly improves the vascularity of the flap and allows closure of larger defects.

Bilobed flaps are most useful for defects of the lower two-thirds of the nose. As the defect site is moved cephalically into the upper third of the nose, necessary recruitment of donor skin from the medial canthal or glabellar region begins to limit the applicability of the flap. Defects of the lateral ala also deserve caution when considering bilobed flaps, as important facial contours are lost when a flap traverses the alar crease or alar-facial sulcus. The lobes of the bilobed flap (Burget design) are based on a musculocutaneous blood supply and are preferably based laterally, but a medial base can be appropriate given the generally robust vascular supply of the nasal skin-soft tissue-muscle envelope. A laterally based flap design additionally allows for placement of the standing cutaneous deformity within or parallel to the alar groove for optimal cosmesis.[10,11]

The pivot point is set at a distance of one radius away from the margin of the defect at the desired location, accounting for the standing cutaneous deformity that occurs at this point. Often this is placed within or parallel to the alar groove. Two arcs centered on the previously determined pivot point are then drawn out from the center and periphery of the defect. The distance between these two arcs helps configure the shape and size of the transposition flaps. Each lobe should be nearly the same width of the defect given the relatively inelastic nature of the nasal skin. The first lobe is designed between the greater and lesser arcs, with its linear axis 45° from that of the defect. The second lobe is placed 45° to the axis of the primary lobe and often extends in a triangular fashion beyond the path defined by the arcs to a distance that is twice the height of the primary lobe. This placement serves to facilitate adequate closure of the secondary donor site. The length of the secondary lobe can be modified based on flap location and elasticity of the skin.

Full-thickness incisions are carried out as designed. Dissection is then performed below the nasal superficial musculoaponeurotic system (SMAS) to protect the vascularity of the flap. The flaps can be thinned as required, taking care to preserve the subdermal vascular plexus and as much of the underlying muscle layer as possible. Wide undermining of the surrounding skin soft tissue envelope is then performed to facilitate closure and reduce centripetal contraction. Closure is then performed in layers starting with the point of maximal tension. The order typically followed is closure of the secondary lobe donor site followed by closure of the primary defect. The standing cutaneous deformity at the pivot point is excised, and the excess skin at the tip of the secondary lobe is trimmed during inset into the primary lobe donor site (**Fig. 2**).

Despite the effectiveness of the bilobed flap and its widespread use, a few pitfalls should be kept in mind when mobilizing local tissue for reconstruction. The underlying structure of the nose deserves some consideration. For example, excessive tension near the alar margin can lead to retraction or notching, particularly if the supporting lower lateral cartilages are thin, cephalically positioned, or weak. Distortion of soft tissues under tension in this region may also occasionally contribute to nasal valve problems in patients with weak underlying structure. To help minimize functional compromise, the authors frequently place alar batten grafts or other sidewall grafts to provide extra lateral wall support and prevent airway compromise. Pincushion deformities may develop and should be anticipated and managed with subcutaneous debulking or a secondary procedure. In patients with thicker sebaceous skin, the authors perform primary multiple Z-plasties incorporated into the flap design to lessen the postoperative pincushioning. Scarring at incisional interfaces or changes in thickness after tissue rearrangement can be managed with dermabrasion in the postoperative period. Additionally, scars tend to be long and do not necessarily fall within relaxed skin tension lines or aesthetic subunit junctions. Planning for these factors in advance and balancing them against alternative options such as full thickness skin grafting may help achieve optimal outcomes.

Dorsal Nasal Flap

The dorsal nasal flap as popularized by Rieger[14] was designed as a random-pattern rotation-advancement extension of the glabellar flap, which could be used to cover large defects of the nose in a single-stage reconstruction. Marchac and Toth[15] redesigned Rieger's flap as an axial flap based on a branch of the angular artery. Many variations of the dorsal nasal and glabellar flaps are possible that take advantage of the rich anastomotic blood supply in this region,[16] which has been extensively described and elaborated by multiple dedicated

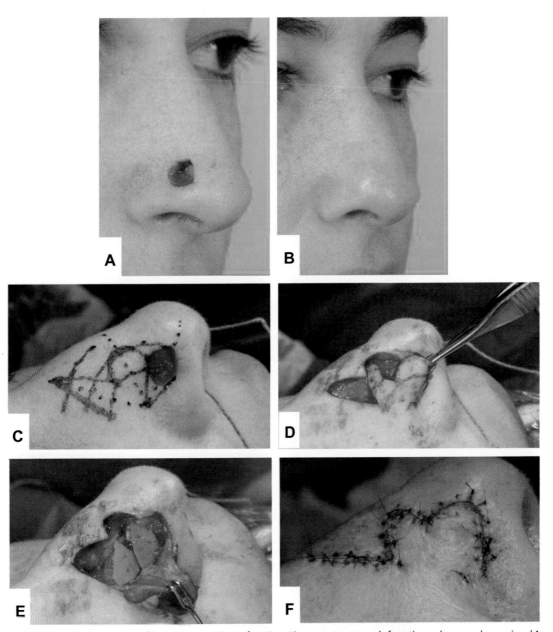

Fig. 2. Bilobed transposition flap reconstruction of a 15 × 12-mm cutaneous defect tip and supra-alar region (A, B). (A) Preoperative and (B) postoperative at 22 months. (C–F) Intraoperative views. (C) Flap geometry is marked. (D) Flap is elevated. (E) Cartilage alar batten grafts are sutured in place. (F) Defect is closed.

vascular studies.[17–20] It is this robust anastomotic network that provides the foundation for nasal reconstruction.

By the design of this flap, glabellar and dorsal nasal skin are recruited to close relatively large defects by mobilizing a large segment of tissue. The upper size limit for defects is 2.5 cm, a limitation set by the degree of skin laxity in the glabellar region.[21,22] The flap is useful for resurfacing defects of the lower third of the nose in a single stage, but

there should be at least 5 mm of native tissue between the defect and the free alar margin to help prevent postoperative retraction. An inverted-V incision is typically placed within the glabellar skin below the height of the medial brow and then is extended inferiorly either ipsilateral or contralateral to the side of the lesion. It is helpful to try to place the incisions in glabellar frown lines superiorly and within the aesthetic boundary at the naso-facial junction to aid in scar camouflage.[23]

The flap is elevated in the subcutaneous plane in the glabellar region but transitions to the submuscular plane over the nasal dorsum to preserve the random blood supply to the flap. Wide undermining is usually required. The flap is then rotated into the defect and closed (**Fig. 3**).

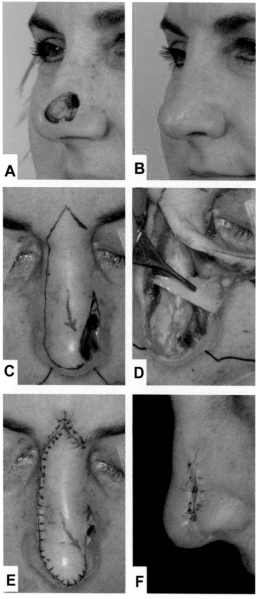

A B C D E F

Fig. 3. Dorsal nasal (Rieger) flap reconstruction of a 22 × 14-mm ala and sidewall defect. (*A*) Preoperative and (*B*) postoperative appearance at 4 months. (*C–E*) Intraoperative photographs. (*C*) The flap is designed with an inverted-V glabellar incision and an ipsilateral pedicle. (*D*) Septal cartilage batten graft. (*E*) Closure before removal of standing cutaneous deformity. (*F*) Subsequent in-office excision of standing cutaneous deformity with closure at 1 month postoperative.

The advantage of this technique is that defects are resurfaced with adjacent skin, with favorable thickness and color match characteristics, in a single-stage reconstruction that can performed under local anesthesia. A wide variety of defects can be closed, including larger defects of the distal third. The flap is well vascularized, and flap failure is exceedingly rare. However, the flap has several drawbacks. De Fontaine and colleagues[24] noted that certain aspects of the original flap design violated the aesthetic subunit principle and proposed modifications to relocate the incisions. Problems also arise in the interbrow and medial canthal regions as these become distorted by flap advancement and skin thickness mismatches. Rohrich and colleagues[25] described a modification of the dorsal nasal flap that omitted the glabellar extension of the incision and instead placed a transverse incision within the radix crease and a lateral extension that approximated the brow tip aesthetic line. Distally, cephalocaudad forces create a tendency for cephalic retraction of the nostril margin or over-rotation of the nasal tip. There may also be a need for postoperative debulking and/or management of standing cutaneous deformities. Dermabrasion can be a useful postoperative adjunct to improve the appearance of the incisional interfaces.[23,25] Thus, the dorsal nasal flap is a robust flap that can cover relatively large defects of the nasal tip but can be difficult to achieve an optimal aesthetic result.

Interpolated Flaps

Interpolated melolabial flaps

Melolabial flaps used in nasal reconstruction take advantage of the mobile, well-vascularized skin of the medial cheek at the melolabial fold. The cheek skin and subcutaneous tissues possess reliable similarity to the nasal tip skin and offer a good qualitative match, whereas the robust vascularity allows for closure of large defects and support of free cartilage grafting, which is an important component of alar reconstruction.[22,26,27] Donor site morbidity is predictable, and the scar is camouflaged within the natural melolabial crease. The ala, lower sidewall, and in some cases the nasal lining are amenable to reconstruction with this flap. In addition to nasal defects, it is ideally suited for reconstruction of the upper lip and medial cheek.

Several different designs using this tissue are possible and have been well described. Two major categorical uses of melolabial flaps are as transposition flaps with the base of the flap adjacent to the defect and as interpolated flaps crossing over intervening normal tissue. With regard to cutaneous nasal defects, the interpolated flap offers distinct advantages in reconstruction of the alar lobule and represents its most powerful application in nasal reconstruction. The flap is designed as a superiorly pedicled random-pattern flap based on the rich subdermal vascular plexus supplied by perforators of the angular artery.[22,26] The skin paddle is composed of the thicker, more sebaceous cheek skin lateral to the melolabial groove. The contralateral normal ala serves as a 3-dimensional template for design of the skin paddle. The pedicle is then developed as either a cutaneous (peninsular) or subcutaneous (island) pedicle. The cutaneous pedicle design has a narrower pedicle that allows for greater effective reach of the skin paddle but causes more distortion of the donor site than the subcutaneous pedicle design. The subcutaneous pedicle design contains a potentially more robust pedicle but requires a deeper and wider dissection and subsequently places midfacial branches of the facial nerve at an increased risk of inadvertent injury.[27] One of the major advantages of the subcutaneous pedicle design is that the complex triangular cutaneous area just lateral to the alar lobular insertion into the cheek at the superior most aspect of the nasolabial crease can be preserved. Bridging the interpolated flap over this

triangular subunit allows a more inconspicuous repair. Reconstruction is performed in 2 stages with a delayed inset, typically performed 3 weeks after flap elevation (**Fig. 4**).

The design of this flap as an interpolated flap is ideal for reconstruction of the lower third of the nose, particularly the ala, because the alar-facial groove can be completely preserved[28] (**Fig. 5**). The junction between the alar lobule, upper lip, and medial cheek is a complex topographic region that can be impossible to restore in a completely natural way. If this area is uninvolved in the cancer ablation, the apical triangle within 5 mm of the alar-facial junction is preserved during flap elevation so that it will remain undistorted after reconstruction. If the alar-facial sulcus is involved in the ablation, a cheek flap is advanced into the sulcus in order to recreate the boundary between distinct subunits.[26] Because this region also comprises the external nasal valve, the use of cartilage grafting and reconstruction of the nasal lining is required for full-thickness reconstruction of the alar subunit in order to preserve its contour and function. The melolabial flap in these circumstances is used to resurface the skin or, alternatively, as a hinge flap to reconstruct the vestibular lining in

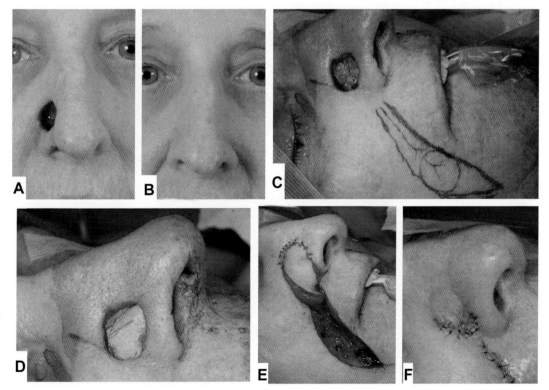

Fig. 4. Interpolated melolabial flap reconstruction of a 14 × 15-mm ala and lateral wall defect (*A, B*). (*A*) Preoperative and (*B*) postoperative view at 6 months. (*C–F*) Intraoperative photographs. (*C*) Flap design. (*D*) Septal cartilage alar batten graft. (*E*) Flap elevated with interpolated subcutaneous pedicle. (*F*) Second-stage flap inset.

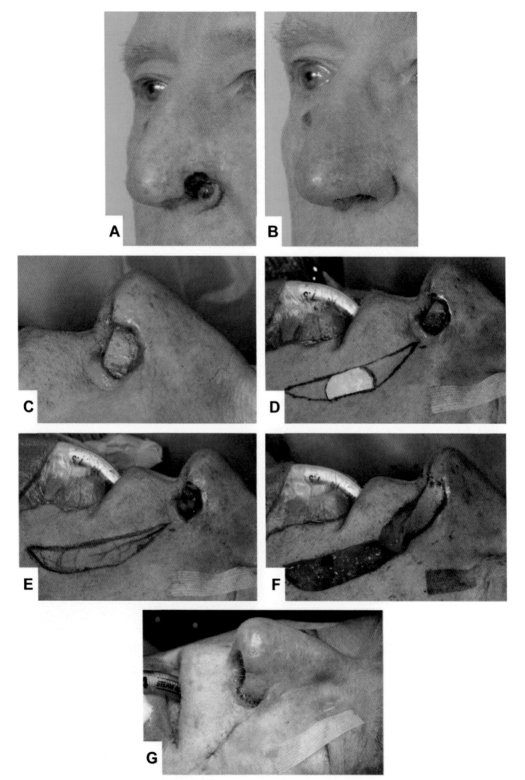

Fig. 5. Alar reconstruction with preservation of alar-facial sulcus. (*A*) Preoperative defect of alar subunit. (*B*) Postoperative appearance after interpolated melolabial flap reconstruction at 11.5 months. (*C–F*) Intraoperative flap design. Note preservation of the complex triangular cutaneous area just lateral to the alar lobular insertion into the cheek at the superior most aspect of the nasolabial crease. (*C*) A nonanatomic free cartilage graft is placed to support the reconstructed alar lobule. (*D*) Template used to design skin paddle. (*E*) Elevation of flap with interpolated pedicle. (*F*) Flap rotated into defect. (*G*) Inset at second stage.

conjunction with skin graft resurfacing.[22,26] It can also be used for reconstruction of the columella in conjunction with structural cartilage grafting. Nonanatomic free cartilage grafting, typically from a contralateral auricular donor site, can be used for cutaneous defects to provide resistance to scar contracture and cephalic movement of the alar margin.

Probably the most significant disadvantage of this reconstructive technique is that it requires 2 stages, which may be undesirable for certain patients. Alternative flap designs allow for single-stage flap transfer, including tunneling the flap subcutaneously across the alar-facial junction, or a single-stage transposition with a superiorly based cutaneous pedicle. These techniques are not generally favored because they typically result in blunting of the sulcus and, therefore, violate the aesthetic boundary between the ala, cheek, and upper lip.

Interpolated paramedian forehead flaps

The interpolated paramedian forehead flap is the most versatile flap for reconstruction of the nose and is the true workhorse flap of this discipline. Numerous variations of this flap design have an extensive history of use in nasal reconstruction, including complex subtotal and total nasal defects. The paramedian design of the modern forehead flap has evolved from the earlier median flap design in which bilateral supratrochlear vessels were captured in the pedicle. These modifications have allowed a longer and narrower pedicle with greater reach and a true axial design.[29,30] The robust vasculature of this flap is ideal for nourishing free structural grafts frequently required during nasal reconstruction. Forehead donor tissue provides a good skin color and texture match with the recipient site, and the thickness of the donor skin can be controlled to provide an appropriate thickness match.

Numerous studies have established the robust anastomotic network of the vessels of the forehead and glabellar region[17–20,30,31] (**Fig. 6**). The forehead flaps are designed as an axial pattern flap inferiorly pedicled on a unilateral supratrochlear artery, but a rich series of anastomoses with branches of the supraorbital and dorsal nasal vessels in the medial canthal region provides additional blood supply. The pedicle is reliably located 1.7 to 2.2 cm from the midline as it exits the supratrochlear foramen. A Doppler ultrasound probe can assist in its accurate identification, which in turn permits more precise narrowing of the pedicle for optimal flap geometry, though many surgeons find this to be unnecessary. After piercing the orbital septum, the vessels travel superiorly in a

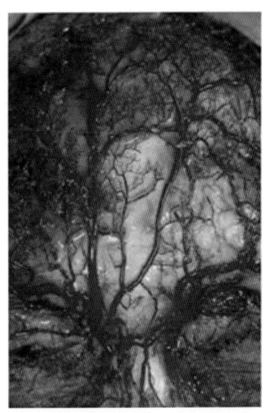

Fig. 6. Forehead and paranasal vascular supply. A rich anastomotic network involving branches of the angular, dorsal nasal, supratrochlear, and supraorbital vessels supplies the flaps used in nasal reconstruction.

paramedian position in the plane deep to the orbicularis oculi but superficial to the corrugator muscle. The pedicle then pierces the frontalis muscle at a point 2 cm above the orbital rim to travel in a more superficial plane within the subcutaneous and subdermal tissue cephalically.

Intraoperatively, the pedicle is identified and marked and centered at the medial brow. The width at the base can be as narrow as 10 to 15 mm to facilitate rotation. In some patients, the cutaneous portion of the flap can be completely removed allowing maximal rotation of the flap. If this is done, the free subcutaneous pedicle must be protected to prevent desiccation and loss of the vascular pedicle. A split-thickness skin graft or acellular dermis can be used to protect the pedicle. The defect is then assessed, and subunit resection is planned if appropriate. A 3-dimensional template is created of the planned defect before subunit resection. The template is reversed and brought to the forehead to plan the precise shape of the flap. A paramedian design places the skin paddle on a vertical path above the supratrochlear notch in line with the vascular pedicle. An alternative design known as the midline forehead flap places the skin paddle in the precise midline, medial to the pedicle to improve donor site scarring.[32] The required length is assessed, and the flap template is moved accordingly until the placement is precise. Incisions are performed through the scalp tissues to the subgaleal plane. The flap is then elevated in the subgaleal plane from superior to inferior. Near the base of the flap, the corrugator muscle can be divided or dissection performed in a subperiosteal plane to increase the length of the flap. Extensions of the incisions below the medial brow should be performed superficially, through skin only.

The flap can be thinned in the subcutaneous or muscular plane near the hairline to create an appropriate thickness that matches the recipient site. Frontalis muscle and subcutaneous tissue are routinely removed from this portion of the flap. More proximal debulking should be staged to protect the pedicle. The skin paddle itself is designed in the forehead skin adjacent to the hairline and can be oriented obliquely to avoid crossing into the hairline. If a large skin paddle is needed, crossing into the hair-bearing scalp may be unavoidable and reconstruction should be accompanied by depilating procedures. An alternative design involves midline positioning of the skin paddle, which may provide a donor scar better aligned with the facial aesthetic units.[32] Forehead flap skin paddles can also be extended to include segments purposed for resurfacing of the columellar skin or turn in flaps that can be used to reconstruct the caudal vestibular lining (**Fig. 7**).

Management of the pedicle during the period of flap interpolation requires some attention. Many surgeons use skin grafts or acellular dermis to resurface the exposed portion of the pedicle. The authors have used a cyanoacrylate adhesive to cover the exposed pedicle with great success. At the end of the first stage of transposition, the exposed area of the forehead flap is covered with the cyanoacrylate adhesive to prevent desiccation. Care is taken to avoid gluing the flap to surrounding structures. Over the first 2 weeks after surgery, the pedicle will heal allowing the cyanoacrylate adhesive to be removed. Use of the cyanoacrylate adhesive protective covering eliminates the need for harvesting a skin graft to cover the pedicle (**Fig. 8**).

The procedure is typically performed as either a 2- or 3-stage operation. In a 2-stage operation, the pedicle is divided at 3 weeks postoperatively and the flap is subcutaneously debulked and inset. The senior author (DMT) prefers a 3-stage operation in which debulking is performed as an intermediate stage. Leaving the vascular pedicle intact at the second stage permits more aggressive contouring for an optimal aesthetic outcome. Some surgeons reserve a 3-stage approach for difficult cases in which the vascularity of the flap is in question, such as in smokers or patients with other vascular disease. When the pedicle is divided at either the second or third stage, a small triangular flap of skin is preserved and used to reconstruct the interbrow region at the pivot point to restore the normal glabellar contour and medial brow position. This small triangular flap is at high risk for pincushioning. This risk can be minimized by using multiple Z-plasties to break up the scar, minimize pincushioning, and provide camouflage (**Fig. 9**).

CUTANEOUS RECONSTRUCTION BY SUBUNIT
Dorsum and Sidewalls

The dorsum and sidewalls are well suited to many reconstructive techniques. Skin grafting can be done with good cosmetic results, particularly in the thin skin over the nasal dorsum. Bilobed and other transposition flaps or even primary closure can be performed in this region for appropriate defects without undue anatomic distortion in many cases. Dorsal nasal and glabellar flaps can cover larger defects of the entire length of the dorsum. Paramedian forehead flaps are optimal for larger and deeper cutaneous defects. Defects of the underlying framework and mucosal lining must be simultaneously reconstructed with the cutaneous defect.

Nasal Tip

Cutaneous defects of the tip can be reconstructed using a variety of techniques based on characteristics of the defect. Small superficial defects can be managed with bilobed transposition of local tissue. Larger defects are amenable to paramedian forehead flap reconstruction and can also be reconstructed in a single stage with a dorsal nasal flap. Full-thickness skin grafts are a viable option in the tip provided a reasonable match between donor and recipient skin can be achieved. Structural grafting of tip support structures should be performed as needed (**Fig. 10**).

Columella and Soft Tissue Facets

Management of defects of the columella and soft tissue facets can become quite complex. Cutaneous defects can be managed with full-thickness skin grafts or auricular composite

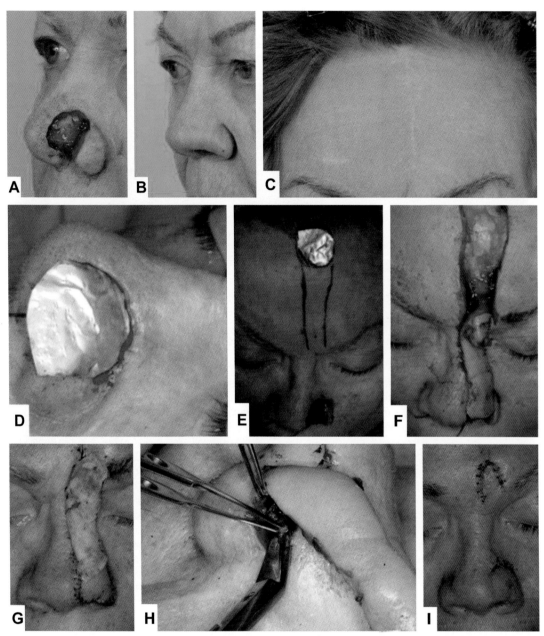

Fig. 7. Interpolated paramedian forehead flap reconstruction of a 20 × 21-mm tip, ala, sidewall defect (*A–C*). (*A*) Preoperative and (*B*) postoperative view at 6 months. (*C*) Donor site at 6 months. (*D–G*) First stage of paramedian forehead flap procedure. (*D*) Defect template created. (*E*) Flap design. (*F*) Flap elevated. (*G*) Closure of first stage with interpolated pedicle. (*H*) Second stage subcutaneous debulking. (*I*) Third stage inset of flap with glabellar closure.

grafts. Larger defects will typically require restoration of structural support and nasal vestibular lining. Unilateral or bilateral interpolated melolabial flaps can be used in conjunction with free cartilage grafting to reconstruct the columella. Alternatively, composite septal chondromucosal flaps can also provide support and reconstruct the vestibular lining.[22]

Ala

The anatomy of the alar subunit is unique and has special implications for reconstruction. It is important to understand that the alar lobule is essentially suspended in space by the structural framework of the nose and maxilla. It is composed of soft tissue only and does not

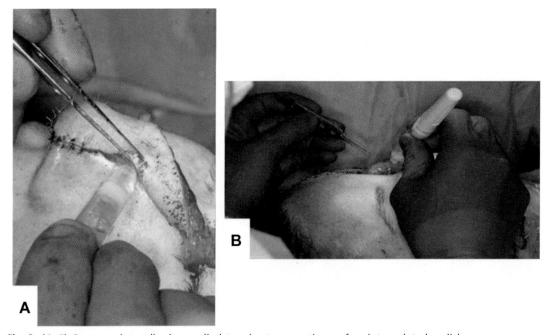

Fig. 8. (*A*, *B*) Cyanoacrylate adhesive applied to subcutaneous tissue of an interpolated pedicle.

contain any cartilage or other structural elements. It is mainly supported at its cephalic edge by the caudal margin of the lateral crura, the strength and quality of which are considerably variable. The position and contour of the free margin are, therefore, easily disturbed. The transition between external skin cover and internal lining occurs within this subunit and is a critical factor to consider during reconstruction. Functionally, the alar subunit is a component of the external nasal valve. These factors make the ala a very delicate subunit, susceptible to distortion and functional problems that can be difficult to manage.[33]

Very small, superficial defects of the concavities that surround the alar subunit may be allowed to heal by secondary intention, but larger defects heal with webbed scars that obliterate these contours. Primary closure is a poor option as the skin in the alar lobule lacks sufficient laxity and will create distortion. A subcutaneously based V to Y island advancement flap designed along the alar crease can be used for smaller defects. Interpolated melolabial flaps are the workhorse flaps for reconstruction of the alar subunit and are usually required for larger or deep defects (**Fig. 11**).

Free cartilage and composite grafting play an important role in reconstructing the alar subunit.[34,35] In cases whereby the internal lining is intact, free cartilage grafts are placed in a nonanatomic position within the reconstructed alar lobule

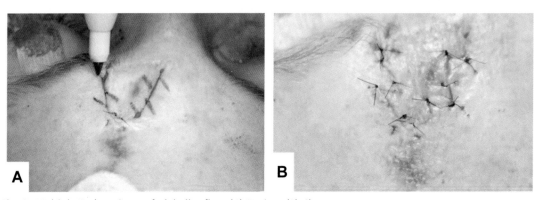

Fig. 9. Multiple Z-plasty inset of glabellar flap. (*A*) Design. (*B*) Closure.

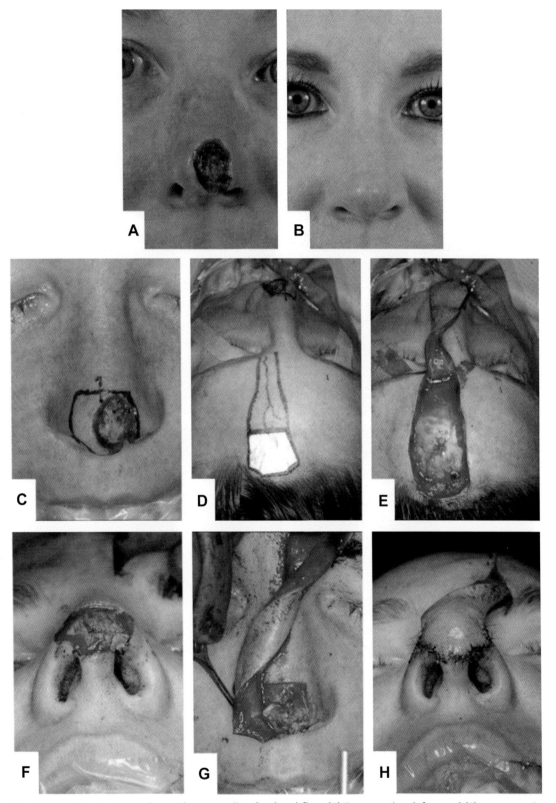

Fig. 10. Nasal tip reconstruction with paramedian forehead flap. (*A*) Preoperative defect and (*B*) postoperative appearance at 6.5 months. (*C–H*) Intraoperative photographs. (*C*) Defect and planned subunit resection. (*D*) Flap designed marked with precise placement of template. (*F*) Composite graft for soft tissue facet reconstruction. (*G*) Free cartilage graft for tip reconstruction. (*H*) Paramedian forehead flap rotated into defected and sutured in place.

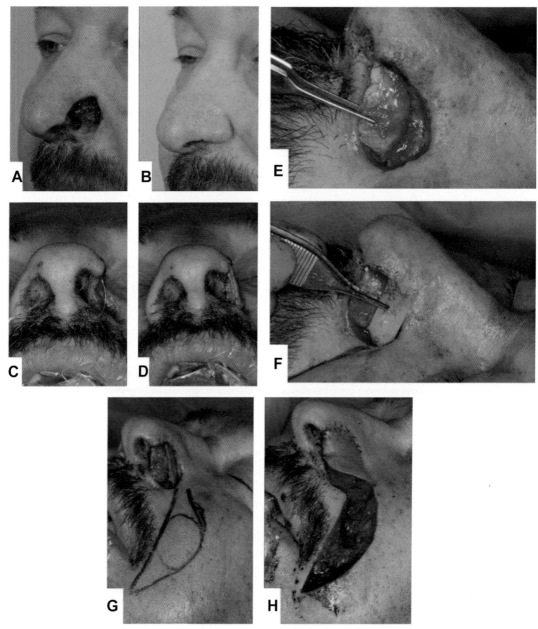

Fig. 11. Alar reconstruction. (*A*) A 22 × 20-mm full-thickness defect; (*B*) 6 months' postoperative appearance. (*C–H*) Intraoperative photographs. (*C*) Full-thickness defect base view. (*D*) Lining reconstructed with auricular composite graft. (*E*) Cartilage component of composite graft provides support to alar margin. (*F*) Alar batten graft placed for support of nasal sidewall. (*G*) Interpolated melolabial flap design. (*H*) Elevation of flap with rotation into defect to provide external cover.

and covered with vascularized tissue, such as a melolabial or paramedian forehead flap. Free cartilage grafts can also be placed during full-thickness skin graft reconstruction of the alar skin provided they are a few layers deep to the vascularized wound bed that will receive the skin graft.[6] This method of reconstruction helps to maintain the

contour and position of the subunit against the forces of contracture. These grafts are typically procured from the contralateral concha, which most closely matches the convexity of the alar subunit.

Auricular chondro-cutaneous composite grafts can be used to restore both structural support as well as external skin and internal lining. They can also be effectively used in revision cases whereby contraction of the nostril has resulted in vestibular stenosis. Composite grafts are delicate, have high metabolic requirements, and critically depend on vascular imbibition and inosculation for survival. Therefore, they are typically kept small, generally less than 1 cm, to mitigate the risk of necrosis and graft failure. Grafting techniques in which perichondrium is left intact over the area of cartilage extending beyond the cutaneous portion of the graft can considerably improve the take rate by increasing the surface area of donor microcirculation. This increase enables the surgeon to occasionally use larger grafts (**Fig. 12**). A small amount of dissection between the skin and cartilaginous portion of the graft at the periphery of the skin island aids in graft inset by creating a cuff of cutaneous tissue that can be everted during closure. Small full-thickness skin grafts harvested from the postauricular sulcus are generally used to resurface the auricular donor site defect. Both donor and recipient site require the application of bolster dressings to prevent shearing forces that could contribute to graft failure.

Internal Lining and Nasal Framework

Adequate reconstruction of the nose after Mohs surgery is not limited to cutaneous reconstruction. Local reconstructive options for restoring the internal lining include several mucosal flaps. These flaps include bipedicled vestibular skin advancement, septal mucoperichondral flaps, septal composite flaps, and turbinate flaps. Septal chondro-mucosal composite flaps can also be manipulated to simultaneously restore the nasal framework of the dorsum, sidewalls, or columella.[22] External cover skin can be *turned in* to reconstruct lining,[36] or similarly turn-in flaps can be incorporated into the design of paramedian forehead flaps for caudal lining deficits. Chondro-cutaneous composite grafts can address small deficits of internal lining and provide a degree of structural integrity to the alar lobule. More distant options include interpolated melolabial flaps or even microvascular free tissue transfer.

Free cartilage grafting is an essential tool for restoring the nasal framework. Anatomic cartilage grafts are used whenever normal structural elements have been violated by the resection. Nonanatomic grafts are used whenever the alar subunit is reconstructed or as alar batten grafts to preserve or augment the nasal valve. Costal cartilage grafts can be used in the upper third of the nose to restore the bony nasal vault. Free grafts should be nourished by adequate vascularized soft tissue, such as native tissue or well-vascularized flaps. A full discussion of framework and lining reconstruction is beyond the scope of this article.

POSTOPERATIVE CARE

Vigilant postoperative care is important for a successful outcome. The care should be patient and technique specific. Maintaining a moist local wound environment is critical. Occlusive or semi-occlusive dressings can promote reepithelialization over areas healing by secondary intention. Bolster dressings should be applied when skin grafts and composite grafts are used to prevent shearing and graft loss. The exposed tissue of an interpolated flap pedicle is dressed with a simple petrolatum gauze or a layer of cyanoacrylate adhesive. The authors typically administer a short course of oral antibiotic prophylaxis and antibiotic ointment for all patients undergoing cutaneous reconstruction.

Certain adjunctive procedures can greatly improve the aesthetic outcome. Local flaps are commonly plagued by pincushion deformities. These deformities can be managed with subcutaneous debulking or thinning of the flap in the primary surgery to improve contour but frequently needs to be accomplished in a staged fashion. The senior author (DMT) performs a second-stage debulking procedure routinely as part of a 3-stage paramedian forehead flap procedure 3 weeks before transection of the pedicle and inset of the flap. This practice allows for a more aggressive procedure with reduced risk of compromising the flap, a technique that has enormous value in patients who smoke or who have other vascular risk factors. Wide undermining at the time of closure in conjunction with thinning of the flap can help prevent or reduce the pincushion deformity.

Steroid injections are useful adjuncts to reduce fibrosis and excessive formation of scar tissue. Injections are placed subdermally, typically using triamcinolone acetonide at 10 mg/mL. This technique can be used to initially manage pincushion deformities, although a second procedure may be required in which excessive scar tissue is excised. Where scars are uneven, particularly at the incisional interfaces, subsequent dermabrasion can be performed 6 weeks after the primary surgery. Some surgeons advocate aggressive, early, and routine dermabrasion in their nasal reconstructive practice.[4] Some scars may be better managed with excision and closure with multiple Z-plasties. Silicone scar sheeting can improve postoperative appearance and is frequently used in the authors' practice.

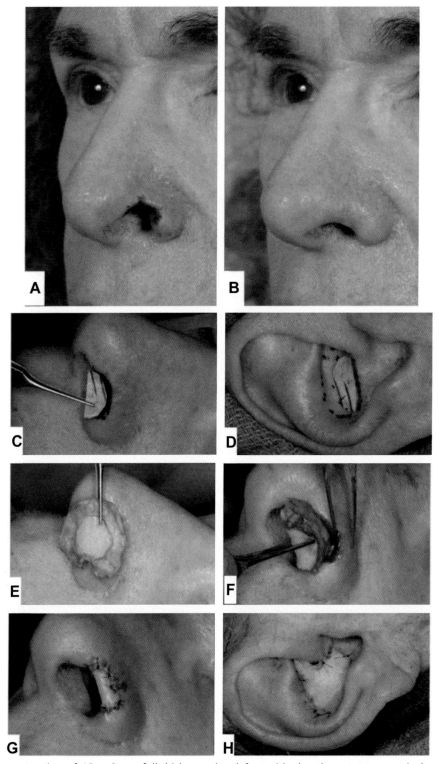

Fig. 12. Reconstruction of 16 × 6-mm full-thickness alar defect with chondro-cutaneous auricular composite graft. (*A*) Preoperative and (*B*) postoperative appearance at 5 months. (*C–H*) Intraoperative views. (*C*) Defect template. (*D*) Template transferred to auricular donor site. Note larger size of cartilaginous portion relative to skin paddle. (*E*) Graft harvested with intact perichondrium. (*F*) Graft inset into defect after subcutaneous undermining and (*G*) sutured in place. (*H*) Full-thickness skin graft resurfacing of donor site.

SUMMARY

The paranasal region permits several flap designs and multiple variations thereof based on the well-established pattern of anastomoses between the major vessels of the central face. These flaps form the foundation of cutaneous nasal reconstruction. Defect characteristics, such as size and location, as well as the principles of subunit reconstruction as outlined by Burget and Menick[2] guide the surgeon in choosing the most appropriate type of reconstruction. Elderly patients have increased skin laxity, which improves the ability to obtain tension free closure and minimize distortion when using local tissue. Full-thickness skin grafts have a valuable place in the management of cutaneous defects of the nose, including the lower third, if applied correctly in appropriate patients. The workhorse interpolated flaps remain indispensable options for managing larger defects and can be tailored to several situations. The nasal ala has unique structural properties that make reconstruction a challenge for even experienced surgeons; special considerations of lining, framework, and nonanatomic cartilage grafting all come in to play in this subunit. Dermabrasion, steroid injections, and staged debulking or scar revision procedures can be valuable tools in the postoperative period and can greatly improve results.

REFERENCES

1. Bailey BJ, Johnson JT, Newlands SD, editors. Head and neck surgery-otolaryngology. 3rd edition. Philadelphia: Lippincott Williams & Wilkins; 2001.
2. Burget GC, Menick FJ. The subunit principle in nasal reconstruction. Plast Reconstr Surg 1985; 76(2):239–47.
3. Burget GC, Menick FJ. Aesthetic reconstruction of the nose. St Louis (MO): Mosby; 2002.
4. Rohrich RJ, Griffin JR, Ansari M, et al. Nasal reconstruction – beyond aesthetic subunits: a 15 year review of 1334 cases. Plast Reconstr Surg 2004; 114(6):1405–16.
5. Zitelli JA. Secondary intention healing: an alternative to surgical repair. Clin Dermatol 1984;2(3):92–106.
6. Sapthavee A, Munaretto N, Toriumi DM. Skin grafts vs local flaps for reconstruction of nasal defects a retrospective cohort study. JAMA Facial Plast Surg 2015;17(4):270–3.
7. Jacobs MA, Christenson LJ, Weaver AL, et al. Clinical outcome of cutaneous flaps versus full thickness skin grafts after Mohs surgery on the nose. Dermatol Surg 2010;36(1):23–30.
8. McCluskey PD, Constantine FC, Thornton JF. Lower third nasal reconstruction: when is skin grafting an appropriate option? Plast Reconstr Surg 2009; 124(3):826–35.
9. Jewett BJ. Skin and composite grafts. In: Baker SR, editor. Local flaps in facial reconstruction. 3rd edition. Philadelphia: Mosby; 2014. p. 339–67.
10. Baker SR. Bilobe flaps. In: Baker SR, editor. Local flaps in facial reconstruction. 3rd edition. Philadelphia: Mosby; 2014. p. 187–205.
11. Steiger J. Bilobed flaps in nasal reconstruction. Facial Plast Surg Clin North Am 2011;19:107–11.
12. Esser JF. Gestielte locale nasenplastik mit zweizipfligem lappen decking des sekunaren detektes vom esten zipfel durch den zweiten. Dtsh Z Chir 1918; 143:385.
13. Zitelli JA. The bilobed flap for nasal reconstruction. Arch Dermatol 1989;125:957.
14. Rieger RA. A local flap for repair of the nasal tip. Plast Reconstr Surg 1967;40(2):285–93.
15. Marchac D, Toth B. The axial frontonasal flap revisited. Plast Reconstr Surg 1985;76(5):686–94.
16. Seyhan T. The figure of eight radix nasi flap for medial canthal defects. J Craniomaxillofac Surg 2010;38(6):455–9.
17. Mangold V, Lierse W, Pfeifer G. The arteries of the forehead as the base is of nasal reconstruction with forehead flaps. Acta Anat (Basel) 1980; 107:18.
18. McCarthy JG, Lorenc ZP, Cuting L, et al. The median forehead flap revisited: the blood supply. Plast Reconstr Surg 1985;76:866.
19. Shumrick KA, Smith TL. The anatomic basis for the design of forehead flaps in nasal reconstruction. Arch Otolaryngol Head Neck Surg 1992;118:373.
20. Park SS. Reconstruction of nasal defects larger than 1.5 centimeters in diameter. Laryngoscope 2000; 110(8):1241–50.
21. Johnson TM, Swanson NA, Baker SR, et al. The Rieger flap for nasal reconstruction. Arch Otolaryngol Head Neck Surg 1995;121(6):634–7.
22. Baker SR. Reconstruction of the nose. In: Baker SR, editor. Local flaps in facial reconstruction. 3rd edition. Philadelphia: Mosby; 2014. p. 415–80.
23. Zimbler MS, Thomas JR. The dorsal nasal flap revisited: aesthetic refinements in nasal reconstruction. Arch Facial Plast Surg 2000;2:285–6.
24. De Fontaine S, Klaassen M, Soutar DS. Refinements in the axial frontonasal flap. Br J Plast Surg 1993; 46(5):371–4.
25. Rohrich RJ, Muzaffar AR, Adams WP. The aesthetic dorsal nasal flap: rationale for avoiding a glabellar incision. Plast Reconstr Surg 1999;104(5):1289–94.
26. Baker SR. Melolabial flaps. In: Baker SR, editor. Local flaps in facial reconstruction. 3rd edition. Philadelphia: Mosby; 2014. p. 231–67.
27. Yellin SA, Nugent A. Melolabial flaps for nasal reconstruction. Facial Plast Surg Clin North Am 2011;19: 123–9.

28. Baker SR, Johnson TM, Nelson BR. The importance of maintaining the alar facial sulcus in nasal reconstruction. Arch Otolaryngol Head Neck Surg 1995; 121(6):617–22.

29. Millard DR Jr. Reconstructive rhinoplasty for the lower half of a nose. Plast Reconstr Surg 1974; 53(2):133–9.

30. Baker SR. Interpolated paramedian forehead flaps. In: Baker SR, editor. Local flaps in facial reconstruction. 3rd edition. Philadelphia: Mosby; 2014. p. 268–316.

31. Reece EM, Schaverein M, Rohrich RJ. The paramedian forehead flap: a dynamic anatomical vascular study verifying safety and clinical implications. Plast Reconstr Surg 2008;121(6):1956–63.

32. Thomas JR, Griner N, Cook TA. The precise midline forehead flap as a musculocutaneous flap. Arch Otolaryngol Head Neck Surg 1988;144(1):79–84.

33. Bloom JD, Ransom ER, Miller CJ. Reconstruction of alar defects. Facial Plast Surg Clin North Am 2011; 19:63–83.

34. Immerman S, White WM, Constantinides MW. Cartilage grafting in nasal reconstruction. Facial Plast Surg Clin North Am 2011;19:175–82.

35. Burget GC, Menick FJ. Nasal reconstruction: seeking a fourth dimension. Plast Reconstr Surg 1986;78:145.

36. Park SS, Cook TA, Wang TD. The epithelial "turn in" flap in nasal reconstruction. Arch Otolaryngol Head Neck Surg 1995;121:1122–7.

Reconstruction of Mohs Defects of the Lips and Chin

Yuna C. Larrabee, MD, Jeffrey S. Moyer, MD*

KEYWORDS

- Lip reconstruction • Chin reconstruction • Cutaneous defects • Lip neoplasms • Local flaps
- Cutaneous malignancy • Mohs micrographic surgery

KEY POINTS

- The cutaneous and mucosal lips are critical structures of the face performing a vital role in oral function and competence as well as overall facial aesthetics.
- Attention to the aesthetic boundaries of the lip, cheek, and nasal subunits will result in the best reconstructive outcomes of the perioral region.
- Revision surgery, including Z-plasty, is often necessary to achieve the best long-term results.

INTRODUCTION

The lips are prominent facial features important for both functional and aesthetic aspects of daily life. Defects from Mohs micrographic surgery can alter the normal lip appearance and impact patients' self-image and their quality of life. Successful repairs encompass both functional and aesthetic concerns. The goals of reconstruction are the restoration of oral competence, maintenance of oral opening, restoration of normal anatomy, and provision of an acceptable aesthetic outcome.[1]

Defects of the lip are challenging to reconstruct for several reasons. There is an increase in the risk of anatomic distortion through increased wound contraction due to the lack of a substantial fibrous framework. The area is under constant motion, and wound contracture can lead to poor functional and aesthetic outcomes. As the lips are within the observational center of the face, even minor lip defects require meticulous reconstruction to minimize the distraction caused by the defect.[2] A review by Coppit and colleagues[1] in 2004 found no major advances in lip reconstruction but,

rather, continued advances in already accepted techniques. When reconstructing the cutaneous lip, it is preferable to confine tissue movement within the aesthetic region of the lips, unless this causes distortion of adjacent structures, such as the melolabial crease.[3] Local flaps generally provide the best match for the quality of the skin and mucosa of the lips. The focus of this article is on local tissue transfer for primarily cutaneous defects after Mohs surgery.

ANATOMIC CONSIDERATIONS

The lips are a major component of the lower third of the face. The lip encompasses the area from the subnasale to the mental crease and from commissure to commissure (**Fig. 1**). The lips are divided into the cutaneous, vermilion, and mucosal parts. Vermilion is specialized mucosa that covers the lips. Vermilion is divided into the dry (external) and wet (internal) vermilion. The white lip, or cutaneous lip, is made up of the non-vermilion skin surrounding the lip. The cutaneous lip extends from the nasal base superiorly, to the

Disclosure Statement: The authors have nothing to disclose.

Division of Facial Plastic and Reconstructive Surgery, Department of Otolaryngology–Head and Neck Surgery, University of Michigan, Taubman Center Floor 1 TC1904, 1500 East Medical Center Drive, Ann Arbor, MI 48109, USA

* Corresponding author.

E-mail address: Jmoyer@med.umich.edu

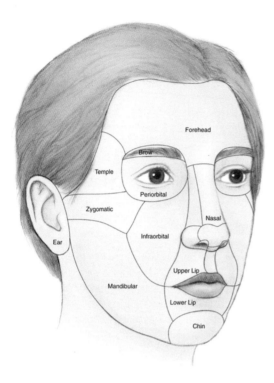

Fig. 1. Aesthetic units of the face. (*From* Bradley DT, Murakami CS. Reconstruction of the cheek. In: Baker SR, editor. Local flaps in facial reconstruction. 2nd edition. St Louis (MO): Mosby; 2007. p. 526; with permission.)

by the philtral groove. The upper lip consists of a medial and 2 lateral subunits, demarcated by the philtral ridges and the nasolabial folds (**Fig. 2**).

Each lip is composed of the orbicularis oris muscle that is invested by skin and subcutaneous tissue externally, by mucosa and submucosa intraorally, and the vermilion over its free edge. The lips contain a circular muscular structure, the orbicularis oris, that is pulled into an oval by radially oriented cheek suspensory muscles (**Fig. 3**).[4] All of these muscles are innervated by the facial nerve. The second division of the trigeminal nerve via the infraorbital nerve provides sensory innervation to the upper lip, and the third division of the trigeminal nerve via the inferior alveolar nerve provides sensory innervation to the lower lip and chin. The arterial supply of the lips is the labial artery, which is a branch of the facial artery. Veins follow the arteries.

Functional considerations for repair include maintenance of oral competence for facilitation of oral intake, containing secretions, articulation, kissing, smiling, and expressing emotion. The lips are essential for phonation of the letters M, B, and P. Aesthetic considerations include symmetry, normal anatomic proportions, presence of a philtrum, normal oral commissures, and the presence of a vermilion-cutaneous white border. Other considerations are the age, general state of health of patients, previous treatment, tissue laxity, and dental status.[1]

labiomental crease inferiorly, and the nasolabial folds laterally. The lower lip acts as a dynamic dam to retain saliva and prevent drooling.[4] The lips are defined by the red-white vermilion-cutaneous border. The white roll separates the skin and vermilion, whereas the red line separates the dry vermilion from the wet vermilion or intraoral labial mucosa. Cupid's bow is composed of the apices of the upper lip and central depression and is of variable prominence. The medial upper lip vermillion prominence is the tubercle. The philtral columns extend up to the columella, separated

PRIMARY REPAIR

The preferred method for reconstruction of most cutaneous tumors of the lip is fusiform excision and primary wound repair. Small defects of the cutaneous lip can be closed with elliptical excision with primary closure. The fusiform excision should be oriented with its long axis parallel to the relaxed skin tension lines if possible (**Fig. 4**). M-plasty can aid in closure that does not cross aesthetic borders of the lips or into the vermilion.

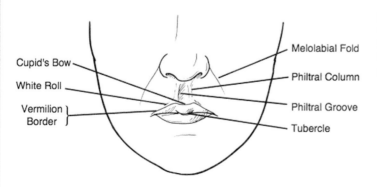

Fig. 2. Surface anatomy of the lip. (*From* McCarn KE, Park SS. Lip reconstruction. Facial Plast Surg Clin North Am 2005;13:302; with permission.)

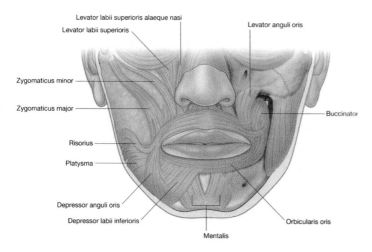

Fig. 3. Lip musculature. (*From* Drake RL, Vogl W, Mitchell AWM. Gray's anatomy for students. Philadelphia: Churchill Livingstone; 2005; with permission.)

Mucosal Lip

Labial mucosal advancement flap

Defects involving the vermilion only can be reconstructed with a labial mucosal advancement flap (**Fig. 5**). Mucosal incisions are made toward the gingivobuccal sulcus, and mucosa is elevated off of the orbicularis oris muscle.[2] The flap has a 2:1 length-to-width ratio, and a back cut is included if needed to allow for advancement of the flap into the defect.[5] A pedicled orbicularis oris flap can be rotated into the base of the defect if muscle was removed with tumor and the mucosal flap does not provide sufficient bulk.[2] A free buccal mucosal flap can be used for coverage of nonvisible portions of the mucosal defect and for coverage of the mucosal donor site.[2]

Central Cutaneous Lip

Advancement flap

Cutaneous lip advancement flaps are most commonly used to reconstruct central cutaneous lip defects.[3] Dissection is in the subcutaneous plane superficial to the orbicularis oris and facial

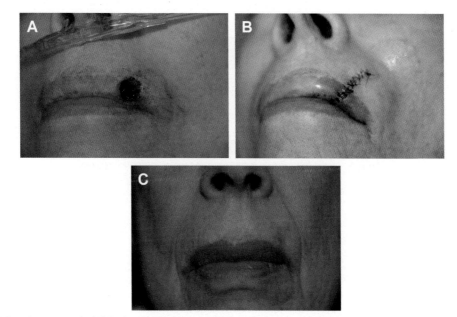

Fig. 4. Lip primary repair. (*A*) Patient with a 1 cm defect of the left upper lip that is crossing the vermilion. (*B*) A mucosal advancement flap was created in the lower lip by dissecting the mucosa off of the orbicularis oris circumferentially around the defect. Undermining was also performed circumferentially around the cutaneous portion of the defect. The vermillion was matched precisely, and standing cutaneous deformities were removed superiorly in the skin and inferiorly in the mucosal portion of the lip. (*C*) Postoperative appearance.

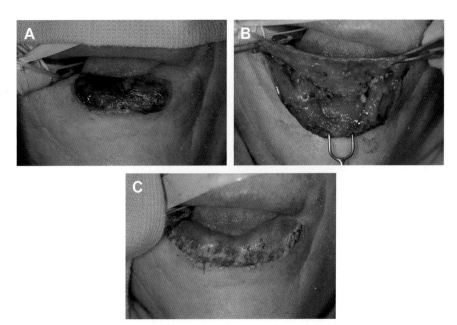

Fig. 5. Lip mucosal advancement flap. (*A*) Patient with a 4.3 cm × 2.0 cm lip defect after Mohs micrographic surgery for a squamous cell carcinoma of the midline lip. (*B*) A large mucosal advancement flap was elevated down to the gingivolabial sulcus. Standing cutaneous deformities were removed in the leading edge laterally. (*C*) The wound was closed with interrupted 4-0 chromic, and then a running 5-0 fast gut was used to attach the skin to the mucosa.

muscles.[3] As the flap is advanced medially, its base often overlaps the oral commissure; this redundancy of skin may require excision.[3] With medial advancement of the flap, the oral commissure may be pulled superiorly or inferiorly. The displacement of the oral commissure may be self-correcting as the natural pulling of the lip musculature causes a corrective adjustment over time (**Fig. 6**).[3]

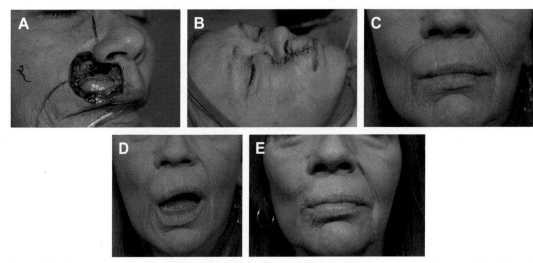

Fig. 6. Lip advancement flap. (*A*) Patient with extensive squamous cell carcinoma of the right upper lip with perineural involvement. (*B*) The closure of the full-thickness central portion of the defect was performed with mucosal advancement flaps. The lip defect was closed with a large lateral lip and cheek advancement flap with the standing cutaneous deformity being removed superiorly in the peri-alar region. (*C, D*) Postoperatively, a lip asymmetry was present from loss of buccal nerve function. (*E*) Two years postoperatively after a right scar revision Z-plasty and cheek lift to reestablish right melolabial crease. Four years postoperatively after the original lip advancement.

H-plasty (bilateral unipedicled advancement flaps)

An H-plasty is another option if primary closure or advancement does not provide suitable tissue volume for closure (**Fig. 7**). For the upper lip, incisions for opposing advancement flaps are made along the vermilion-cutaneous border and immediately below the nasal sill (**Fig. 8**).[6] For the lower lip, incisions are placed in the vermilion-cutaneous border and the mental crease.[6] The skin of the lip must be dissected off of the underlying orbicularis oris. Removal of a Burrow triangle from the vermilion is usually necessary to prevent excess bunching with approximation of the opposing borders of the two advancement flaps.[6]

Lateral Cutaneous Lip

V-Y flap

V-Y subcutaneous tissue pedicle island advancement flaps are ideal for repair of defects of the lateral cutaneous upper lip and take advantage of the mobility of the fat and skin in the lower, lateral face.[6] The flap is designed as a loose variation of an isosceles triangle, whereby the base is adjacent to the defect and the equal sides of the triangle are designed to meet in the melolabial crease inferiorly and laterally.[6] The base of the triangle is the height of the defect, and the height of the triangle is 2 times the width of the defect (**Fig. 9**). The perimeter of the skin island is incised to the level of subcutaneous tissue laterally, and the flap is freed from orbicularis oris muscle attachments near the commissure. Dissection is continued through subcutaneous tissue surrounding the skin island, beveling slightly away from the skin island down to the level of the fascia overlying the facial musculature.[6] The pedicle can be narrowed to aid in advancement of the skin island toward the defect. Narrowing of the pedicle is performed by back-cutting the peripheral borders of the flap in a subcutaneous plane, leaving at least the central one-third of the total flap surface attached to the underlying subcutaneous tissue

to allow for adequate perfusion of the flap.[6] Thinning of the leading border of the flap may be performed to match the recipient site. Subcutaneous undermining is performed at the recipient site of the skin adjacent to the flap if puckering of the peripheral facial skin occurs with flap mobilization.[6] After advancing the flap into the recipient site, the secondary defect is closed by advancement in a horizontal vector.[6] A vertical vector should be avoided to prevent upward distortion of the vermilion (**Fig. 10**).[7]

O-T flap

An O-T flap is a modification of the H-plasty flap (**Fig. 11**). Instead of 2 parallel incisions, only one incision is made on opposing sides of the defect. The two flaps are advanced and slightly pivoted toward each other to repair the defect, leaving a standing cutaneous deformity on the opposite side of the two incisions. The cutaneous deformity is excised and the wound repaired with a final suture line forming a T configuration. The vertical limb of the T represents the excision of the standing cutaneous deformity. The main advantage is that the horizontal limb of the O-T flap can be placed parallel to important aesthetic boundaries or structures (ie, the vermillion border, eyebrow, and so forth) without causing movement or distortion (**Fig. 12**). The O-T flap has just one incision with fewer scars than the parallel incisions for used in an H-plasty flap.

An O-T flap is an effective method of reconstructing lateral cutaneous lip defects adjacent to the vermilion.[6] With an O-T flap repair of cutaneous lip defects, excision of standing cutaneous defects of the vermilion are not always necessary and may be distributed in the horizontal closure by slightly lengthening the incision. Most of the incision lines remain on the cutaneous lip. Bilateral incisions are made along the vermilion margin at the defect base, which comprise the two horizontal limbs of the O-T flap. The superior border of the defect opposite the vermilion is excised to remove

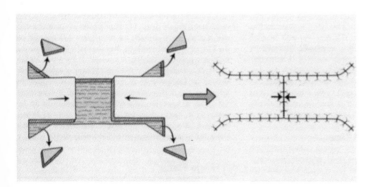

Fig. 7. H-plasty design. Bilateral advancement flaps combined to repair a defect resulting in an H-shaped wound. The arrows indicate the direction of maximum tension. (*From* Baker SR. Flap classification and design. In: Baker SR, editor. Local flaps in facial reconstruction. 2nd edition. St Louis (MO): Mosby; 2007. p. 91; with permission.)

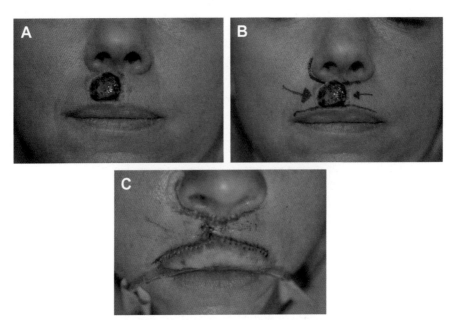

Fig. 8. Lip H-plasty flap. (*A*) Patient with a 2 cm (in diameter) right upper lip Mohs defect. (*B*) Planned incision lines marked along the vermilion-cutaneous border and immediately below the nasal sill and on the right extending into the alar facial sulcus. The *arrows* depict the vectors of advancement. (*C*) Vertical mattress sutures using 5-0 Prolene were placed to close the vertical limb of the H-plasty.

a triangle of tissue, which represents the standing cutaneous deformity that will form from advancement of the two flaps.[6] This excision converts the round defect into a triangular one. Wide undermining in the subcutaneous plane of adjacent skin lessens wound closure tension and minimizes the risk of philtrum distortion.[6] After the flaps have been advanced and secured, the Burrow triangles are excised, if required, at the most medial and lateral aspects of the horizontal flap limbs.[6]

Rotation flap

Cutaneous lip rotation flaps are most frequently used to reconstruct lateral lip defects.[3] Skin is moved medially from the area immediately lateral to the defect. The rotation advancement flap is designed so the lateral border of the flap is in or parallel to the melolabial crease. The inferior aspect of the flap can extend below the level of the oral commissure. The width of the flap should provide sufficient tissue to reconstruct

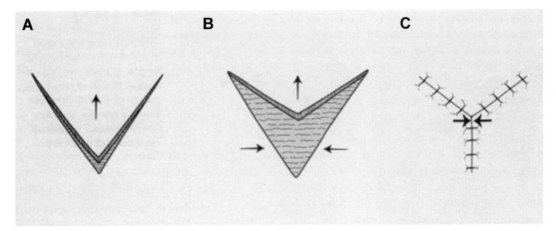

Fig. 9. V-Y advancement flap design. (*A, B*) The V-Y advancement flap achieves advancement by recoil or by being pushed forward. It is not stretched or pulled toward the defect. The wound closure forms a Y-shaped configuration. (*C*) The arrows indicate the direction of maximum tension. (*From* Baker SR. Flap classification and design. In: Baker SR, editor. Local flaps in facial reconstruction. 2nd edition. St Louis: Mosby; 2007. p. 92; with permission.)

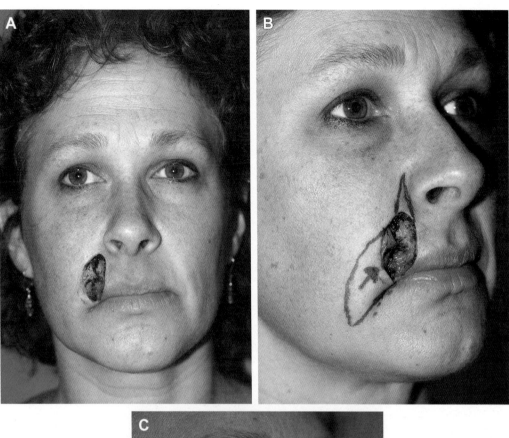

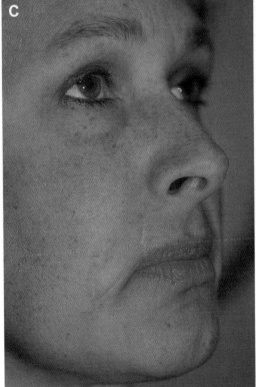

Fig. 10. V-Y advancement flap. (*A*) Patient with a right upper lip Mohs defect measuring 3.3 cm × 3.0 cm. (*B*) A standard V-Y advancement flap was designed. The *arrow* depicts the vector of advancement. The standing cutaneous deformity is also marked in the nasal facial crease. Portions of the mucosal lip were then advanced to recreate the vermillion cutaneous border. (*C*) Postoperative appearance.

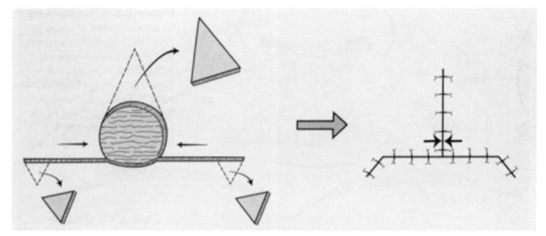

Fig. 11. O-T flap (or T-plasty) design. O-T flaps require 2 flaps advanced toward each other. Standing cutaneous deformity excised at the vertical limb of the T. Arrows represent the point of greatest wound tension. (*From* Baker SR. Advancement flaps. In: Baker SR, editor. Local flaps in facial reconstruction. 2nd edition. St Louis (MO): Mosby; 2007. p. 161; with permission.)

the vertical height of the lip.[3] Adequate flap width is obtained by extending the lateral border of the flap laterally into the cheek. Dissection is in the subcutaneous tissue plane superficial to the orbicularis oris and facial muscles.[3] The lateral wound border is longer than the medial wound border, which can be remedied by equally dividing the skin redundancy during closure.[3] If

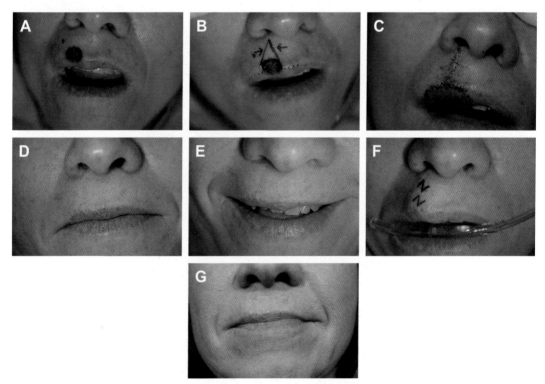

Fig. 12. O-T flap. (*A*) Patient with a 1.3 cm × 0.9 cm defect of the upper cutaneous and dry vermilion. (*B, C*) An O to T advancement flap was created to close the cutaneous portion of the defect. The *arrows* depict the vectors of advancement. The standing cutaneous deformity was removed superiorly up to the nasal sill. A mucosal advancement was elevated over the orbicularis oris muscle to repair the vermilion defect. (*D, E*) Postoperative appearance showing a slightly depressed scar and malalignment of the vermilion cutaneous junction. (*F*) Two Z-plasties designed for scar revision. Direct excision of scar at the vermilion-cutaneous junction. (*G*) Postoperative appearance 2 years after the scar revision and 3.5 years after the O-T plasty.

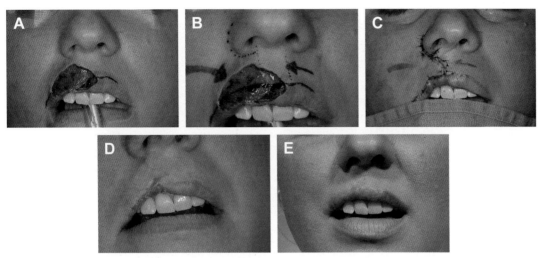

Fig. 13. Lip rotation-advancement flap. (*A*) Patient with a cutaneous and mucosal lip defect measuring 3.4 cm × 1.3 cm. (*B*) Markings showing planned mucosal advancement flap, with *arrows* depicting the vectors of advancement; left lip advancement flap closure of the 1 cm × 1 cm left medial lip defect; rotation advancement flap closure from the right cheek of a 2.4 cm × 0.5 cm cutaneous lip defect of the right lip lateral to the right philtral column. (*C*) Closure closed deeply with 5-0 Monocryl; vertical portion of the lip was closed with vertical mattress of 5-0 nylon, and then the peri-alar crescent in the right alar groove was closed with a combination of vertical mattress and 5-0 nylon. (*D*) Postoperative appearance before surgeries done to correct lip volume. (*E*) Postoperative appearance 4 months after an upper lip implant and lip expander.

required, small Burrow triangles can be excised (**Fig. 13**).

Note flap

A note flap is a transposition flap that can be used to repair lateral cutaneous lip defects. This flap for lip repair takes advantage of the mobile skin and fat in the inferomedial cheek. The note flap was described by Walike and Larrabee, Jr[8] as an angular transposition flap with a design that resembles a musical eighth note. A note flap allows closure of a circular defect with a triangular transposition flap (**Fig. 14**). An advantage of note flaps is a decreased likelihood

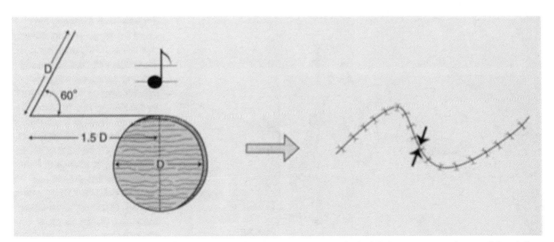

Fig. 14. Note flap design. The note flap is designed to look like a musical eighth note. It can be used for defects that are less than 2 cm in size. One side of the flap is drawn parallel to relaxed skin tension lines and in a tangent to the defect. This line should measure 1.5 times the diameter of the defect. The second side of the flap forms a 50° to 60° angle with the first side and is the same length as the diameter of the defect. The arrows indicate the direction of maximum tension. (*From* Baker SR. Transposition flaps. In: Baker SR, editor. Local flaps in facial reconstruction. 2nd edition. St Louis (MO): Mosby; 2007. p. 137; with permission.)

of trap door defects because of the angular closure.

The flap is designed by drawing a tangent on one side of the circle parallel to relaxed skin tension lines.[9] The length of the tangent is 1.5 times the diameter of the circular defect.[9] The angle of the note flap is 50° to 60°, and the second side of the flap has a length equal to the diameter of the circle.[10] The flap is transposed into the defect. Clinical judgment is necessary in using this flap, as the note flap is designed to be 25% less than the area of the defect.[9] The greatest wound closure tension is at the closure of the donor site and approximately perpendicular to the tangent line.[9] The pivotal arc is 45°; thus, a minimal standing cutaneous deformity develops that may not require excision (**Fig. 15**).[9]

Full-Thickness Defects

Small-sized full-thickness lip defects

In general, if a full-thickness lip defect involves less than 30% of the width of the lip, reconstruction can consist of a *wedge excision and primary repair*. Success of this technique is increased if cutaneous lip is excised along with vermilion lip for tension-free closure (**Fig. 16**).[4] Primary repair of the upper lip often requires excision of perialar crescents to facilitate medial movement of the labial edges.[4] The apex of lower lip excisions should not pass the mental crease, whereas the apex of upper lip excisions should not pass the melolabial crease.[1] An M-plasty can be quite useful in either of these situations to prevent the standing cutaneous deformity from extending past important anatomic borders. Mucosa, muscle, and skin are re-approximated in a 3-layer

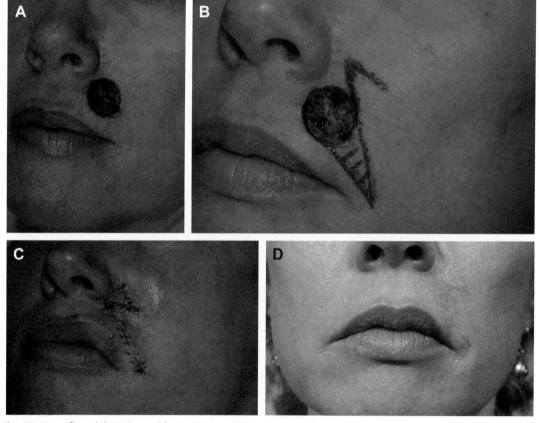

Fig. 15. Note flap. (*A*) Patient with a 1.5 cm × 2.0 cm Mohs defect of the left upper lip. (*B*) Note flap design. Striped area depicts the standing cutaneous deformity requiring excision. (*C*) The defect was widely undermined, and then a laterally based note flap was elevated and transposed into place. Standing cutaneous deformity was then taken along the left melolabial fold. (*D*) Postoperative appearance 2 months after a scar revision for a widened scar and 11 months after the note flap.

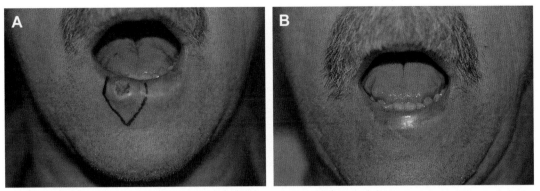

Fig. 16. Lip wedge excision with primary repair. (*A*) Wide local excision measuring 1.5 cm × 3.0 cm. A 0.5 cm margin was marked around the right lower lip squamous cell carcinoma in a wedge-shaped fashion. The muscle layer was closed using 5-0 interrupted PDS (polydioxanone suture). (*B*) Postoperative appearance.

closure. The vermilion edges must be re-approximated precisely as even small irregularities can be conspicuous.[2] Before wedge excision, it is helpful to mark the vermilion.[1] Closure begins with placement of the suture to re-approximate the vermilion border.[2] The orbicularis muscle is closed with absorbable suture, and the exposed and intraoral components of the red lip can be closed with chromic suture.[2]

Medium-sized full-thickness lip defects

The ideal reconstruction of a lip defect that is between 30% and 60% of the horizontal lip is an *Abbe* or *Estlander flap*. The advantage of these flaps is the similarities of tissue texture, muscular composition, and appearance of the donor and recipient site. The Abbe flap is used for defects medial to the oral commissure. The Estlander flap is used for defects involving the oral commissure.

After full-thickness resection from the lower lip, the upper lip triangular full-thickness flap is designed to have the same height as the defect with a width one-half to two-thirds of the defect size.[2] The blood supply to the flap is from the labial artery, which should be preserved when raising the flap. After insetting the flap, the division of the pedicle can be performed after 14 to 21 days (**Fig. 17**).[2]

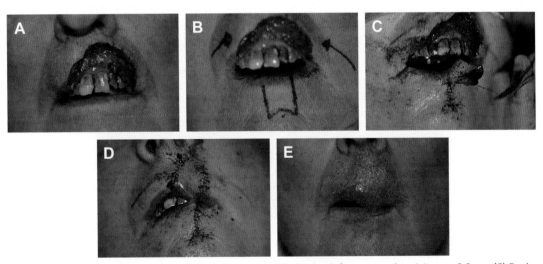

Fig. 17. Abbe flap. (*A*) Patient with a full-thickness upper lip Mohs defect measuring 4.1 cm × 2.3 cm. (*B*) Design of an inferiorly based Abbe flap based medially. Bilateral advancement flaps were used to decrease the width necessary for the lower lip secondary defect. *Arrows* depict the vectors of advancement. (*C*) The lower lip full-thickness Abbe flap on its pedicle is shown. The inferior lip was closed with an M-plasty. (*D*) Inset of Abbe flap. (*E*) Postoperative appearance before the detachment of the flap performed 21 days later.

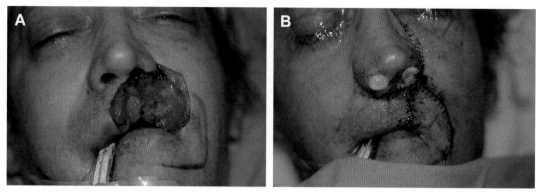

Fig. 18. Estlander flap. (*A*) Patient with a left upper lip basal cell carcinoma with defect measuring 4.5 cm × 4.0 cm. A unilateral Estlander-type flap was designed along the left lip. (*B*) Immediate postoperative result.

The upper lip anatomy is more complex than that of the lower lip. Thus, upper lip defects require special attention. For defects involving more than 50% of the subunit, the entire subunit should be reconstructed.[2] The flap is designed using a template from the intact contralateral subunit (**Fig. 18**).

Large-sized full-thickness lip defects
The Gilles fan flap can reconstruct full-thickness defects involving 70% to 80% of the lip. This flap uses a full-thickness pedicle, allowing for redistribution of the remaining lip (**Fig. 19**).[2] Karapandzic modification uses incisions through only skin and mucosa to preserve the musculature (**Fig. 20**).[2]

Muscle is released as required for closure of the defect by spreading parallel to the muscle fibers.[2]

Commissuroplasty and other revision surgery
Commissuroplasty is performed to correct microstomia or rounding of the commissure that can occur after lip reconstruction. For example, commissuroplasty is generally required after an Estlander flap because the flap causes the commissure to be blunted and rounded. The simplest method of commissuroplasty was originally described by Converse and Wood-Smith[11] as a horizontal full-thickness incision at the blunted commissure extending laterally to have the same horizontal extension as the contralateral side (**Fig. 21**).[3]

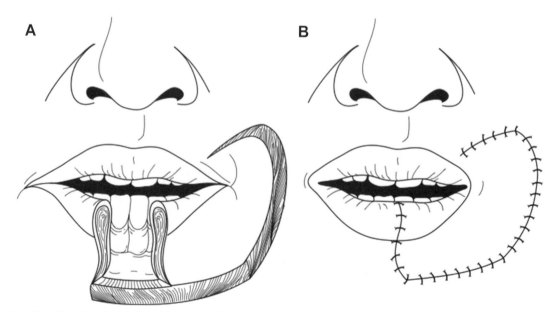

Fig. 19. Gilles fan flap design. (*A*) Defect of the lower lip has been excised. A full-thickness pedicle allows for redistribution of the remaining lip. (*B*) Closure of the incision lines. (*From* Ishii LE, Byrne PJ. Lip reconstruction. Facial Plast Surg Clin North Am 2009;17:451; with permission.)

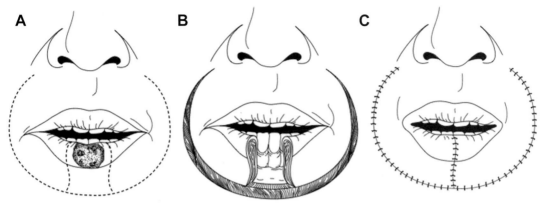

Fig. 20. Karapandzic flap design. (*A*) Planned incision lines with excision of central lower lip defect. (*B*) The incision is placed through only skin and mucosa to preserve the musculature. (*C*) Closure of incision lines. (*From* Ishii LE, Byrne PJ. Lip reconstruction. Facial Plast Surg Clin North Am 2009;17:451; with permission.)

Mucosa is advanced to restore the vermilion. A small triangle of skin and subcutaneous tissue from the commissuroplasty may be removed for a more natural result. However, caution must be taken to avoid oral incontinence.[3]

Scar revision surgery is quite common and is often necessary to achieve the best results after lip reconstructive surgery. Almost all perioral scars can be improved with dermabrasion. Long, vertical scars of the lip in the absence of other rhytids are quite

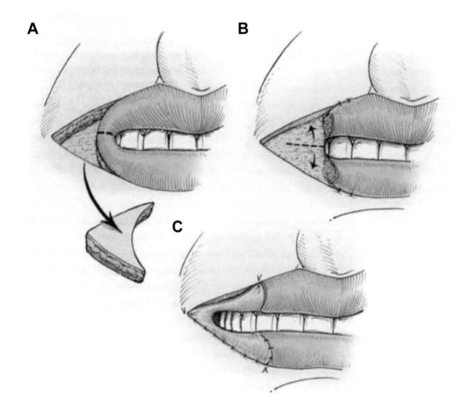

Fig. 21. Commissuroplasty design. (*A*) Small triangle of skin may be excised lateral to distorted commissure. (*B*) Horizontal incision placed through blunted commissure. (*C*) Mucosa advanced superiorly, inferiorly, and laterally to restore vermilion of lips and commissure. (*From* Renner GJ. Reconstruction of the lip. In: Baker SR, editor. Local flaps in facial reconstruction. 2nd edition. St Louis (MO): Mosby; 2007. p. 513; with permission.)

noticeable and are distracting. Z-plasty followed by dermabrasion can be very helpful in improving the final appearance of these scars (see **Fig. 6**E).

CHIN DEFECTS
Anatomy

The chin is the aesthetic unit that confers strength to the face.[12] The lower lip and chin compose two-thirds of the lower portion of the face. The mento-labial sulcus separates the cutaneous lower lip from the chin. The chin is a single subunit of the face and is bordered superiorly by the mentolabial sulcus, inferiorly by the inferior border of the osseous chin, and laterally by the mentolabial crease. The chin is structured by skin, subcutaneous tissue, and the chin muscles. The skin of the chin is the thickest skin of the face with an average thickness of 2.6 mm. This thickness results in poorer scars than other parts of the face with more depressed scarring. The arterial supply to the chin consists mainly of the mental artery, the labiomental artery, and the terminal branch of the submental artery. Motor innervation to the chin is by the facial nerve. Sensation to the chin is from branches of the mental nerve (third division of the trigeminal nerve).

H-Plasty

The classic chin repair for central chin defects is an H-plasty. If possible, one of the horizontal incisions is placed in the mentolabial crease for scar camouflage. One of the disadvantages of H-plasty for chin defects is the lack of naturally occurring skin creases in which to place incisions. H-plasty of the chin is designed in the same fashion as that described earlier for the lip with Burrow triangles excised from the lateral aspect of each flap (**Fig. 22**).

O-T

Central chin defects may be repaired using an O-T flap with a central vertical limb as described earlier for lip defects. Lateral chin defects can also be closed by designing an O-T flap with flaps that are asymmetrical such that more advancement occurs from the lateral chin than the medial chin (**Fig. 23**).

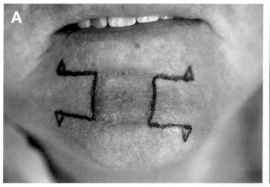
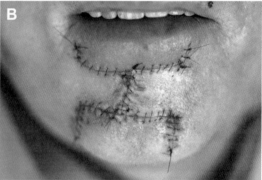
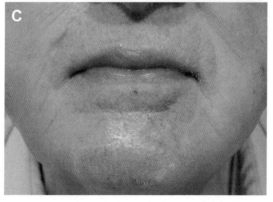

Fig. 22. Chin H-plasty. (*A*) Patient undergoing an excision of anterior chin melanoma measuring 2.5 cm × 2.5 cm. Design of H-plasty with Burrow triangles marked. (*B*) Bilateral advancement flaps elevated and adjacent tissue widely undermined and advanced into the defect. (*C*) The 11-month postoperative appearance.

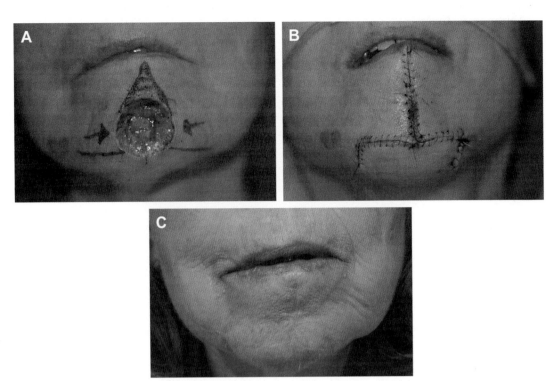

Fig. 23. Chin O-T flap. (*A*) Patient with a 2.8 cm × 2.5 cm defect of the central chin. An O to T closure was designed with the lateral limbs being placed along the jaw line. The striped portion shows a standing cutaneous deformity being removed up toward the lip. The *arrows* depict the vectors of advancement. (*B*) This area was then widely undermined. The vertical incision in the midportion of the chin was at the greatest tension and was closed with vertical mattress sutures to achieve skin eversion. (*C*) The 9-month postoperative appearance.

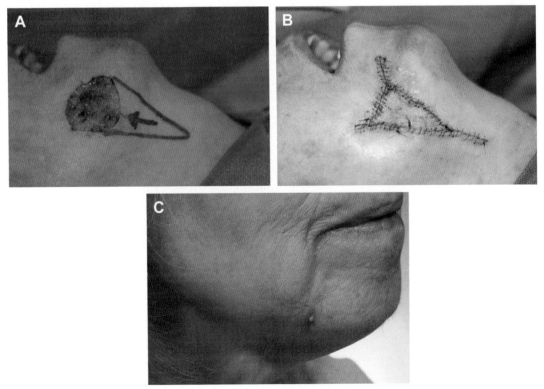

Fig. 24. Chin V-Y flap. (*A*) Patient with a right lower chin Mohs defect measuring 3.0 cm × 2.5 cm. A standard V-Y advancement flap is designed from skin advancing from the neck. The arrow depicts the vector of advancement. (*B*) After wide undermining, the flap was advanced into the defect. (*C*) The 8-month postoperative appearance.

V-Y

V-Y flaps can be used for lateral chin defects. V-Y flaps for chin defects have the disadvantage of fewer natural creases in which to hide an incision. This disadvantage is in contrast to the V-Y flaps explained earlier for lip defects whereby one of the incisions can be placed in the melolabial crease (**Fig. 24**).

SUMMARY

Reconstruction of defects of the lips after Mohs micrographic surgery needs to encompass both functional and aesthetic concerns. The lower lip and chin compose two-thirds of the lower portion of the face. Various flaps exist for repair of cutaneous defects after Mohs surgery. For small defects, elliptical excision with primary closure is a viable option. Lip repair should reconstruct the layers of the lip, including mucosa, muscle, and the vermillion or cutaneous lip. It is especially important to realign the vermillion border precisely for optimal results. Chin defect repair is made challenging by the thicker nature of the skin and tendency for depressed scarring. Reconstructions with local flaps can be improved on by scar revision for optimal results.

REFERENCES

1. Coppit GL, Lin DT, Burkey BB. Current concepts in lip reconstruction. Curr Opin Otolaryngol Head Neck Surg 2004;12:281–7.
2. Ishii LE, Byrne PJ. Lip reconstruction. Facial Plast Surg Clin North Am 2009;17:445–53.
3. Renner GJ. Reconstruction of the lip. In: Baker SR, editor. Local flaps in facial reconstruction. 2nd edition. St Louis (MO): Mosby; 2007. p. 476–524.
4. Langstein HN, Robb GL. Lip and perioral reconstruction. Clin Plast Surg 2005;32:431–45, viii.
5. Nakamura N, Kawano S, Nakao Y, et al. An alternative method for vermilion reconstruction after resection of hemangiomas of the lip. J Oral Maxillofac Surg 2005;63:1239–43.
6. Baker SR. Advancement flaps. In: Baker SR, editor. Local flaps in facial reconstruction. 2nd edition. St Louis (MO): Mosby; 2007. p. 157–87.
7. Skouge JW. Upper lip repair–the subcutaneous island pedicle flap. J Dermatol Surg Oncol 1990;16:63–8.
8. Walike JW, Larrabee WF Jr. The 'note flap'. Arch Otolaryngol 1985;111:430–3.
9. Baker SR. Transposition flaps. In: Baker SR, editor. Local flaps in facial reconstruction. 2nd edition. St Louis: Mosby; 2007. p. 133–56.
10. Larrabee WF Jr. Design of local skin flaps. Otolaryngol Clin North Am 1990;23:899–923.
11. Converse JM, Wood-Smith D. Techniques for repair of defects of the lips and cheeks. In: Converse JM, editor. Reconstructive plastic surgery. Philadelphia: W.B. Saunders Company; 1977. p. 1544–94.
12. Ridley MB, VanHook SM. Aesthetic facial proportions. In: Papel ID, editor. Facial plastic and reconstructive surgery. 3rd edition. New York: Thieme; 2009. p. 119–33.

Reconstruction of Cheek Defects Secondary to Mohs Microsurgery or Wide Local Excision

John E. Hanks, MD[a], Jeffrey S. Moyer, MD[b], Michael J. Brenner, MD[b],*

KEYWORDS

- Cheek • Skin cancer • Mohs reconstruction • Local flap • Facial reconstruction • Melanoma
- Basal cell carcinoma • Squamous cell carcinoma

KEY POINTS

- Cheek tissue is heterogeneous, with differences in skin thickness, mobility, and contour that influence reconstruction approach as a function of individual patient characteristics, and anatomic zone.
- Appreciation of functional and aesthetic regions relative to anatomic location (medial, lateral, periorbital) will improve surgical planning and outcomes.
- Respecting mobile structures (eyelids, lips, and nose), aesthetic landmarks (melolabial fold, orbital rim, malar eminence, hairlines), and vascular supply to the reconstruction are all of paramount importance.
- A diverse array of adjacent tissue transfer maneuvers is available, allowing for artistry in achieving aesthetic facial reconstruction.

INTRODUCTION

When considering the optimal reconstructive options for a particular cheek defect, familiarity with the basic anatomy of the face is critical, including both surface anatomy and contour arising from the underlying bony structures and soft tissues. The general borders of the cheek include the temple, infraorbital rim and lower eyelid, preauricular sulcus (Including borders with the tragus/helix/lobule), mandible, lateral nasal wall, nasal ala, and melolabial fold (upper lip).[1–3] It is also important to consider the physical properties of the skin and underlying tissues to be rearranged, as improper planning may lead to unsightly distortion of facial anatomy.[2,3] This consideration is especially important for the facial creases of the cheek and the regions of the cheek adjacent to the lower eyelid, nasal ala, and lips.[3] As with any facial defect, anatomic subunits and relaxed skin tension lines (RSTLs) play a key role in the selection and orientation of local flap repair for cheek defects. Based on anatomic and structural properties, the cheek may be divided into aesthetic subunits.

Disclosure Statement: The authors have nothing to disclose.
a Department of Otolaryngology–Head and Neck Surgery, University of Michigan Health System, 1500 East Medical Center Drive, Ann Arbor, MI 48109, USA; b Division of Facial Plastic and Reconstructive Surgery, Department of Otolaryngology-Head and Neck Surgery, University of Michigan Medical Center, 1500 East Medical Center Drive SPC 5312, 1904 Taubman Center, Ann Arbor, MI 48109-5312, USA
* Corresponding author.
E-mail address: mbren@med.umich.edu

Facial Plast Surg Clin N Am 25 (2017) 443–461
http://dx.doi.org/10.1016/j.fsc.2017.03.013
1064-7406/17/© 2017 Elsevier Inc. All rights reserved.

Over the years, different investigators have offered various patterns by which the aesthetic units of the cheek may be defined. For instance, Weerda[4] has described division of the cheek into 6 anatomic units, including the upper, medial, and lateral divisions of the medial and lateral cheeks, whereas Bradley and Murakami have partitioned the cheek into medial, lateral (mandibular), zygomatic, and buccal divisions.[3,5] Menick[2] posits that aesthetic cheek units vary from individual to individual and are dynamic based on age, hairline, hairstyle, facial hair, and facial expression. Given the diversity of the cheek subunit, the primary reconstructive goals of cheek defects include restoration of skin color and texture, which are more conspicuous than variations in contour and subunit outline.[2]

We have divided the cheek into the following regions with functional and aesthetic significance: medial cheek, perilabial (buccal) cheek, lateral cheek, and zygomatic cheek. Menick[2] advocates that the subunit principle should be followed whenever possible in reconstruction of aesthetic regions of the face, although slight variations from "normal" are much more forgiving in cheek reconstruction when compared with the nose, lips, and eyelids. Moreover, subtle asymmetries in color, texture, and surface topography are generally less obvious in the cheek because direct visual comparison of one cheek to its paired contralateral unit is limited in most views aside from the direct anterior view.[2] However, if possible, the surgeon should use the contralateral normal subunit as a template to recreate symmetry and the optimal cosmetic outcome.[6] The benefit of en bloc reconstruction of entire aesthetic subunits and/or use of strategic scar placement at aesthetic borders is that resultant raised or depressed scars tend to be more subtle within the natural contours, shadows, and accents of the native facial structure that define subunit borders.[7]

If placement along subunit borders is impossible, defects should be closed with incisions parallel to RSTLs, inherently minimizing skin tension closure, because RSTLs are determined by the elasticity of the underlying tissue and resultant tension on the skin.[3,8] Although skin of the medial and buccal cheek is thicker and mobile, skin of the superolateral cheek is relatively affixed to fascia lying beneath. This fixation owes to various retaining ligaments anchoring the skin of the cheek to underlying bone.[1] Overlying skin is very tightly fixed to the zygoma due to particularly robust retaining ligaments called the McGregor patch.[1,3] The labiomandibular crease is another point of dense ligamentous attachment that is formed from attachments from the mandibular retaining ligament to the overlying skin.[1,3] The topography of the cheek is determined from the aforementioned retaining ligaments and fibrous attachments to the superficial musculoaponeurotic system (SMAS), as well as the underlying facial skeleton, malar fat pad, and the muscles of facial expression.[1,3] In general, larger reconstructions often yield better outcomes due to more robust subdermal pedicle and via en bloc subunit repair. Likewise, deliberate standing cutaneous deformity excision commonly yields optimal results.

The vascular supply to the cheek skin is derived primarily from branches of the external carotid artery and is of critical importance when considering flap design to optimize potential flap viability. The primary arterial supply to the cheek skin is the facial artery and its angular branch.[1,3] Additional arterial contributions to the cheek include the infraorbital branch of internal maxillary artery and the transverse facial branch of superficial temporal artery. There are frequently anastomotic connections between these arteries as well.[3] Branches of these named arteries ultimately supply the dermal and subdermal plexuses that perfuse the cheek skin. The venous drainage of the cheek largely mirrors its arterial supply, including facial vein, superficial temporal vein, and retromandibular vein with drainage into the internal and external jugular venous systems.[3]

If the reconstructive surgeon is also responsible for locoregional control, such as in management of certain cutaneous malignancies, familiarity with lymphatic drainage of the cheek is important for situations in which sentinel lymph node biopsy, neck dissection, or adjuvant therapy is considered. First-echelon lymphatic drainage from the cheek includes submandibular, preauricular, and submental lymph nodes.[3,9] Furthermore, second-echelon lymphatic drainage from the cheek consists of superficial jugular lymph nodes.[3,9]

Until margin status can be determined, avoidance of wound bed/margin distortion is strongly recommended. For lesions with high risk of local recurrence (eg, melanoma, Merkel cell carcinoma, dermatofibrosarcoma protuberans) or in need of immunohistochemistry to confirm the diagnosis, a 2-blade square technique for confirming margins can be used to avoid an open wound while awaiting margin status. Sophisticated tissue rearrangements should be reserved until confirmation of clear margins, particularly in melanomas managed with sentinel lymph node biopsy whose accuracy may be altered via disruption of dermal lymphatics and tissue rearrangement.[2] The wound may be dressed with a bolster or closed via techniques that do not distort the wound margin, including primary closure, healing by secondary intention, or full-thickness or split-thickness skin graft.[2] On the other hand, most nonmelanoma skin cancers, including squamous cell and basal cell carcinoma, have a favorable cure rate with microsurgery, and can be reliably reconstructed during a single-stage procedure.[3] Simpler reconstructive options also may be optimal in patients at high risk for flap or graft failure (for example, heavy smokers, diabetic individuals, patients with severe vasculopathy, or patients at risk of hematoma, such as patients on high-dose antiplatelet or anticoagulant medications) or in patients at risk of developing additional primary lesions at or near the reconstruction (such as immunosuppressed patients or those with strong genetic predisposition to cutaneous malignancies, eg, xeroderma pigmentosa). However, in general, the optimal reconstructive option is often determined based on the location, size, and depth of the cheek defect.

A secondary function of the cheek and upper lip is to serve as a platform for the nose. In general, if cheek defects also involve the adjacent nasal and upper lip subunits, the cheek and upper lip should be reconstructed before and independent from the nasal defect to reestablish the base for nasal reconstruction.[2] Flaps and grafts should be designed with their borders terminating at the nasofacial and alar-facial sulci. Subsequently, portions of the defect involving the nasal sidewall or ala are best reconstructed once the nasal platform is reestablished and healed, allowing any potential distortion from wound contraction to have already declared itself before nasal reconstruction.[2] One exception to this general guideline is the shark island pedicle flap (SIPF), discussed later in this article, which allows single-stage reconstruction of the medial cheek and nasal ala with a single advancement flap without blunting critical sulci.[10]

WOUND PREPARATION

For optimal tissue apposition and eversion of the incisional closure, wound edges are prepared by orienting the wound's incisional axis perpendicular to the skin surface.[3] Following Mohs micrographic surgery, the excisional bed is often saucerized and commonly leaves wound edges oriented at an obtuse angle to the skin surface. These beveled edges are excised at a 90° angle to the skin surface at a depth appropriate for the proposed recipient flap or graft. For defects comprising more than 50% of an aesthetic subunit, the remainder of the subunit may be excised for optimal scar placement along the subunit border although this is done infrequently in practice.[3]

Depending on the defect's size, shape, depth, and location (including the subunits involved with and adjacent to the defect), several aesthetically pleasing reconstructive options are available to the reconstructive surgeon for defects of the cheek. One advantage of skin and soft tissue defects of the cheek is the inherent elasticity and mobility of these tissues in this area, allowing adjacent tissue recruitment, which in general lends to a high degree of reconstructive flexibility.[11–13]

TISSUE HANDLING, FLAP SURVIVAL, DISSECTION DEPTH

The dissection plane of local flaps of the cheek is typically within the subcutaneous plane, with blood supply based on the subdermal and subcutaneous plexus.[14] Alternatively, depending on the desired flap thickness or wound tension, elevation of the flap may be performed in a sub-SMAS plane based on transverse facial artery perforators. For example, Jacono and colleagues[14] demonstrated superior distal flap survival in deep-plane (sub-SMAS) cervicofacial advancement flap elevation in Mohs repair, thereby reducing the risk of distal edge necrosis and potential distortion of adjacent structures from suboptimal scarring. The sub-SMAS technique may also be used to reduce superficial wound tension.[3,14] The study by Jacono and colleagues[14] implied improved flap survival with deep-plane elevation in repair of larger defects, as well as the possibility of improved flap survival in active smokers due to more robust vascular supply. The dissection plane is also critically important in terms of identification and protection of the facial nerve. If the dissection plane is maintained superficial to the parotidomasseteric fascia, the nerve is typically well-protected, although once the flap is elevated anteriorly to the anterior border of the parotid gland, the nerve emerges from the parotid tissue and necessitates careful dissection and identification.[15] For interpolated flaps, V-to-Y flaps, and other circumferential flap designs, preservation of musculocutaneous perforators is also critical.

Flap survival and cosmesis are improved with a variety of basic soft tissue techniques, which include atraumatic tissue handling, such as using sharp skin hooks and sharp retractors for gentle tissue retraction, tissue handling with toothed forceps to avoid crushing, preparation of the wound bed, and maintaining flap moisture with periodic application of moist gauze.[16] Furthermore, the risk of distal wound necrosis also can be limited with avoidance of wound closure under tension, closure of the incisions in layers, and use of pulley sutures when appropriate. Undue tension at the distal point of a large flap may be avoided by anchoring the flap with more proximal tacking sutures before inset of the distal flap. This technique is also particularly helpful in avoiding necrosis. Finally, care should be taken during repair such that wound edges are everted (for which interrupted vertical mattress sutures can be particularly useful), and superficial nonabsorbable sutures should be promptly removed (ideally within 7–10 days) to avoid crosshatching.[16]

HEALING OF CHEEK DEFECTS BY SECONDARY INTENTION, PRIMARY CLOSURE, AND SCAR PLACEMENT ALONG AESTHETIC BOUNDARIES

In general, healing by secondary intention has a limited role, as it tends to lead to suboptimal aesthetic outcomes in cheek defect repair. This approach is generally reserved almost exclusively for small defects of the nasofacial, melolabial, preauricular, or alar-facial sulci. Resultant scars from secondary intention tend to contract and lack requisite convexity to reconstruct defects of the remainder of the cheek, thereby making contracture and discoloration more conspicuous.[17] Conversely, the relative concavity of these prominent sulci often conceals scars well. Primary closure provides an excellent option for small (<1 cm) cheek defects, those nearing aesthetic subunit borders (especially within the nasofacial, melolabial, preauricular, or alar-facial sulci), or those able to be closed parallel to RSTLs.[3]

The amenability of a lesion to primary closure is largely dependent on tissue laxity, but in general is a viable option for defects consisting of 30% or less of the total aesthetic subunit. On the other hand, larger defects often rely on recruitment of tissue from the adjacent cheek or from the neck.[2,15] Elliptical closure can be used to accomplish ideal scar orientation in circular or ovoid defects that commonly arise from micrographic resection.[3,18] Because ample undermining is required to close increasingly large defects, differential or asymmetric undermining is one technique that is often useful to avoid disturbing the natural positions of facial anatomy and for preferential incisional placement within sulci or aesthetic borders.[3] Furthermore, extending incisions to obscure standing cutaneous cones within aesthetic borders is also useful, as is incising intervening tissue between a defect and the nearest anatomic boundary.[3] Primary closure is a good option for defects bordering the nasal sidewall that obscures the closure within the nasofacial sulcus. Likewise, the preauricular crease is useful to conceal lateral cheek defects, and the lateral rhytids offer additional disguise for small superolateral cheek defects with proximity to the lateral

canthus.[3] To better plan for incisional placement in the zygomatic region, the patient can exaggerate the lateral rhytids by clenching the eyes preoperatively, which accentuates the wrinkles along which the closure's linear axis will lie.[3] Additionally, for defects of the medial zygomatic subunit threatening to impinge on the lids or lateral canthus, an M-plasty may be used to shorten the length of the incision, thereby preventing it from distorting the eyelid.[3] In general, flaps transposed, advanced, or rotated toward the eyelids and lateral canthus transmit lateral tension on the lateral canthus and eyelids. This tension and the tissue distortion that results can be lessened by anchoring the flap to the static underlying periosteum surrounding the orbit.[3]

The melolabial fold, the prominent sulcus serving as the boundary between the medial cheek and upper lip, represents another vastly important aesthetic landmark. Although in certain circumstances the melolabial fold provides a reconstructive challenge, it also allows for camouflage of primary closure of small defects. Differential undermining also may be used to preferentially position scars in aesthetically optimal locations.[3] These techniques may be useful for closure of medium-sized perilabial and perinasal cheek defects adjacent to aesthetic boundaries and facial creases or oriented parallel to RSTLs.[3]

Much like primary closure, the leading border of advancement, transposition, or rotational flap closures can be strategically placed within the nasofacial, melolabial, preauricular, and alar-facial sulci by means of excision of intervening tissues to position standing cones and incisions along these borders. The inherent elasticity and mobility of medial cheek tissue adjacent to the defect allows closure of the defect without appreciable tension or distortion of surrounding anatomy while conserving tissue and positioning incisions along aesthetic boundaries. The nasofacial sulcus, alar-facial sulcus, and melolabial crease often provide ideal opportunities to hide defects using this technique.

PERIORBITAL CHEEK DEFECTS AND CONSIDERATIONS FOR LOCAL FLAPS BORDERING THE ORBIT AND LOWER LID

When it comes to maintaining both functional and aesthetic outcomes in cheek reconstruction, eyelid considerations are paramount. Therefore, when planning repair of cheek defects adjacent to the inferior orbital rim, lower eyelid, medial canthus, and/or the lateral canthus, one should anticipate risk for distortion of the eyelid or canthi, as appropriate planning to avoid major functional and aesthetic implications. As a general rule, a vertical downward vector is avoided in proximity of the lower lid. When a local flap is transferred near the eyelids or orbital rim, the border of the flap should be anchored to the underlying periosteum at the orbital rim, medial canthus, and/or lateral canthus to alleviate unwanted tension and reduce the risk of ectropion and lid traction.[3]

For large defects adjacent to the nasal ala, lateral nasal wall, and inferior orbital rim, large cervicofacial flaps and rotational/advancement flaps are often required, and scar concealment presents a unique challenge. In young patients with adequate orbicularis oculi tone, the subciliary line often offers optimal scar camouflage for defects of the perinasal and periocular cheek. In such cases, both the resultant tension vectors imposed by flap transfer as well as the physical properties exhibited by the transferred tissue are primary concerns. Care must be taken in such cheek advancements to avoid ectropion, inferior lid retraction, and chronic lower lid edema. Elderly individuals lacking lower lid tone and robust lymphatic drainage are particularly susceptible to persistent edema.[3] Therefore, patient selection to determine preoperative lid laxity is crucial to avoid functional and aesthetic abnormalities. Neglect of such considerations carries risk of corneal abrasion, keratitis, and even blindness.[3,19]

Several techniques have been described to assess lid laxity, most of which were initially developed for use during preoperative assessment before blepharoplasty.[20] Two such tests include the eyelid distraction test and the eyelid snap test, and these also may be used to screen patients who may be suited for subciliary advancement flaps. In the eyelid distraction test, the lower lid is pulled away from the eyeball and the distraction of the lid from the eyeball should not exceed 6 mm.[20] Alternatively, the eyelid snap test estimates eyelid muscular tone and consists of pulling the lower lid toward the lower orbital rim. A lower eyelid with adequate orbicularis tone should return to the resting position spontaneously. A lower lid with significant laxity may require one or more blinks to return to resting position.[20] An eyelid with normal eyelid snap test should tolerate postoperative scar healing without significant eyelid retraction following advancement flap closure involving the subciliary line. For patients thought to be poor candidates for subciliary advancement flap closure, an alternative option for incisional placement includes the inferior bony orbital rim. This option also maintains aesthetic boundaries (medial cheek and lower eyelid borders) while still placing the incision in an aesthetically inconspicuous location.

Moreover, routine concurrent lateral canthopexy or temporary tarsorrhaphy have also been advocated for advancement flap closures nearing the lower lid to further prevent retraction.[21] Irrespective of the ultimate incisional placement for superomedial cheek defects, the use of suspension sutures to anchor the flap to the infraorbital rim periosteum is recommended to alleviate inferior traction on the eyelid.[3] For further medial support, the superomedial tip of the advancement flap may be deepithelialized and secured to the periosteum of the medial canthal region with dermis-to-periosteum anchoring sutures.[3]

DEFECTS OF THE MEDIAL CHEEK, INCLUDING PERINASAL CONSIDERATIONS

When considering local flap reconstruction for defects of the medial cheek, adjacent skin is most frequently recruited from the inferior and lateral cheek. The medial cheek skin has the most mobility of any skin on the face, which also facilitates tissue advancement and transposition.[3] The most important anatomic considerations for reconstruction of the perinasal and perilabial cheek are avoidance of blunting or distortion of the melolabial crease, nasal ala, alar-facial sulcus, lower lid, and upper lip. Tissue should not be transposed across aesthetic unit borders or anatomically prominent sulci.[17] The importance of the alar-facial sulcus is that it represents the border between 3 independent aesthetic facial units, including the nose, medial cheek, and upper lip.[17] If defects of the nasal ala are improperly reconstructed, such as with transposition of tissue recruited from the medial cheek, both the nasoalar and the alar-facial sulci become blunted, making the natural concavity of these sulci exceedingly difficult to restore.[17]

For defects adjacent to the nasal ala, V-to-Y subcutaneous pedicled advancement closure is particularly useful to maintain the alar-facial sulcus as well as the apical triangle of the upper lip and to camouflage the trailing limb of the closure within the melolabial fold.[12,18] The flap is designed by creating a V-shaped skin flap adjacent to the defect with a subcutaneous tissue pedicle.[7,22] The flap design relies on the well-vascularized subcutaneous fat in the medial cheek.[3] The width of the triangular base should be equal to the width of the defect at its widest point, and the length of the skin triangle should be twice the defect height. However, the length required may be decreased in areas with very mobile skin, such as the lower third of the face, for example in the jowl region. The apex of the triangle is placed within the melolabial crease, and the vector of the flap advancement as well as trailing edge of the resultant Y-closure is oriented parallel or ideally within the melolabial crease. The skin flap is incised to the subcutaneous plane and undermining is carried out to the surrounding 2 cm adjacent to the planned recipient site.[22] The surrounding subcutaneous tissue is dissected down to the level of the fascia enveloping the muscles of facial expression. At least one-third of the skin flap remains attached to the underlying subcutaneous tissue pedicle to maintain adequate vascular supply from perforating vessels. The leading edge is advanced and the trailing edge is then closed in a Y fashion[22] (**Fig. 1**). Considerable advancement of the skin island can be achieved by using the subcutaneous fat pedicle, although the inferior orbital rim is generally considered the superior limit of the V-to-Y flap advancement.[3] One potential downside of V-to-Y advancement closure is its tendency to result in trapdoor deformity, which may require revision in some cases. On the other hand, a major benefit of the V-to-Y design is that apposition of the skin edges of the Y's trailing limb minimizes wound tension at the leading edge. In fact, closure of the V-shaped wound defect into a Y-shape shifts the apex of the defect toward its base and thereby effectively pushes the advancement flap forward. Additionally, Cvancara and Wentzell[10] described the SIPF for single-staged reconstruction of combined nasal alar and melolabial defects. The SIPF is a modified V-to-Y advancement flap, named due to its resemblance to the outline of a shark, that allows for simultaneous reconstruction of a cheek and adjacent nasal defect with preservation of the nasofacial sulcus, apical triangle, and the so-called "perialar concavity." The flap is designed largely in the same fashion as the previously described

V-to-Y closure; however, the advancement flap is designed to encompass the superolateral aspect of the oval defect, which forms the shark flap's "mouth." The flap is advanced and inset by folding of the flap at the at the junction of the medial cheek and ala, which acts to close the shark's "jaws" and thereby recreating the perialar concavity (**Fig. 2**).[10]

Advancement flap closure for defects in the perinasal and perilabial cheek may be used by recruiting skin from the lateral and/or inferior cheek (**Fig. 3**). Tissue advancement is a particularly useful technique that takes advantage of the inherent elasticity and mobility of the cheek skin, which arises from ample subcutaneous fat.[3] Flaps are elevated most commonly within the subcutaneous plane, although they may be elevated in the sub-SMAS plane, as previously discussed.[14] Much like in the alar-facial sulcus or along the melolabial sulcus, the primary goal in reconstructing defects bordering the nasofacial sulcus is to maintain its natural concavity. Consequently, tissue should not be transferred across aesthetic subunits to reconstruct the medial cheek and nasal sidewall, for risk of blunting the nasofacial sulcus.[2] One technique used to maintain the nasofacial sulcus includes attachment of the leading edge of the advancement flap skin to the underlying periosteum in the sulcus using long-lasting tacking sutures.[3]

Local cheek flaps are also useful for reconstructing the medial cheek, including rotational, transposition, or rotational/advancement flaps. For rotational flap closure, the radius and length of the rotational arc, point of pivotal rotation, vector of wound closure tension, and positioning of potential Burow triangles should be carefully planned.[23] In general, to minimize standing cutaneous deformities, the radius of the rotational

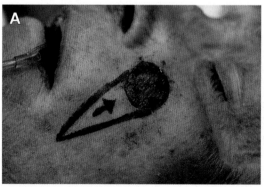
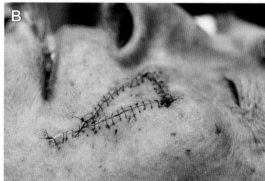

Fig. 1. V-to-Y advancement flap closure of defect using the melolabial fold. (*A*) Flap design displaying advancement vector within melolabial fold. (*B*) Following undermining of defect, at least one-third of the mobilized skin paddle remains attached to the underlying subcutaneous fat pedicle. The leading (superior) edge is advanced across the defect resulting in a Y-shaped configuration. The inferior closure of the "Y" serves to push the flap superiorly and minimizes wound tension on the remainder of the flap.

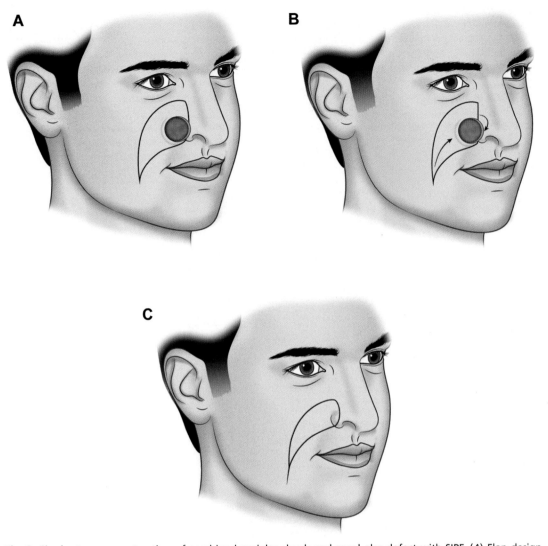

Fig. 2. Single-stage reconstruction of combined perialar cheek and nasal alar defect with SIPF. (*A*) Flap design with height of shark's "snout" denoted by distance *x*, which corresponds with the distance from the native alar sulcus to the medial-most aspect of the wound. (*B*) Modified V-to-Y design with "snout" rotated medially and trailing edge closed within the melolabial sulcus. Rotation of the snout and medial advancement of the remainder of the flap closes the "jaws" of the shark and recreates the alar sulcus. (Not shown) Standing cutaneous deformity is excised superior to the wound to further aid with recreation of the sulcus. (*C*) Flap after inset: incision line arising from medial rotation of the superolateral snout and its apposition with the trailing "lower jaw" demarcates and prevents blunting of the alar sulcus while allowing simultaneous reconstruction of the nasal alar and medial cheek anatomic subunits.

flap should be 2.5 to 3.0 times the width of the defect, and the outer length of the rotational arc is estimated at 4.0 times the diameter of the defect.[3,23] Circular defects are converted to triangular defects with a height approximately equal to the rotational arc's radius to aid with rotational closure. If the rotational flap's pivotal point is moved along a line perpendicular to the defect's vertical axis, the flap assumes a greater advancement component and less rotation, which tends to lessen the development of standing cutaneous deformities. This phenomenon arises because a purely rotational flap relies on closure of 2 incongruent arcs (the arc of the rotational flap is shorter than the recipient arc due to removal of tissue corresponding to the defect).[22] The varying contribution of flap advancement versus rotation is also important in determining the vector of maximal wound closure tension. For rotational flaps with a significant advancement component,

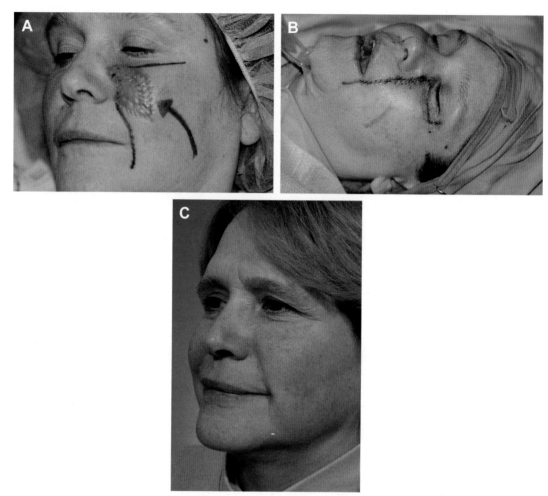

Fig. 3. Advancement flap closure of medial cheek defect. Medial cheek defect closed with inferolaterally based advancement flap. Optimal cosmesis is ensured by incisional placement along cosmetic borders of inferior orbital rim, nasofacial sulcus, and melolabial fold. Risk of ectropion and distortion of mobile facial structures is lessened by use of permanent tacking sutures to the underlying periosteum. (*A*) Square excision for melanoma in situ with design. (*B*) Flap inset. (*C*) Postoperative result.

the maximal tension lies on the distal closure along the base of the flap, whereas for rotational closures lacking advancement, the primary tension vector is tangent to the long rotational arc.[24] Another advantage to the addition of an advancement component to an otherwise strictly rotational flap is that the length of the incision is reduced, which is crucial for cosmesis of the cheek. Another important consideration for rotational flaps is that the base of the arc should be designed inferiorly whenever possible to prevent flap edema that results from transecting the inferiorly based cutaneous lymphatic drainage.[22] Rotational flaps designed specifically for repair of medial cheek defects use an incision extending from the nasofacial sulcus to the melolabial crease (**Fig. 4**).[3] The flap is undermined in the subcutaneous or sub-

SMAS plane, and the standing cutaneous deformity is excised as it develops corresponding to the point of pivotal rotation.[3] To account for the standing cutaneous deformity, additional Burow triangle(s) may be excised. Conversely, Z-plasty and/or back-cuts also may be used to accomplish tissue advancement while obviating or reducing the need for Burow triangle excision (**Fig. 5**).[3] Positioning of the eyelid is a principal consideration for rotational advancement flaps. Therefore, anchoring of the flap with periosteal sutures is highly recommended at both the infraorbital rim as well as at the medial canthal region following deepithelialization of the flap's medial tip. Furthermore, concurrent lateral canthopexy also may be useful to supplement periosteal suturing in prevention of lid retraction.[21]

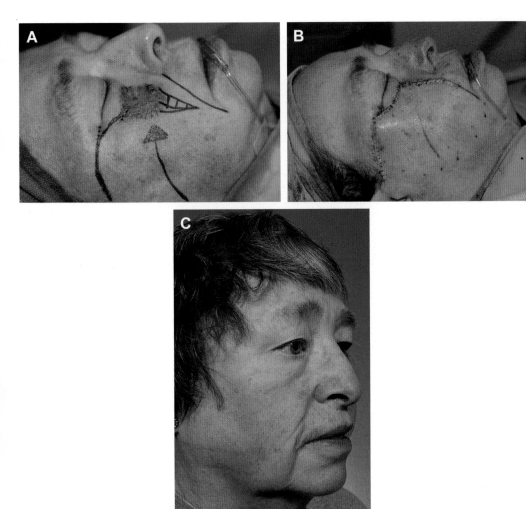

Fig. 4. Advancement flap closure of medial cheek defect with periorbital involvement. (*A*) Flap design demonstrating advancement/rotation of tissue from the lateral cheek and neck with inferiorly based standing cutaneous deformity (effectively converting the defect to a triangle). Optimal cosmetic outcome emphasized via use of subunit borders for incisional placement including the border between the zygomatic cheek and temple, the lateral rhytids, the infraorbital rim, and the melolabial fold. (*B*) Intraoperative flap inset. Horizontal advancement vector and permanent tacking sutures to the periosteum at the infraorbital rim and at the leading edge of the flap near the nasofacial sulcus reduces distortion of lower lid and other anatomically sensitive structures. (*C*) Postoperative maintenance of melolabial fold and nasofacial sulcus and without lower lid tension/ectropion.

For medial cheek defects of in excess of 3 cm, tissue is commonly recruited from laterally in the form of a rotational advancement flap, recruiting large amounts of skin from the lateral cheek and superior neck.[3] When faced with a large defect requiring the recruitment of a large lateral and inferiorly based rotational flap, the resultant curvilinear incision is long and can be challenging to camouflage along aesthetic borders unless planned very carefully. For large cervicofacial flaps, the planned flap incision typically uses the preauricular crease and neck for the arc of rotation, and inferiorly based standing cutaneous deformity is excised and concealed within the melolabial crease.[2,3]

The superomedial aspect of the incision is carried onto either the subciliary line or the inferior orbital rim.[3] For the subciliary incision, the incision is extended laterally to a position above the lateral canthus. This placement accomplishes 2 goals: hiding the incision in the lateral rhytids and providing support for the lower lid against retraction, especially when combined with a lateral canthopexy.[3] The incision is extended from the limb adjacent to the lateral canthus laterally, either outlining or passing through the sideburn before passing in front of the preauricular crease, and finally curving beneath the lobule.[15] At this point, the incision may be carried onto the medial neck

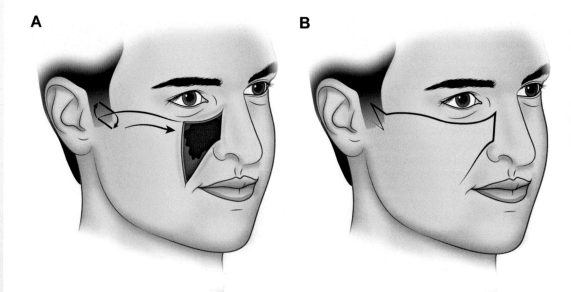

Fig. 5. (*A*) Cervicofacial advancement flap design to address medial cheek defect bordering the infraorbital rim and nasofacial sulcus. Flap design drawn using Z-plasty to assist with flap advancement and standing cutaneous deformity camouflage. (*B*) Cervicofacial flap following advancement and inset, utilizing the nasofacial sulcus, melolabial sulcus, and infraorbital rim to camouflage scar. Buried anchoring sutures to periosteum also recommended to reduce distal wound tension.

or extended into the postauricular sulcus and along the posterior hairline; that is, with use of a facelift incision (**Fig. 6**).[2,3]

For very large defects, the flap may be fashioned as a modified bilobe flap, although this has the disadvantage of introducing an additional suture line if both flaps are transferred to the cheek.[25] The flap derives its blood supply primarily from the subdermal plexus, so the flap may be incised and elevated in either the subcutaneous or sub-SMAS plane depending on the desired thickness and the extent of the contour defect of the recipient site.[3,14] The flap is widely elevated surrounding the defect and including the cheek, chin, postauricular region, and neck down to the level of the clavicle.[15] The flap may be then transferred to the face, and the inferior standing cutaneous deformity can be excised either primarily or at a second-stage procedure. As always, the flap should be anchored to periosteum at the important aesthetic boundaries of the cheek, including the inferior orbital rim, nasofacial sulcus, and near the medial canthus.[3] Additional wound tension and standing cutaneous deformity at the base of the flap can be addressed via Z-plasty, back-cut, or Burow triangle excision.[3]

An additional consideration in planning primarily rotational, advancement, or combination rotational/advancement flap closures, is the number and orientation of the standing cutaneous

deformities. Flaps that rely entirely on an inferiorly based unilateral advancement design develop bilateral inferiorly based standing cutaneous cones. On the other hand, standing cutaneous deformities that arise from rotational advancements occur lateral to the defect and superior to the flap's leading edge, which provides the opportunity to use the subciliary line or the border between the lower lid and cheek at the infraorbital rim for scar camouflage.[3]

For small to moderate-sized cheek defects, transposition flaps offer an additional useful technique that take advantage of the inherent elasticity and mobility of the medial cheek skin.[3] In contrast to advancement flaps, transposition flaps instead minimize distal wound tension by placing the greatest wound tension on the donor site[24,26] (**Fig. 7**).

DEFECTS OF THE PERILABIAL (BUCCAL) CHEEK

Buccal cheek reconstructions often use skin superior to and lateral to the defect. Defects of the buccal cheek not amenable to primary closure are frequently closed with advancement or transposition flaps.[3] Several variations of rhombic transposition flaps may be used for perilabial cheek defects, including the Limberg rhombic flap, as well as the Dufourmental and Webster

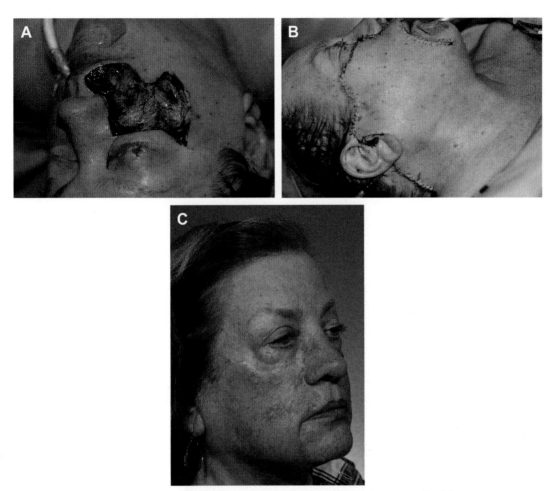

Fig. 6. Cervicofacial advancement flap repair of large multiunit facial defect using facelift incision. (*A*) Large cheek and upper lip defect with periorbital and perinasal involvement. (*B*) Inset of large cervicofacial advancement flap using facelift incision extended to posterior hairline, preauricular sulcus, lateral rhytids, infraorbital rim, alar-facial sulcus, and melolabial fold. Careful dissection maintaining perforating arterial supply improves flap survival and diminishes risk of distal tip necrosis. Diligent respect of the subunit principle yields acceptable cosmetic result. (*C*) Postoperative result with satisfactory scar camouflage and without lower lid tension or distortion of nasal sidewall, ala, upper lip, or oral commissure.

modifications of the Limberg flap.[3] For all rhombic flaps, the defect is first modified to a rhombus shape. It is straightforward to conceptualize the final positioning of scars, and the vector of maximal wound tension can be planned carefully to minimize unwanted tension on cosmetically and functionally sensitive facial structures. The scars are linear and multidirectional, such that some but not all can be oriented at aesthetic boundaries or parallel to RSTLs, potentially crossing the center of anatomic subunits.[27] Scar camouflage is often imperfect in rhombic flaps. However, when unable to place scars in the cosmetically ideal orientation parallel to RSTLs, cosmetic outcome is alternatively optimized by instead orienting the flap borders parallel to lines of maximal extensibility (LME). LMEs run perpendicular to RSTLs and allow the incision to be closed under the least tension, which decreases the likelihood of scar widening and distal flap loss.[28] Finally, an additional technique to optimize final cosmetic outcomes in rhombic flaps that also uses LMEs is to design the flap so that the vector of maximal tension is parallel to LMEs, and this technique may generally be applied to all local flaps.[29]

For the classic Limberg rhombic flap, the defect consists of a rhombic shape with equilateral sides and sets of 2 opposing 60° and 2 opposing 120° angles.[30] The resulting rhombus can be divided into 2 equilateral triangles whose collective base is formed from the defect's short diagonal, which

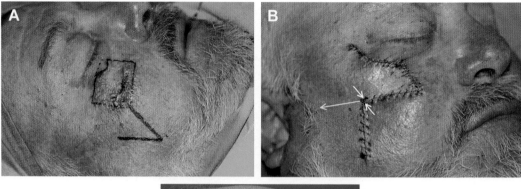

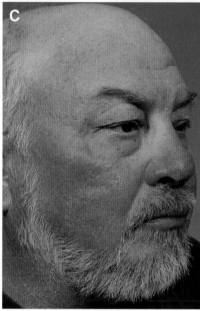

Fig. 7. Limberg (rhomboid) flap repair of periocular cheek defect. (*A*) Rhombic flap design. (*B*) Flap transposed and inset to defect. Point of maximal wound closure tension is indicated by the opposing white arrows. The approximate vector of wound tension is indicated by the yellow arrow. Flap designed with minimal inferior wound tension on the lower eyelid, making the risk of ectropion negligible. (*C*) Postoperative result with preserved eyelid position.

bisects the opposing internal 120° angles.[27,31] Flap design is initiated by drawing a line extending from the short diagonal of the defect to a length equal to itself (which is also equal to the length of all of the other sides of the rhombus). Flap design is continued by drawing a second line parallel to and equal in length to an adjacent side of the defect. The final flap forms a 60° angle at the flap apex and is identical in size to the defect.[27] In total, 1 rhombic defect can be repaired with a potential of 4 different rhombic flaps. The donor site possesses the point of maximal wound tension, whose vector can be approximated as roughly parallel to the side of the defect that is contiguous with the harvest site closure.[27,32] Alternatively, prior calculations have shown donor site tension primarily lies 20° from the defect's short

diagonal.[31] There is minimal tension on other aspects of the flap following inset.[27,33]

An important variant of the classic Limberg flap that is very useful for medium-sized buccal cheek defects is the Dufourmental variant. Whereas the Limberg flap relies on flap design with strict 60° and 120° internal angles, the Dufourmental flap is designed with any combination of paired internal angles.[27,34,35] This flexibility allows more catering of flap design to the shape of the defect and in turn requires less excision of normal tissue to execute the flap.[3] Flap design begins with drawing an extension from the short diagonal and a second extension from one of the sides of the defect. The angle between these extensions is bisected to form the vector of the first side of the flap, whose length is equal to the sides of the defect. Drawn adjacent to the first side of the flap, the second side is equal in length to the first side and defect sides, and is drawn parallel to the long diagonal of the defect. The primary benefit of using the Dufourmental variant compared with the Limberg flap includes reliance on a smaller pivotal arc. This diminishes resultant standing cutaneous deformities, limits resultant wound closure tension, and reduces the potential for unwanted tension on surrounding tissues.[27]

The Webster variant (or 30° rhombic flap) also may be used on the perilabial cheek. The design has components of both the Limberg and Dufourmental flaps. The defect consists of opposing 60° and 30° angles and an opposing set of 135° angles. The 30° angle is drawn opposite the angle that will accept the desired transposition flap. This 30° angle within the defect is frequently modified into an M-plasty that serves to both diminish the height of the defect and to decrease the flap's pivotal movement, thereby reducing the resultant standing cutaneous deformity.[27] This forms an "M" or "W" with two 30° angles separated by a 30° peninsular skin flap.[36] The first limb of the transposition flap is oriented in the same fashion as the Dufourmental variant by drawing an extension from the short diagonal of the defect and a second extension from the side of the defect adjacent to the M-plasty. The surgeon then bisects the angle between these extensions to define the direction of the first side of the flap, whose length is equal to the sides of the defect corresponding to the 60° angle. The angle between the first limb of the flap incision and the defect should be at least 110° to maintain vascular supply to the flap and surrounding tissues.[31] The transposition flap is designed with a 30° apex, and the second limb is drawn to a length equal to the first limb. The aforementioned design of the 30° transposition flap establishes a flap base whose width is approximately 50% of the defect's largest width, and the resultant shape is half of an equilateral triangle.[37] The transposition flap and M-plasty flap are both mobilized and inset into the defect. The 30° angle of the transposition flap allows even distribution of wound closure tension at the donor site. However, the resultant surface area discrepancy between the flap and the recipient site leads to an increased tendency to distort adjacent tissues. This tendency arises because closure requires undermining and advancement of surrounding tissue toward the center of the defect.[32,36]

The note transposition flap approximates a modified rhombic flap that offers an additional reconstructive option for defects of the medial cheek, which is ideally suited for circular defects smaller than 1.5 cm but is useful for defects up to 3.0 cm in size.[3] A benefit of the note flap is that it allows transposition of adjacent tissue while requiring excision of less normal tissue than a rhomboid flap. Design of the note flap is relatively straightforward and consists of drawing a line tangent to the defect to a length of 1.5 times the defect diameter in addition to a second line of equal length drawn at a 60° angle to the first. Following excision of the standing cutaneous deformity at the base of the defect, the flap may be inset into the defect along with primary closure of the donor site limbs[3] (**Fig. 8**). The note flap may be modified into an O-to-Z-plasty, whose design is very similar to the classic note flap, but differs via the addition of standing cutaneous deformity excision opposite the advancement limb altering the simple transposition flap into a modified Z-plasty.

The bilobed flap, most commonly used in nasal reconstruction, is also a versatile reconstructive option for 3-cm to 6-cm circular defects of the perilabial cheek. The bilobed flap is useful for perilabial cheek defects of this size because the limited availability of remaining immediately adjacent tissues typically prohibits repair of both the defect and the donor site without significant distortion of surrounding tissues.[38] The bilobed flap recruits skin from both the lateral preauricular cheek and the postauricular neck (**Fig. 9**).[38] The bilobed flap may be designed in numerous ways, but in general is a double-lobed pivotal transposition flap whose arc of rotation is ideally 90 to 100°. The first lobe is typically designed 45° from the defect axis, and each subsequent lobe is then designed 45° from the previous lobe.[38] However, because of the abundant adjacent donor skin and laxity in the cheek and neck, the surgeon has much more flexibility and may be somewhat less precise in designing the bilobed flap for cheek repair compared with other areas, such as the nose. Depending on the size and location of the defect, the surgeon may orient lobes based on optimal scar camouflage, degree of skin laxity, and availability of donor tissue. In certain circumstances, the second lobe may be oriented as much as 180° from the axis of the defect, with each limb separated by 90°.[39] The first lobe of the bilobed flap is typically located in the preauricular skin and is designed with a diameter 75% to 100% of the defect diameter. The second lobe is designed in the postauricular region and/or upper neck to close primarily and has a diameter smaller than the first lobe.[38] The lobes' skin flaps are dissected in the subcutaneous or sub-SMAS (where available) plane and transposed into the defect and first lobe donor site. The donor site of the second lobe is closed primarily by

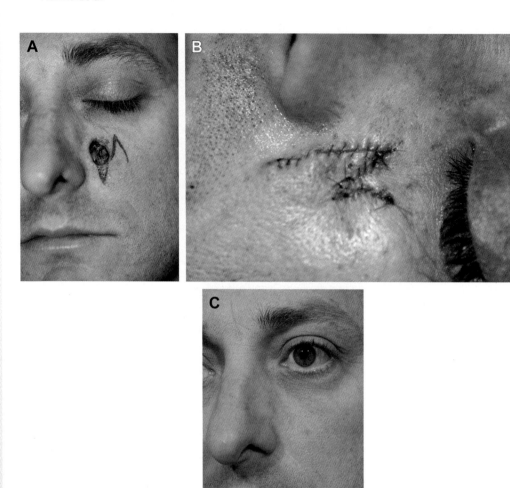

Fig. 8. Closure of small circular medial cheek defect with modified note flap (O-to-Z-plasty variant). (*A*) Design of flap differs from classic note flap with inclusion of inferiorly based standing cutaneous deformity excision. Note flap allows transposition of adjacent tissue while requiring excision of less normal tissue than rhomboid flap. (*B*) Intraoperative flap inset following excision of inferiorly based standing cone and inset. (*C*) Long-term follow-up with well-camouflaged scar.

advancement of adjacent tissues. Much like other transposition flaps discussed for repair of perilabial cheek, the curvilinear flap design, multiple flap limbs, and limited availability of aesthetic boundaries neighboring the subunit create a challenge for discrete scar placement due to irregular incisional borders and relative paucity of options for inconspicuous incisional placement.[38]

Advancement flaps and cervicofacial rotational advancement flaps also may be used for perilabial cheek defects in the fashion previously described for repair of medial cheek defects. Large perilabial cheek defects may be repaired by full-thickness skin grafting if the defect is thought not to be amenable to cervicofacial advancement, rhombic

flap, bilobed flap, or other local flap closure (such as patients lacking sufficient skin quality or laxity). Because skin grafting often lacks good color and texture match to the cheek, a combination of local flap closure and skin grafting may be used to reduce the size of the skin graft needed.[3] Often such skin grafts are excised at later stages to improve tissue match.

DEFECTS OF THE LATERAL/PREAURICULAR CHEEK

The lateral/preauricular cheek is often less conspicuous but presents its own challenges in reconstruction. First, the lateral cheek contains less

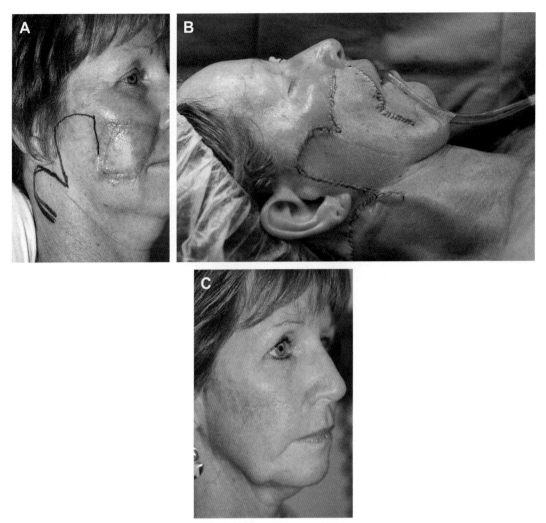

Fig. 9. Bilobed flap repair of large buccal cheek defect. (*A*) Large perilabial cheek defect following square procedure with flap design using a double transposition flap with recruitment of skin from lateral cheek and postauricular neck. (*B*) Flap inset: bilobed flap's double transposition design allows recruitment of large amounts of nonadjacent tissue to repair large defect. Defect's proximity to several high-risk mobile structures including the nasal ala, upper lip, and oral commissure requires large tissue transfer without excessive lateral traction. (*C*) Postoperative following minor surgical revisions including decrease of inferiorly based standing cutaneous deformity.

redundant skin, less subcutaneous fat, and is far less mobile than the medial and perilabial subunits due to underlying retaining ligaments and adherence to underlying parotidomasseteric fascia, as well as the proximity of the ear, which itself is fixed.[1,3,22] On the other hand, the preauricular crease is an ideal border at which scars can be hidden via primary closure, advancement flap closure (including using asymmetric undermining, elliptical closure, and/or excision of intervening normal tissue between the defect and the crease), and transposition flap repair for small lateral cheek defects (<1 cm).[3] The preauricular crease has the added benefit that it often becomes deeper and more pronounced with age, offering added camouflage. Alternatively, the beard-line offers an additional inconspicuous location for scar placement in men, whereas horizontally oriented scars may be routinely hidden within the inferior border of the pretragal sideburn in both men and women.[3]

Lateral cheek defects are often closed with advancement, rotational, or transposition flaps. For defects adjacent to the auricle, the defect may be converted to a vertical ellipse. The surrounding tissue is undermined and closed primarily within the preauricular crease. Similarly, defects not directly bordering the pretragal crease can be enlarged to border the crease and similarly excised via elliptical closure along this border.

Linear advancement flaps of the lateral cheek are designed by advancing superior cervical skin upward, and/or superolateral cheek flap downward, with the posterior incision resting within the preauricular crease. The flap is advanced in the subcutaneous plane, and standing cutaneous deformities at the base of the flap(s) are addressed with the Burow triangle excision, Z-plasty, or back-cuts.[3] Rotational cervicofacial advancement flap closure of medium or large (>3 cm) defects of the lateral cheek relies on advancement of skin from the infra-auricular cheek and the superior neck. Placement within the lateral neck crease affords more mobility of the flap and allows easier closure of the donor site, whereas placement of the incision along the posterior hairline yields superior scar camouflage.[3] The standing cutaneous deformity is excised inferior to the defect along the radius of the flap's arc of rotation. Additional wound tension and the standing cutaneous deformity at the base of the flap can be addressed via Z-plasty, back-cut, or Burow triangle excision.

O-to-T-plasty may be used for medium-sized circular defects or A-to-T-plasty for triangular defects of the lateral cheek. The O-to-T flap is designed using opposing modified bilateral advancement flaps, using only 1 incision tangent to the defect serving as the flap base (ideally positioned within the preauricular crease).[3,13,40] The primary standing cutaneous deformity is excised opposite the flap base and forms the "vertical" limb of the "T," and additional standing cutaneous

deformities that form along the base of the advancement flaps may be addressed as necessary.[13] Whereas the base of the flap is hidden well within the preauricular crease, the "vertical" aspect of the "T" is oriented toward the medial cheek and is not within aesthetic boundaries. However, this limb may be hidden within the lateral rhytids or within the sideburn in some patients with superolateral cheek defects (**Fig. 10**).[3] Alternatively, lateral cheek lesions may be repaired via V-to-Y advancement flaps in a similar manner to those previously discussed.

DEFECTS OF THE ZYGOMATIC CHEEK

The zygomatic cheek subunit covers the zygoma and malar eminence and is bordered by the temple superiorly, the lateral periorbital and perilabial subunits anteriorly, lateral cheek subunit inferiorly, and the ear posteriorly.[3,22] Skin over the zygoma is highly adherent and relatively immobile due to the presence of robust retaining ligaments (McGregor patch).[1] Therefore, donor skin for repair of zygomatic defects is most commonly harvested either superiorly from the temple or from the adjacent perilabial cheek subunit. Importantly, flap design must take both the preoperative position of the lateral canthus and the expected course and depth of the temporal branch of facial nerve as it crosses the zygomatic arch into close account. Extreme care should be taken to avoid placing the vector of maximal wound closure of a flap

A   **B**

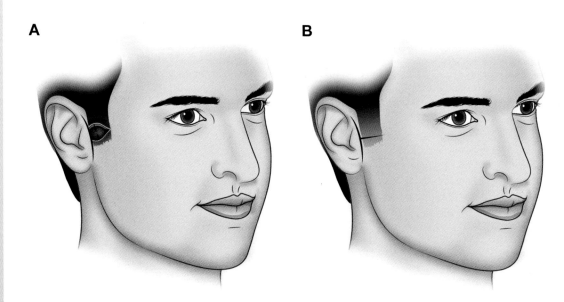

Fig. 10. (*A*) O-to-T-plasty design for closure of lateral cheek defect. Designed to utilize sideburn and preauricular crease to camouflage scars. (*B*) O-to-T-plasty following bilateral advancement and inset.

reconstruction in such a way that distorts the lateral canthus. Furthermore, knowing intricacies of the facial nerve course, its depth, and its branching patterns is also of paramount importance to avoid injuring the nerve. The temporal branch primarily controls the frontalis muscle of the ipsilateral forehead, and deficits include flaccidity of the forehead and ptosis of the eyebrow, which may lead to asymmetric appearance and obstruction of upward visual gaze on the ipsilateral eye.[41] The temporal branch course in the zygomatic region is contained within a triangle with points at the lobule of the ear, lateral brow, and temporal hairline. There are several established landmarks to predict the course of facial nerve as it crosses the zygomatic arch, which represents the most superficial point in its course, including 2 cm posterior to the anterior aspect of the

zygomatic arch, 1.8 cm anterior to the anterior helical rim, or approximately at the mid aspect of the zygomatic arch.[3] The depth of the plane in which the temporal branch runs throughout its course also must be known intimately before operating in the zygomatic region, temple, and forehead regions. The temporal branch courses over the zygoma in the sub-SMAS plane superficial to temporalis fascia and continues in this plane as it passes over the temple before it finally dives deep after piercing the frontalis muscle over the lateral forehead.[41] The dissection plane of flaps in this region is developed within the subcutaneous fat superficial to the temporoparietal fascia and frontalis muscle to prevent nerve injury.[3]

Transposition flaps of the zygomatic cheek also may be performed with success, using techniques such as note flap or rhombic flap closure (**Fig. 11**).

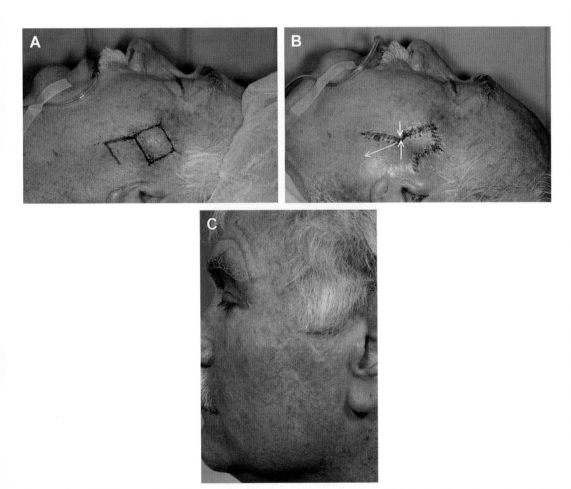

Fig. 11. Rhomboid flap repair of diamond-shaped zygomatic cheek defect. (*A*) Rhombic flap designed with first side of flap extending from short diagonal of defect equal in length to sides of defect. Second line drawn at 60° angle from first and equal in length to defect sides. (*B*) Flap transposed and inset to defect. Point of maximal wound closure tension is indicated by the opposing white arrows. The approximate vector of wound tension is indicated by the yellow arrow. (*C*) Postoperative result. In this individual prone to scarring, changes were most evident at point of maximal tension.

However, the size of the flap should be equal the size of the recipient site due to the relatively immobile skin surrounding the zygoma and malar eminence, as well as the risk of distortion of the periorbital unit. This prevents unwanted wound tension, the need to secondarily advance tissues surrounding the eye, and the risk of flap necrosis in the anatomically sensitive periorbital region.[26] Moreover, the resultant wound tension vector and standing cutaneous deformity orientation should be considered carefully when choosing which flap to use and its potential orientation to minimize distortion and place incisions in the optimal aesthetic location.[3] Care must be taken to avoid recruiting skin from the periorbital region due to risk of eyelid distortion.[3]

Zygomatic defects larger than 3 cm can be closed with a similar array of flaps used to close large defects in other regions of the cheek, such as transposition flaps (eg, bilobed flap), linear advancement flaps, or cervicofacial rotational advancement flaps.[3]

SUMMARY

Across the different regions of the cheek, there is far more variability, in skin thickness, mobility, and contour, than is commonly recognized. This anatomic heterogeneity has important implications for reconstruction after skin cancer removal. Cornerstones of successful cheek reconstruction include deep respect for the eyelid and other readily distorted structures, which is coupled with an appreciation for aesthetic facial units and vascular anatomy. Equipped with an understanding of functional and aesthetic anatomy of the cheek, the surgeon can successfully reconstruct the range of cheek defects with excellent cosmetic and functional outcomes.

REFERENCES

1. LaTrenta, Gregory S. Atlas of Aesthetic Face & Neck Surgery. Philadelphia: Saunders; 2004.
2. Menick FJ. Reconstruction of the cheek. Plast Reconstr Surg 2001;108(2):496–505.
3. Bradley DT, Murakami CS. Reconstruction of the cheek. In: Baker SR, editor. Local flaps in facial reconstruction. Philadelphia: Mosby Elsevier; 2007. p. 521–56.
4. Weerda H. Special techniques in the reconstruction of cheek and lip defects. Laryngol Rhinol Otol (Stuttg) 1980;59:630–40.
5. Kuehnemund M, Bootz F. Reconstruction of the cheek. Facial Plast Surg 2011;27(3):284–90.
6. Menick FJ. Defects of the nose, lip, and cheek: rebuilding the composite defect. Plast Reconstr Surg 2007;120(4):887–98.
7. Burget GC, Menick FJ. The subunit principle in nasal reconstruction. Plast Reconstr Surg 1985;76(2):239–47.
8. Piérard GE, Lapière CM. Microanatomy of the dermis in relation to relaxed skin tension lines and Langer's lines. Am J Dermatopathol 1987;9(3):219–24.
9. Veer V. Surgical anatomy of the head and neck. Janfaza, Nadol Jr, Galla, Fabian, Montgomery. Harvard University Press, 2011. J Laryngol Otol 2012;126(10):1081.
10. Cvancara JL, Wentzell J. Shark island pedicle flap for repair of combined nasal ala-perialar defects. Dermatol Surg 2006;32(5):726–9.
11. Juri J, Juri C. Cheek reconstruction with advancement-rotation flaps. Clin Plast Surg 1981;8:223.
12. Bennett RG. Local skin flaps on the cheeks. J Dermatol Surg Oncol 1991;17(2):161–5.
13. Baker SR. Advancement flaps. In: Baker SR, editor. Local flaps in facial reconstruction. Philadelphia: Mosby Elsevier; 2007. p. 157–87.
14. Jacono AA, Rousso JJ, Lavin TJ. Comparing rates of distal edge necrosis in deep-plane vs subcutaneous cervicofacial rotation-advancement flaps for facial cutaneous Mohs defects. JAMA Facial Plast Surg 2014;16(1):31.
15. Mureau MAM, Hofer SOP. Maximizing results in reconstruction of cheek defects. Clin Plast Surg 2009;36(3):461–76.
16. Wu T. Plastic surgery made easy simple techniques for closing skin defects and improving cosmetic results. Aust Fam Physician 2006;35(7):492–6.
17. Baker SR, Johnson TM, Nelson BR. The importance of maintaining the alar-facial sulcus in nasal reconstruction. Arch Otolaryngol Head Neck Surg 1995;121(6):617–22.
18. Johnson-Jahangir H, Stevenson M, Ratner D. Modified flap design for symmetric reconstruction of the apical triangle of the upper lip. Dermatol Surg 2012;38(6):905–11.
19. Özkaya Mutlu Ö, Egemen O, Dilber A, et al. Aesthetic unit-based reconstruction of periorbital defects. J Craniofac Surg 2016;27(2):429–32.
20. Nerad JA. "Diagnosis and Treatment of Ectropion." Techniques in Ophthalmic Plastic Surgery: A Personal Tutorial. Edinburgh: Saunders Elsevier; 2010. p. 81–98.
21. Jelks GW, Jelks EB. Prevention of ectropion in reconstruction of facial defects. Otolaryngol Clin North Am 2001;34(4):783–9.
22. Baker SR. Flap classification and design. In: Baker SR, editor. Local flaps in facial reconstruction. Philadelphia: Mosby Elsevier; 2007. p. 71–105.
23. Murakami C, Nishioka G. Essential concepts in the design of local skin flaps. Facial Plast Surg Clin North Am 1996;4:458.
24. Angel MF, Kaufman T, Swartz WM, et al. Studies on the nature of the flap/bed interaction in rodents Part

I: flap survival under varying conditions. Ann Plast Surg 1986;17(4):317–22.

25. Cook TA, Israel JM, Wang TD, et al. Cervical rotation flaps for midface resurfacing. Arch Otolaryngol Head Neck Surg 1991;117(1):77–82.

26. Jewett BS. Complications of local flaps. In: Baker SR, editor. Local flaps in facial reconstruction. Philadelphia: Mosby Elsevier; 2007. p. 690–722.

27. Park SS, Little S. Rhombic flaps. In: Baker SR, editor. Local flaps in facial reconstruction. Philadelphia: Mosby Elsevier; 2007. p. 212–30.

28. Borges AF. The rhombic flap. Plast Reconstr Surg 1981;67(4):458–66.

29. Larrabee WF, Bloom DC. Biomechanics of skin flaps. In: Baker SR, editor. Local flaps in facial reconstruction. Philadelphia: Mosby Elsevier; 2007.

30. Limberg A, Wolf S. The planning of local plastic operations on the body surface: theory and practice. Br J Surg 1984;71(11):920.

31. Bray D. Rhombic flaps. In: Baker S, editor. Local flaps in facial reconstruction. St Louis (MO): Mosby; 1995. p. 151.

32. Larrabee WF, Trachy R, Sutton D, et al. Rhomboid flap dynamics. Arch Otolaryngol Head Neck Surg 1981;107(12):755–7.

33. Park S. Local and regional cutaneous flaps. In: Papel I, editor. Facial plastic and reconstructive surgery. 2nd edition. New York: Thieme; 2002. p. 528.

34. Lister GD, Gibson T. Closure of rhomboid skin defects: the flaps of Limberg and Dufourmentel. Br J Plast Surg 1972;25:300–14.

35. Dufourmental C. An L-shaped flap for lozenge-shaped defects. Transactions of the Third International Congress of Plastic Surgery. Amsterdam: Excerpta Medica; 1964.

36. Webster RC, Davidson TM, Smith RC. The 30-degree transposition flap. Laryngoscope 1978;88:85.

37. Larrabee WF. Design of local skin flaps. Otolaryngol Clin North Am 1990;23:899–923.

38. Baker SR. Bilobe flaps. In: Baker SR, editor. Local flaps in facial reconstruction. Philadelphia: Mosby Elsevier; 2007. p. 188–211.

39. Baker SS. Transposition flaps. In: Baker SR, editor. Local flaps in facial reconstruction. Philadelphia: Mosby Elsevier; 2007. p. 138–56.

40. Salasche SJ, Grabski WJ, Look EG. Flaps for the central face. Plast Reconstr Surg 1990;86(5):1036.

41. Siegle RJ. Reconstruction of the forehead. In: Baker SR, editor. Local flaps in facial reconstruction. Philadelphia: Mosby Elsevier; 2007. p. 557–79.

Scar Revision and Recontouring Post-Mohs Surgery

Eric W. Cerrati, MD*, J. Regan Thomas, MD

KEYWORDS

- Scar revision • Steroid injection • Dermabrasion • Laser resurfacing • Z-plasty
- Mohs reconstruction

KEY POINTS

- The ideal scar is narrow, flat, level with surrounding skin, and difficult for the untrained eye to see due to incision placement and color match.
- Dermabrasion should extend down to the papillary dermis with careful attention not to injure the reticular dermis because additional scarring can result.
- Laser resurfacing is an alternative to dermabrasion, either of which can be performed early in the healing process.
- Some scars are best treated with surgical revision followed by the nonsurgical adjuncts to achieve the ideal result.
- Serial Z-plasty is often useful for trap-door deformity of a prior local flap.

INTRODUCTION

To achieve the optimal results following Mohs reconstruction, the surgeon has many available options. First, it is important to realize that, despite the surgeon's best efforts, it is impossible to erase a scar because all wounds and incisions result in scar formation. The techniques outlined by Dr Halsted in 1929 should be applied to all wound closures. These include gentle handling of tissue, aseptic technique, sharp anatomic dissection of tissue, careful hemostasis, obliteration of dead space, avoidance of tension, and reliance on rest.[1] Beyond these considerations, the patient's individual factors determine the speed and effectiveness of wound healing. The wound will progress through the classic 3 stages (inflammation, proliferative, remodeling) with the final appearance being reached approximately 1 year after the initial surgery.[1–5]

Several factors contribute to poor scar formation. These include, but are not limited to, tissue ischemia, traumatic tissue handling, infection, and poor flap design. Some of these factors are preventable, whereas others are not.[6] For example, excessive tension causes widened scars. Also, inadequate wound edge eversion predisposes to depressed scars. Other technical causes include uneven approximation of wound edges, insufficient undermining, or lack of deep closure; all of which can lead to suboptimal scars.[7] Patient factors that the surgeon cannot control include diabetes, Accutane use, radiation therapy, sun exposure, tobacco use, and poor nutritional status.

Conflicts of Interest: None.
Funding: None.
Department of Otolaryngology–Head and Neck Surgery, College of Medicine, University of Illinois at Chicago, 1855 West Taylor Street, Chicago, IL 60611, USA
* Corresponding author.
E-mail address: ecerrati@gmail.com

Facial Plast Surg Clin N Am 25 (2017) 463–471
http://dx.doi.org/10.1016/j.fsc.2017.03.014

For analysis, the ideal scar is narrow, flat, level with surrounding skin, and difficult for the untrained eye to see due to incision placement and color match.[2–4,6,8] Generally, surgeons wait to revise or consider alternative treatment modalities at least 6 to 8 weeks following initial reconstruction. At that time, the wound has rebuilt enough tensile strength to withstand the additional treatments.[3,4,9] In general, the nonsurgical options can be performed at an earlier date, whereas surgical revisions are recommended after a period of 3 to 6 months.[8]

INTRALESIONAL STEROID INJECTIONS

Although triamcinolone injections are commonly used for the treatment of hypertrophic scars and keloids, they are also effective adjuncts during the initial stages of wound healing to reduce tissue edema. Triamcinolone preparation comes in 2 concentrations: 10 mg/mL and 40 mg/mL. The application of these injections is extremely variable in the literature and largely depends on individual surgeon's preferences. The senior author advocates using small amounts of triamcinolone 10 mg/mL injected intralesionally at intervals of 2 to 4 weeks. The amount injected is usually on the order of 0.05 mL to 0.5 mL, depending on the targeted area. The rationale for serial injections using small quantities of triamcinolone is to limit the side-effect profile of the treatment. Intralesional steroid injections can cause thinning of the dermis with subcutaneous fat atrophy, resulting in a skin divot. Additionally, pigmentation changes (especially in darker individuals) and the creation of surrounding telangiectasias have been described.[4,8] Once these side effects occur, they can be very difficult to address; it is recommended that treatment be performed in a conservative manner.

DERMABRASION

An effective scar treatment that has been in use since 1500 BC is mechanical resurfacing, also known as dermabrasion.[10] It is a minimally invasive procedure aimed at smoothing small surface irregularities resulting in a softer scar appearance. It has been studied extensively. Compared with laser resurfacing, it has a lower cost, a better safety profile, and can be used in almost any outpatient setting.[8] Dermabrasion is ideally performed 6 to 8 weeks following the initial surgical procedure. At this point in the wound healing process, tensile strength is essentially maximized at 80% and can withstand the stresses of the procedure.[11–13] Of note, dermabrasion can also be

performed at a later date with similarly effective results.

Preoperative Consideration

In addition to taking a full medical history, surgeons should be particularly careful in obtaining a medication history. Ideally, the use of anticoagulants should be discontinued 2 weeks before the procedure. Isotretinoin (Accutane) should be discontinued for 6 to 12 months prior due to the concern of causing hypertrophic scarring and keloid formation.[9] If a patient has a history of herpes simplex virus (HSV) outbreaks, he or she should be treated prophylactically with antivirals. Some surgeons advocate treating all patients with antivirals regardless of history. Although the senior author typically does not prescribe preoperative medications for localized treatment, 2 medications have been studied in the context of facial resurfacing to prevent hyperpigmentation: hydroquinone and retinoic acid. Hydroquinone inhibits melanocyte conversion of tyrosine to dihydroxyphenylalanine (DOPA), causing a reversible lightening of the skin. It is typically prescribed as a 4% topical cream or gel that is applied twice daily.[14] Retinoic acid, a vitamin A derivative, has been shown to result in accelerated re-epithelialization when applied daily starting 2 weeks before dermabrasion.[9]

Equipment

A variety of dermabrasion equipment brands are available (**Fig. 1**). Of significant help is a dermabrasion unit that allows foot control, reversible direction, and variable speed. Typically, for facial scars, diamond fraises of variable coarseness are used. Wire brush heads are avoided on the face as they tend to cause unintended deep dermis injury.

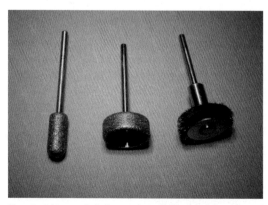

Fig. 1. Diamond fraises of variable coarseness and shapes are available. Typically, wire brushes are avoided for facial scars.

Procedure

Universal precautions should be used by all staff because the treated tissue and blood products can be spread into the air. This includes gowns, gloves, and surgical masks with eye protection. The targeted area is then anesthetized, usually with local injection of 1% lidocaine with 1:100,000 epinephrine. If a larger area is being treated, then the addition of a nerve block can be used. The skin is then prepped in a sterile fashion and the superficial skin can be inked to provide a reference for the surgeon. The targeted area is then treated until diffuse punctate bleeding is noted. This finding signifies that the depth of injury is within the papillary dermis. The reticular dermis, which has a yellow chamois color and visible collagen strands, houses the adnexal structures (sweat glands, hair follicles, sebaceous glands) that are necessary for re-epithelialization. If these deeper structures are injured, scarring is likely to occur (**Fig. 2**).

Postoperative Care

The senior author applies antibiotic ointment and covers the area with an occlusive dressing for 24 hours. After that time, the dressing can be removed but the patient is instructed to keep ointment over the treated area for 1 week. Re-epithelialization is typically complete by day 7. Postprocedural erythema is expected and can last for several weeks. Sun avoidance and frequent application of sunscreen is critical for proper wound healing (**Fig. 3**).

Complications

Although the procedure is generally viewed as having a high safety profile, the most worrisome complications are scarring and hyperpigmentation. Fortunately, these are usually avoidable with good technique and careful attention to patient history. Other complications include milia, bleeding, and infection (*Staphylococcus aureus*, candida, and HSV).

LASER RESURFACING

Another option for minimally invasive scar management is laser resurfacing. Before discussing the different types of lasers and their applications, it is important to understand the principles of selective photothermolysis, which transformed the field in 1983, by Anderson and Parrish.[15] They explained that the laser wavelength, pulse duration, and fluence allow targeted treatment with minimal surrounding tissue damage.[15–18] Each laser has a specific wavelength that is preferentially absorbed by tissue chromophores, allowing precise targeting of thermal destruction. The fluence, or energy density, must be high enough to cause the desired effect. The pulse duration, or break in energy, must be shorter than the thermal relaxation time of the targeted tissue.[18]

With respect to atrophic scar treatment, the traditionally used lasers are the ablative types such as carbon dioxide (CO_2) and erbium:yttrium-aluminum-garnet (Er:YAG) lasers.[8,16,18,19] The CO_2 laser has a wavelength of 10,600 nm and the Er:YAG laser has a wavelength of 2940 nm; however, both target the chromophore water, which exists in the intracellular tissue. The mechanism of action is similar to that of dermabrasion. In the same manner that the depth of dermabrasion is paramount to proper wound healing, the stacking of laser pulses (multiple passes over the same area) increases the depth of penetration, which can lead to scarring when the reticular dermis is injured.[20] In general, the same preoperative and postoperative care as dermabrasion can be applied.

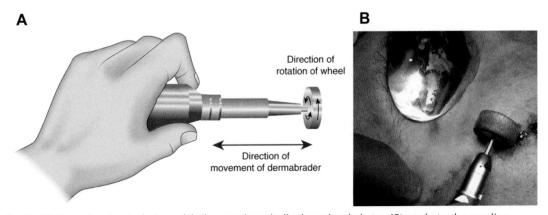

A

Direction of rotation of wheel

Direction of movement of dermabrader

B

Fig. 2. (*A*) Dermabrasion technique. (*B*) The area is typically dermabraded at a 45° angle to the scar line.

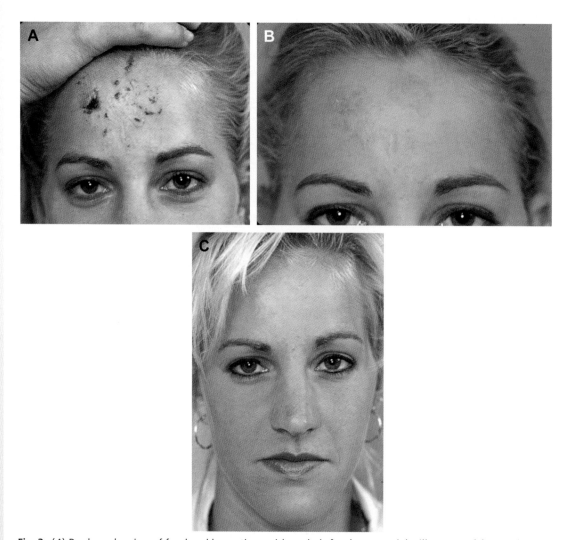

Fig. 3. (A) Predermabrasion of forehead lacerations with asphalt foreign material still present. (B) 2 weeks postdermabrasion. (C) 2 months postdermabrasion.

The slight differences in wavelength between the 2 lasers contribute to their application and side-effect profile. The CO2 laser can penetrate to a depth as much as 1 mm. Although this allows targeted collagen remodeling, it is also the cause for persistent erythema that can last up to 6 months or longer. The ideal application is for irregularly contoured and elevated scars. The Er:YAG laser has a shallower depth of penetration so there is no effect on the collagen matrix. Additionally, its hemostatic abilities are much less than CO2. The ideal application is for depressed or atrophic scars.[16,18,19]

In 2004, the concept of fractional photothermolysis was introduced, referring to the treatment of a fraction of the overall surface area by sparing intervening areas of skin. By having viable tissue surrounding the columns of thermal injury, the rate of re-epithelialization is significantly improved. Additionally, the risk of pigmentation changes and prolonged erythema are significantly decreased.[17] This technology allows scars to be treated at a greater depth without increasing the potential risks.

SCAR REVISION SURGERY

Despite the minimally invasive options, some scars are best addressed surgically. These include

- Widened scars
- Depressed scars
- Scars with uneven edges
- Scars needing reorientation
- Scars needing irregularization.

Although revision surgery replaces the old scar with a new scar, the goal is to create a narrower and flatter scar that is less conspicuous.[2–4,8] When it comes to surgical management, the least complex form of therapy with acceptable results is frequently the best option.

Excisional Techniques

Excisional techniques include

- Shave excision
- Fusiform excision
- M-plasty
- Serial partial excision.

The simplest form of scar excision is a shave excision. With this technique, a superficial irregularity is tangentially shaved using a scalpel (typically an 11-blade). The resulting wound is then allowed to heal by secondary intention. The deep dermis should not be violated with this procedure. Shave excision can be used in isolation or in conjunction with other techniques.

If the scar lies in a favorable position such as within a relaxed skin tension line (RSTL), then a simple fusiform excision is best. The opposing angles should be 30° or less. Particular attention to beveling the scalpel away from the scar will assist in everting the skin edges while closing. A variation of this technique is an M-plasty. This is particularly useful when trying to avoid long fusiform incisions

and in situations that require angles between 30° and 60°.

With all of these techniques, generous undermining of the adjacent tissue allows tension-free closure. Furthermore, thickened scar tissue beneath the flap can be effectively thinned at this stage. The subcutaneous and dermal layers are closed in a buried interrupted fashion using 5–0 polydioxanone (PDS) suture. The superficial layer is reapproximated with 5–0 or 6–0 polypropylene (prolene) suture, which is typically removed at day 7.

Irregularization Techniques in Flaps

Irregularization techniques include

- Z-plasty
- W-plasty
- Geometric broken line closure (GBLC).

Z-plasty

The Z-plasty technique is a powerful tool in scar revision because it has many different applications. Traditionally, 2 flaps are created from 3 equal limbs and 2 same-degree angles. Once the flaps have been transposed, the result is a scar that has been rotated and lengthened. Using angles of 30°, 45°, and 60° will lengthen the incision

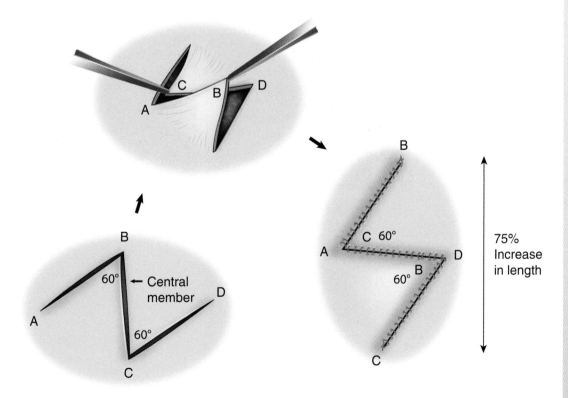

Fig. 4. Z-plasty technique.

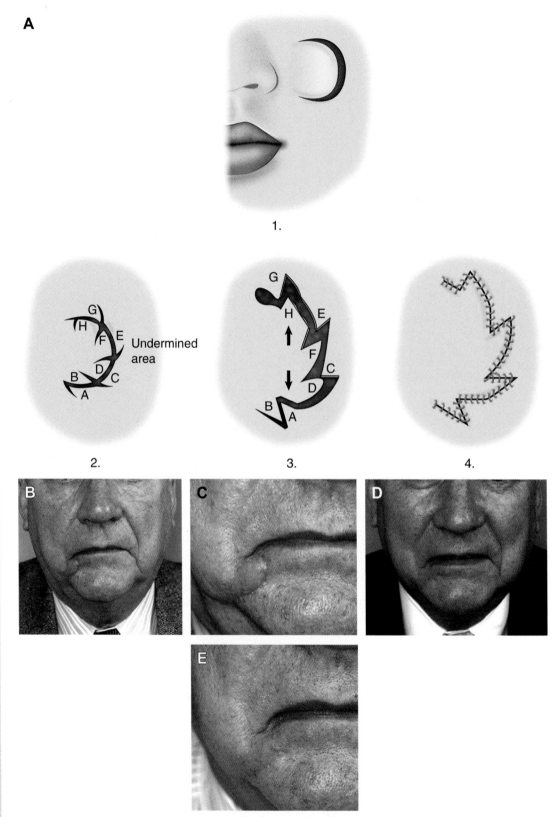

Fig. 5. (*A*) Technique of applying multiple z-plasties to correct a trap door scar deformity. (*B*) Trap door scar deformity resulting from a flap located on the lower lip, lower face photo and (*C*) up close. (*D*) The appearance after multiple Z-plasties have been performed to the periphery of the flap, lower face photo and (*E*) up close.

by 25%, 50%, and 75%, respectively, and will rotate the resulting incision by 45°, 60°, and 90°, respectively. Angles less than 30° places flap viability at risk and angles greater than 60° lead to standing cone deformities after transposition (**Fig. 4**).

Common in post-Mohs reconstruction is the trap-door deformity or pin-cushioning appearance as a result of semicircular incisions. This is a result of the semicircular scar contracting, which tends to bunch the flap tissue resulting in a thickened or pin-cushioned appearance. In addition to generous undermining, the trap-door deformity is best treated with multiple Z-plasties, which break up the scar and redistribute the tension. Another common applications are the release of contractures and the effacement of webs (**Fig. 5**).

W-plasty

A running W-plasty technique, not to be confused with serial Z-plasties, was first described in 1959 by Borges.[21] It involves the creation of an incision made up of several small Ws on either size of the scar such that, once the scar is excised, the 2 lines will precisely interdigitate to create a new irregular scar. Each limb of the incision should be 5 mm to allow for easy tissue handling without creating obvious incision lines. As opposed to Z-plasty, there is no scar lengthening. This technique is ideal for long, straight scars that are perpendicular to RSTLs. The design should also create incisions that are within RSTLs to give an irregular pattern, making the result less noticeable (**Fig. 6**).

Geometric broken line closure

The most complex scar irregularization procedure is the GBLC. This technique uses a combination of triangles, squares, rectangles, and other shapes to create an irregular pattern. Once the pattern has been placed on 1 side of the scar, the mirror image is placed on the opposite side so that the 2 patterns will precisely interdigitate once the scar is removed. The GBLC is similar in concept to the W-plasty; however, the resulting scar is less noticeable to the untrained eye. The geometric shapes should be between 5 and 7 mm in length. If the shapes are less than 5 mm, tissue handling can become problematic. Conversely, if the shapes are greater than 7 mm, the design becomes more conspicuous (**Fig. 7**).

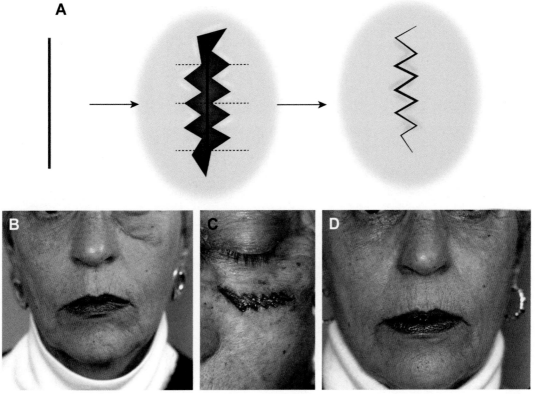

Fig. 6. (*A*) A W-plasty breaks up the scar appearance using interposition flaps. (*B*) Preoperative cheek scar of the face from a Mohs resection. (*C*) The scar has been excised and is ready to close as a W-plasty. (*D*) Postoperative appearance following a W-plasty.

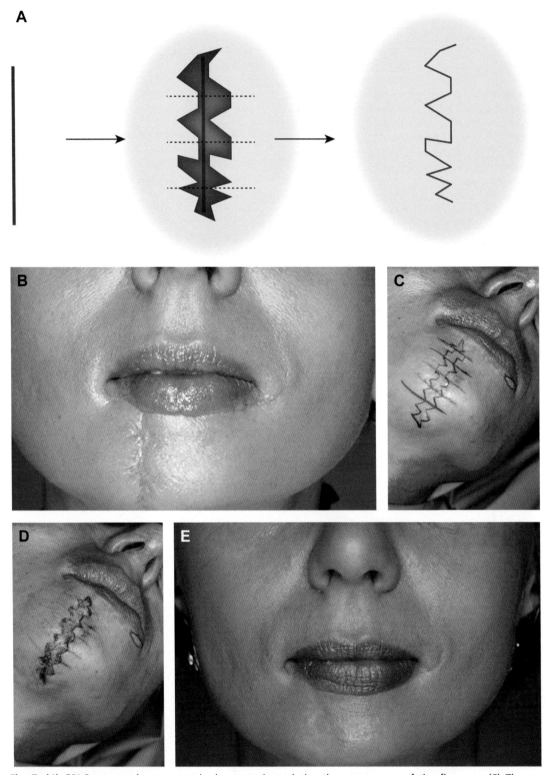

Fig. 7. (*A*) GBLC uses random geometric shapes to irregularize the appearance of the flap scar. (*B*) The scar appearance before revision. (*C*) The GBLC surgical procedure before incision. (*D*) The GBLC surgical procedure after incision. (*E*) The appearance following a GBLC procedure.

For these techniques that rely heavily on the creation of angles and patterns, it is imperative to be extremely meticulous when performing the incisions. Generally, an 11-blade is used for all 3 of the irregularization techniques. The incisions are then closed in the standard fashion with PDS and prolene sutures. Additionally, it is often useful to incorporate dermabrasion at 6 to 8 weeks postoperatively following W-plasty and GBLC.

SUMMARY

Following Mohs reconstruction, scar revision techniques can play a significant role. Depending on timing and the physical examination findings, multiple options are available to the treating physician. These options can begin as early as a few weeks following the initial surgery or up to a year following. Although the scar treatments vary widely among surgeons, the end purpose remains consistent, which is to create a narrow, flat, inconspicuous scar. Patients must also have realistic expectations and understand the risks involved with the various revision procedures. When performed properly and executed meticulously, the results can be dramatic.

REFERENCES

1. Howes EL, Sooy JW, Harvey SC. The healing of wounds as determined by their tensile strength. JAMA 1929;92:42.
2. Thomas JR, Ehler TK. Scar revision. In: Papel ID, Nachlas NE, editors. Facial plastic and reconstructive surgery. St Louis (MO): Mosby; 1992. p. 45–55.
3. Thomas JR, Hochman M. Scar camouflage. In: Bailey BJ, editor. Head & neck surgery-otolaryngology. 2nd edition. Philadelphia: Lippincott-Raven; 1998. p. 2026–33.
4. Thomas JR, Holt GR, editors. Facial scars: incision, revision, and camouflage. St Louis (MO): Mosby; 1989.
5. Goslen JB. Wound healing for the dermatologic surgeon. J Dermatol Surg Oncol 1988;14(9):959–73.
6. Kaplan B, Potter T, Moy RL. Scar revision. Dermatol Surg 1997;23(6):435–42.
7. Zide MF. Scar revision with hypereversion. J Oral Maxillofac Surg 1996;54(9):1061–7.
8. Thomas JR, Prendiville S. Update in scar revision. Facial Plast Surg Clin North Am 2002;10(1):103–11.
9. Surowitz JB, Shockley WW. Enhancement of facial scars with dermabrasion. Facial Plast Surg Clin North Am 2011;19(3):517–25.
10. Lawrence N, Mandy S, Yarborough J, et al. History of dermabrasion. Dermatol Surg 2000;26(2):95–101.
11. Harmon CB, Zelickson BD, Roenigk RK, et al. Dermabrasive scar revision: immunohistochemical and ultrastructural evaluation. Dermatol Surg 1995; 21(6):503–8.
12. Katz BE, Oca AG. A controlled study of the effectiveness of spot dermabrasion (scarabrasion) on the appearance of surgical scars. J Am Acad Dermatol 1991;24(3):462–6.
13. Yarborough JM Jr. Ablation of facial scars by programmed dermabrasion. J Dermatol Surg Oncol 1988;14(3):292–4.
14. Spencer M. Topical use of hydroquinone for depigmentation. JAMA 1965;194(9):962–4.
15. Anderson RR, Parrish JA. Selective photothermolysis: precise microsurgery by selective absorption of pulsed radiation. Science 1983;220(4596):524–7.
16. Newman JB, Lord JL, Ash K, et al. Variable pulse erbium:YAG laser skin resurfacing of perioral rhytides and side-by-side comparison with carbon dioxide laser. Lasers Surg Med 2000;26(2):208–14.
17. Manstein D, Herron GS, Sink RK, et al. Fractional photothermolysis: a new concept for cutaneous remodeling using microscopic patterns of thermal injury. Lasers Surg Med 2004;34(5):426–38.
18. Sobanko JF, Alster TS. Laser treatment for improvement and minimization of facial scars. Facial Plast Surg Clin North Am 2011;19:527–42.
19. Green HA, Domankevitz Y, Nishioka NS. Pulsed carbon dioxide laser ablation of burned skin: in vitro and in vivo analysis. Lasers Surg Med 1990;10(5): 476–84.
20. Fitzpatrick RE, Smith SR, Sriprachya-Anunt S. Depth of vaporization and the effect of pulse stacking with a high-energy, pulsed CO2 laser. J Am Acad Dermatol 1999;40:615–22.
21. Borges AF. Improvement of anti-tension line scars by the "W-plastic" operation. Br J Plast Surg 1959; 12:29.

Index

Note: Page numbers of article titles are in **boldface** type.

Facial Plast Surg Clin N Am 25 (2017) 473–477
http://dx.doi.org/10.1016/S1064-7406(17)30049-4
1064-7406/17

Moving?

Make sure your subscription moves with you!

To notify us of your new address, find your **Clinics Account Number** (located on your mailing label above your name), and contact customer service at:

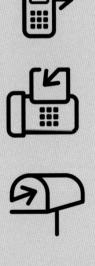

Email: journalscustomerservice-usa@elsevier.com

800-654-2452 (subscribers in the U.S. & Canada)
314-447-8871 (subscribers outside of the U.S. & Canada)

Fax number: 314-447-8029

Elsevier Health Sciences Division
Subscription Customer Service
3251 Riverport Lane
Maryland Heights, MO 63043